A GUIDE TO GLOBAL LANGUAGE ASSESSMENT

A LIFESPAN APPROACH

A GUIDE TO GLOBAL LANGUAGE ASSESSMENT

A LIFESPAN APPROACH

Editor

Mellissa Bortz, PhD, CCC-SLP

Assistant Professor

St. John's University

Queens, New York

Routledge
Taylor & Francis Group
LONDON AND NEW YORK

Designed cover image: Tinhouse Design

First published 2024
by Routledge
605 Third Avenue, New York, NY 10017

and by Routledge
4 Park Square, Milton Park, Abingdon, Oxon, OX14 4RN

Routledge is an imprint of the Taylor & Francis Group, an informa business

ISBN: 978-1-63091-944-3 (pbk)
ISBN: 978-1-003-52447-2 (ebk)

DOI: 10.4324/9781003524472

Typeset in Minion Pro
by SLACK Incorporated

Access the Support Material: www.routledge.com/9781630919443

Dedication

I dedicate this book to my beloved daughter, Maya Thandi Bortz. Mayli, you are the best part of me. You have grown into the woman I wish I was. I am in awe of your values.

My late mother Hannah Bortz. In October 1992 you inscribed the *Concise Oxford Dictionary* that you bought me as I embarked on my master's thesis "May this assist you in your never-ending search for knowledge and excellence." Mamanchikel, thank you so much for this inspirational message and all your constant support, which has resulted in this book.

My other mother/friend/confidant, Happy Modisane. Thank you so much for all the joy and happiness you have brought to our lives.

All the culturally and linguistically diverse children and adults I have assessed who have taught me how to hone my skills to devise reliable and valid assessments with them. Readers, it is my hope that this book will kindle your passion to ensure that we assess and treat all multilingual, culturally and linguistically diverse clients with the equity they deserve.

The late Dr. Jacob, J. M. Semela. Jacob was the first Black speech-language therapist to graduate in South Africa. His perseverance was remarkable. May no colleague ever have to endure the torturous path he did in order to practice their profession.

Contents

Dedication v
Acknowledgments ix
About the Editor xi
Contributing Authors xiii
Preface xvii
Foreword by Yvette D. Hyter, PhD, CCC-SLP, ASHA Honors xxiii

Part I Background 1

Chapter 1 Introduction 3
Mellissa Bortz, PhD, CCC-SLP

Chapter 2 The *International Classification of Functioning, Disability and Health* Framework and Global Assessment 25
Carol Westby, PhD, CCC-SLP

Chapter 3 Language and Language Families 45
Tobias A. Kroll, PhD, CCC-SLP and Dr. phil. Jan Wohlgemuth, MA

Part II Methods of Assessment 67

Chapter 4 Conducting Dynamic Assessments in Culturally and Linguistically Diverse Individuals 69
Samantha Washington, EdD, CCC-SLP and Giselle Núñez, PhD, CCC-SLP

Chapter 5 Ethnographic Assessment of Communication Disorders in Children 91
Elise Davis-McFarland, PhD, CCC-SLP, ASHA Honors

Chapter 6 New Directions in Language Sample Analysis for Multilingual Contexts 111
Hanna Ehlert, PhD; Jeannie van der Linde, PhD; Ulrike Lüdtke, PhD; and Juan Bornman, PhD

Chapter 7 Assessment of Narratives: A Global Perspective 131
Marleen F. Westerveld, PhD, FSPA, CPSP and Carol Westby, PhD, CCC-SLP

Part III Specific Examples of Global Assessments 155

Chapter 8 Partnering to Develop a Community-Based Measure of Expressive Language in Guatemala 157
Lisa Domby, MS, CCC-SLP and Maria Elizabeth Jaramillo, MS, MPH, CCC-SLP

Chapter 9 Drawing on Language Socialization Research to Improve Speech and Language Assessment 177
Keziah Conrad, PhD, MS, CCC-SLP

Chapter 10 Identifying Developmental Communication Milestones in Western Kenya: A Community-Based Approach. 195
Monika Molnar, PhD; David K. Rochus; Rachael Gibson; Florence Omolo; and Lynn Ellwood, MHSc, S-LP(C), Reg. CASLPO

Chapter 11 Assessment of Creole Languages in the Absence of Norms: A Case Study on Guyanese Creole 223
Sulare Telford Rose, PhD, CCC-SLP; Tamirand Nnena De Lisser, PhD; and Anna Monina M. Vanta, MS, CCC-SLP

Chapter 12 The Development of Standardized Language Assessments and Screeners for Mandarin-Speaking Children in China: Lessons for Global Practice 247
Xueman Lucy Liu, AuD/CCC-A/FAAA, MS/CCC-SLP; Wendy Lee, MS, CCC-SLP; Teresa Hutchings, MEd, CCC-SLP; Jill de Villiers, PhD; and Eric Rolfhus, PhD

Chapter 13 The Use of Sentence Repetition Tasks for Culturally and Linguistically Diverse Clients Across the Lifespan. 263
Mellissa Bortz, PhD, CCC-SLP and Christina Valenti, MA, CF-SLP, TSSLD

Part IV Assessment of Language Disorders 273

Chapter 14 Augmentative and Alternative Communication: It Is About Having a Voice 275
Juan Bornman, PhD; Carla van Nieuwenhuizen; and Lebogang Sehako

Chapter 15 Addressing Multicultural and Multilingual Aspects in the Assessment of Individuals With Autism Spectrum Disorder. 289
Kakia Petinou, PhD, SLP; Maria Christopoulou, EdD; and Kyriakos Antoniou, PhD

Part V Adult Language Assessment 305

Chapter 16 Assessment in Aphasia: Global Perspectives 307
Mira Goral, PhD, CCC-SLP and Elizabeth E. Galletta, PhD, CCC-SLP

Chapter 17 Neuropsychological Assessment in Dementia for Global Populations 323
Avanthi Paplikar, PhD, SLP; Aparna Venugopal, MSc, SLP; and Suvarna Alladi, DM Neurology

Glossary 355
Financial Disclosures 371
Index 375

Instructors: *A Guide to Global Language Assessment: A Lifespan Approach* includes ancillary materials specifically available for faculty use. Please visit www.routledge.com/9781630919443 to obtain access.

Acknowledgments

My mentors Professor Mira Goral, Karl Johnson, Distinguished Professor Lorraine Obler, Professor Emerita Yvette Hyter, and the late Professor Emeritus Martin Gitterman. Thank you for always being encouraging and inspirational.

"The family is the first essential cell of human society" (Pope John XXIII)—the constants in my life, the Bortz sisters, "brother" Mark, and their families, Avril, Robin and Celeste, Hans, Lesego, Khutso, Nyakalo, and my "grandson" Shadow. I am also blessed with very caring and supportive friends, Jonathan, Aidan, Edana, Hilary, and Beth, who I have learned so much from.

Thank you to Christina Valenti for her assistance in communicating with all the authors. Thank you to my research students and assistants Lodwica Silva, Christina Valenti, Kayla Aquino, Genesis Barreto, Gabriella Dziwura, Savannah Everett, Raina Richardson, Angelina Russo, Shanell Tufino, and Kate Woo for contributing to the global database of language assessment materials, and Nina R. Amatore, Gianna C. Bovino, Marissa N. Brandl, Alexa M. Brown, Claire Cushing, Cassandra I. DiCosta, Arianna M. Frontera, Ashley N. Golden, Maria S. Gournelos, Jessica L. Mancato, Caitlin E. Olsen, Katerina K. Orisses, Sophia Pedernera, Juliana R. Radulski, and Maria Pia Sapienza, students in CSD 2760 Language Disorders Across the Lifespan, Fall 2021, for completing their Culturally and Linguistically Diverse Assignments, which also added language assessment materials to the database.

It truly has been a privilege and honor to work with all these students. It is very comforting to know that "the torch" of continuing the essential task of developing culturally and linguistic diverse language assessment materials has been lit and will continue in our next generation of speech-language therapists.

About the Editor

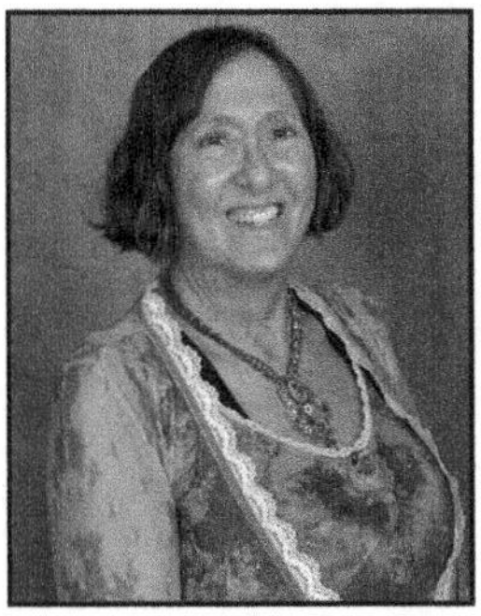

Mellissa Bortz, PhD, CCC-SLP is an Assistant Professor in the Communication Science Disorders Department at St. John's University in New York. Her guiding principles are global engagement as well as diversity, equity, inclusion, and accessibility for all. She teaches undergraduate, graduate, and global exchange courses. Her research focuses on the development of cultural and linguistic multilingual assessment materials. Currently, she is investigating the use of translanguaging in multilingual discourse analysis for children and adults. She also advocates for the expansion of these materials as well as developing repositories for these. She is originally from South Africa where she taught, mentored students, conducted research, and worked as a clinician.

Dr. Bortz is a coordinating committee member of ASHA's SIG 17 Global Issues in Communication Sciences and Related Disorders and SIG 14 Cultural and Linguistic Diversity. She has completed ASHA's Faculty Development Institute 2021—2023, the Leadership Development Program ASHA in April 2017—March 2018, and the Leadership Mentoring Program ASHA in September 2018—March 2019. She is a member of the International Association of Communication Sciences and Disorders and a founding member of African Connections.

Contributing Authors

Suvarna Alladi, DM Neurology (Chapter 17)
Professor and Head of Department of Neurology
National Institute of Mental Health and Neurosciences (NIMHANS)
Bengaluru, Karnataka, India

Kyriakos Antoniou, PhD (Chapter 15)
Post Doctoral Fellow
Department of Rehabilitation Sciences
Cyprus University of Technology
Limassol, Cyprus

Juan Bornman, PhD (Chapters 6 and 14)
Department of Health and Rehabilitation Sciences
Division of Speech-Language and Hearing Therapy
Stellenbosch University
Stellenbosch, South Africa

Maria Christopoulou, EdD (Chapter 15)
Assistant Professor
Program Speech and Language Therapy
European University Cyprus
Nicosia, Cyprus

Keziah Conrad, PhD, MS, CCC-SLP (Chapter 9)
Institute for Human Development
Northern Arizona University
Flagstaff, Arizona

Elise Davis-McFarland, PhD, CCC-SLP, ASHA Honors (Chapter 5)
EDMConsulting, LLC
Charleston, South Carolina

Tamirand Nnena De Lisser, PhD (Chapter 11)
Senior Lecturer of Linguistics
University of Guyana
Georgetown, Guyana

Jill de Villiers, PhD (Chapter 12)
Smith College
Northampton, Massachusetts
Hainan Bo'ao Bethel International Medical Center
Hainan, China

Lisa Domby, MS, CCC-SLP (Chapter 8)
Clinical Associate Professor
University of North Carolina
Chapel Hill, North Carolina

Hanna Ehlert, PhD (Chapter 6)
Department of Speech Language Therapy and Inclusive Education
Leibniz University
Hannover, Germany

Lynn Ellwood, MHSc, S-LP(C), Reg. CASLPO (Chapter 10)
Associate Professor
Department of Speech-Language Pathology
Temerty Faculty of Medicine
University of Toronto
Toronto, Ontario, Canada

Elizabeth E. Galletta, PhD, CCC-SLP (Chapter 16)
NYU Langone Health
NYU Grossman School of Medicine
New York, New York

Rachael Gibson (Chapter 10)
Specialist Speech and Language Therapist and Managing Director
Yellow House Health and Outreach Services
Kenya and the United Kingdom

Mira Goral, PhD, CCC-SLP (Chapter 16)
Lehman College
City University of New York
New York, New York

Teresa Hutchings, MEd, CCC-SLP (Chapter 12)
Hainan Bo'ao Bethel International Medical Center
Hainan, China

Yvette D. Hyter, PhD, CCC-SLP, ASHA Honors (Foreword)
Professor Emerita
Western Michigan University
Owner
Language & Literacy Practices
Kalamazoo, Michigan

Maria Elizabeth Jaramillo, MS, MPH, CCC-SLP (Chapter 8)
University of North Carolina
Chapel Hill, North Carolina

Tobias A. Kroll, PhD, CCC-SLP (Chapter 3)
Texas Tech University Health Sciences Center
School of Health Professions
Department of Speech, Language, and Hearing Sciences
Lubbock, Texas

Wendy Lee, MS, CCC-SLP (Chapter 12)
Hainan Bo'ao Bethel International Medical Center
Hainan, China

Xueman Lucy Liu, AuD/CCC-A/FAAA, MS/CCC-SLP (Chapter 12)
Hainan Bo'ao Bethel International Medical Center
Hainan, China
University of Texas at Dallas
Dallas, Texas

Ulrike Lüdtke, PhD (Chapter 6)
Professor and Head of Department of Speech Language Therapy and Inclusive Education
Leibniz University
Hannover, Germany

Monika Molnar, PhD (Chapter 10)
Department of Speech-Language Pathology
Rehabilitation Sciences Institute
University of Toronto
Toronto, Ontario, Canada

Giselle Núñez, PhD, CCC-SLP (Chapter 4)
Saint Xavier University
Chicago, Illinois

Florence Omolo (Chapter 10)
Parent Liaison Officer
Yellow House Health and Outreach Services
Kenya

Avanthi Paplikar, PhD, SLP (Chapter 17)
Associate Professor
Department of Speech and Language Studies
Research Coordinator
Bangalore Speech and Hearing Research Foundation (BSHRF)
Dr. S. R. Chandrasekhar Institute of Speech and Hearing
Bengaluru, India

Kakia Petinou, PhD, SLP (Chapter 15)
Professor
Department of Rehabilitation Sciences
Director of TheraLab
School of Health Sciences
Cyprus University of Technology
Limassol, Cyprus

David K. Rochus (Chapter 10)
Yellow House Health and Outreach Services
Kenya

Eric Rolfhus, PhD (Chapter 12)
Hainan Bo'ao Bethel International Medical Center
Hainan, China

Sulare Telford Rose, PhD, CCC-SLP (Chapter 11)
Assistant Professor of Speech-Language Pathology
University of District of Columbia
Washington, DC

Lebogang Sehako (Chapter 14)
Centre for Augmentative and
Alternative Communication
Alumni of the
Fofa Youth Empowerment Project
University of Pretoria
Hatfield, South Africa

Jeannie van der Linde, PhD (Chapter 6)
Department of Speech-Language Pathology
and Audiology
University of Pretoria
South Africa

Carla van Nieuwenhuizen (Chapter 14)
Centre for Augmentative and
Alternative Communication
Alumni of the
Fofa Youth Empowerment Project
University of Pretoria
Hatfield, South Africa

Christina Valenti, MA, CF-SLP, TSSLD (Chapter 13)
Kidz Therapy
Garden City, New York

Anna Monina M. Vanta, MS, CCC-SLP (Chapter 11)
Bilingual Speech-Language Pathologist
University of District of Columbia
Washington, DC

Aparna Venugopal, MSc, SLP (Chapter 17)
PhD Scholar
Department of Speech Pathology and Audiology
National Institute of Mental Health and
Neurosciences (NIMHANS)
Bengaluru, Karnataka, India

Samantha Washington, EdD, CCC-SLP (Chapter 4)
Assistant Professor
Southeast Missouri State University
Cape Girardeau, Missouri

Carol Westby, PhD, CCC-SLP (Chapters 2 and 7)
Bilingual Multicultural Services
Albuquerque, New Mexico

Marleen F. Westerveld, PhD, FSPA, CPSP (Chapter 7)
Griffith Institute for Educational Research
Griffith University
Queensland, Australia

Dr. phil. Jan Wohlgemuth, MA (Chapter 3)
Universitas Indonesia, Depok
West Java, Indonesia

Preface

Global Need for Language Assessment Materials

One of the major problems facing the speech therapists in South Africa today is the absence or inadequacy of tests available for use with the Black African population. Educational, cultural, linguistic and environmental factors mean that the tests that are available are generally standardized in England or the United States, on western White middle class populations. This makes them inappropriate and inaccurate for the evaluation of the Black South African populations. New tests must be created to overcome the limitations of translated imported tests and to fill the need for assessment tools for the Black population (Ballentine et al., 1976, p. 5).

The lack of language assessment materials for multicultural and multilinguistic clients is a global challenge facing speech-language therapists.

The unavailability of appropriate language assessment results in many challenges for culturally and linguistically diverse multilingual children and adults who do not speak standard forms of the language of their country. Results of global research in school-aged children give inaccurate overdiagnosis of multilingual Hebrew-and Russian-speaking children with typical language development having developmental language disorder (DLD), as well as the underdiagnosis of children with DLD (Altman et al., 2021). American Indian and Alaskan Native children who are dual language learners are overrepresented in special education (Artiles & Ortiz, 2002) while the misdiagnosis of learning disability in Latino English Learning children could be as high as 9% (Klingner & Artiles, 2003; Kraemer & Fabiano-Smith, 2017). This misdiagnosis may cause an unintended educational disparity between Latino English Learners and Mainstream American English Speakers. Multiple studies conducted for Asian American and Pacific Islander students have found that there are also disparities in this group, resulting in underrepresentation in special education (Cooc, 2019; Sullivan et al., 2020).

Aboriginal and Torres Strait Islander children are likely to be misdiagnosed in Standard Australian English at school if their school does not recognize Aboriginal English as a valid and standard dialect (Pearce & Williams, 2013; Verdon & McLeod, 2015; Zupan et al., 2021). This education policy abrogates Aboriginal-language–speaking students' human rights and results in them being considered as disadvantaged students instead of multilingual speakers (Freeman & Staley, 2018).

Discrimination against students because of the dialect they speak (i.e., a language difference) is all too common in African American English (Craig et al., 2002; Craig & Washington, 2002; Wyatt, 2019). Stockman (2010) reported that African American children score below normative samples of standardized language assessments because they are not included in the standardization samples. According to Wyatt (2019), only 15% of standardization samples on norm-referenced tests are American. The majority of the sample are Mainstream American English Speakers who are from White, middle-class backgrounds.

In a study conducted in South Africa, van Dulm and Southwood (2014) found that service delivery by speech-language therapists to bilingual children was problematic and largely unsatisfactory. The results indicated that the caseloads of speech-language therapists in previously culturally homogenous countries in which a limited number of bilinguals required their services, became steadily more multicultural and multilingual. An example is in Europe, where immigration tripled in the past half century (Levey & Cheng, 2021). This immigration has led to increasingly multilingual school populations in officially monolingual countries like Austria and Greece (Levey & Cheng, 2021). Much research has been conducted to establish the need for changes within the speech-language pathology field in order to provide more appropriate services for the multilingual and multicultural population. However, research indicates that speech-language therapist services provided to these students was less than satisfactory (Roseberry-McKibben et al., 2005; Scheffner-Hammer et al., 2004; van Dulm & Southwood, 2014).

Washington et al. (2019) state that "one of the main difficulties Speech-Language Pathologists face ... is a lack of appropriate assessment tools" (p. 45). While Mdladlo et al. (2019) claim that "the problem of culture-fair assessment is a global problem that has been identified in regions such as Australia (cited Ball & Peltier, 2011), Eastern Europe (cited Moro, 2008), United States (cited Hamilton, 2014), New Zealand (cited Brewer & Andrews, 2016), and Canada (cited Thordardottir, 2011)" (p. 2).

In a more recent study, Newbury et al. (2020) examined the practices of New Zealand speech-language therapists who work with multilingual children. They found that there were marked differences between speech-language therapists' practice when working with multilingual children and best practice guidelines. This could be due to a discrepancy between the languages spoken by the client and the speech-language therapist.

These authors recommend that "speech-language pathologists ... need to become more proficient working across languages. This is particularly applicable in countries where a relatively small number of people speak each minority language, such as New Zealand and Australia" (Newbury et al., 2020, p. 8). Furthermore, "it is evident that unique language situations in different countries and the different scenarios leading to multilingualism will not allow a *one size fits all* approach to assessment and treatment of these children" (Newbury et al., 2020, p. 2).

The purpose of this book is to empower the speech-language therapy[1] profession to assess clients requiring communication-related services, no matter what language they speak or culture they are from. This text shares knowledge of assessment materials, research, and clinical innovation in assessing culturally and linguistically diverse multilingual clients' populations. This book is intended to inspire and encourage speech-language therapists to join in this essential work for our profession so that together we can establish language assessments for our clients in the languages that we speak. This is our professional responsibility.

Author's Positionality Statement

The term *positionality* describes a person's worldview and the positions they adopt about research and social and political context (Darwin Holmes, 2020). Hyter and Salas-Provance (2023) describe the importance of sharing positionality statements "which clearly outline the events that have shaped our thinking and also identify our values and ethical positions" (p. xix).

I identify as a multilingual speaker who has lived as a documented citizen in two countries. I also identify as being a White, educated, industrialized, rich, and democratic (WEIRD; Henrich et al., 2010) South African who was born into and grew up in apartheid South Africa. As such, I had first-hand experiences of the horrors and indignities of overt and systematized racism. At 8 years old I became aware that I was complicit in the system by signing a "special" for our housekeeper "Tall"[2] in the rural town where I grew up. Apartheid required that Black people who wanted to go out after 7:00 pm needed a White person to sign a form that asked for the biographical details of the person, reason, and time of visit. Not only did Tall have to suffer the indignity of asking for the special, she also had to carry her dompas "identity document" allowing Black people to be in "White" areas. Police patrolled the streets regularly and would constantly stop Black people walking in the street. If there was even a minor infraction, the person would be arrested and put in jail. Through my personal development I have navigated the process of learning, unlearning, relearning, and continuing to learn about racism. These experiences have brought me to the discovery of unethical and ineffective language assessment and intervention approaches.

[1]In this book both the identity-first term speech-language therapist, which aligns with the neurodiversity perspective, and speech-language pathologist, which represents the medical model/ableist perspective which is currently used by the American Speech-Language-Hearing Association will be used interchangeably.

[2]Her English name was Elizabeth, but because there was another Elizabeth working in the house she was identified by her appearance. I never knew the name her parents chose for her based on their ethnic group and positive or negative circumstances that they were experiencing at the time of her birth. https://kybeleworldwide.org/baby-naming-customs/

Can a WEIRD Person Develop Language Assessments for Culturally and Linguistically Diverse Populations?

Excerpt from teacher report

Question: What language does the child speak at creche?

Response: Soweto language (Bortz, 1995)

I am not certain of this answer. This citation is one of the many mistakes that I have made when developing culturally and linguistically diverse language materials for the selection of research participants. One of the criteria for selection of participants is that they were required to be first language speakers of isiZulu. I had researched the fact that there was a variety of "Soweto Zulu." This is regarded as an urban-based variety that loans from other languages and is characterized by codeswitching to English, with isiZulu operating as the matrix language (Myers-Scotton, 1993). I had been informed that a particular group of preschools were predominantly isiZulu speaking. However, when conducting pilot testing, the teachers reported that such a criterion did not exist. What a blatant example of lack of cultural humility on my part! A valuable lesson to learn from this is to be culturally responsive as well as to embrace your mistakes and learn from them.

Sadly, the ending of apartheid did not signal speech therapy services for all. Currently South Africa has the dubious reputation of being the most unequal country in the world. Ten percent of the population owns more than 80% of the wealth (World Bank, 2022). This results in large populations of migrants, refugees, and underserved and underserviced populations. What has changed is the belief that collaboration with others and networking can effect change.

To illustrate, I chronicle the journey of a colleague who never gave up despite the enormous and unreasonable challenges he faced. On a freezing day in December 1983 in Chicago, Illinois, far away from the South African summer, Dr. Jacob J. Semela recounted his journey on becoming the first Black speech-language therapist and audiologist in apartheid South Africa. Jacob was a person who stuttered. As a young man he sought out the help of a speech-language therapist, Dr. Peggy Walhaus of the Speech-Language Therapy Department at the University of the Witwatersrand, Johannesburg. The therapy he received inspired him to become a speech-language therapist, which was a 4-year degree course. Apartheid laws decreed that Jacob could take the speech-language therapy courses at the University of the Witwatersrand. However, other required courses, such as psychology, had to be taken at the University of South Africa (UNISA). After he had completed 4 years of this course, regulations required him to retake the UNISA classes at the University of the Witwatersrand. It therefore took Jacob double the amount of time to qualify as a speech-language therapist: 8 years. Jacob and his young family moved to the United States where he completed two PhDs. The Semela family returned to South Africa at the end of apartheid. The post-apartheid period was a challenge for Jacob. Despite the fact that our paths rarely crossed because we were generally on a different continent, Jacob was my lodestar. May no colleague ever have to endure the torturous path he took in order to practice his profession.

While apartheid ran rampant in South Africa majority world country, I became familiar with the same challenges and inequities in the profession, and specifically regarding assessment materials in the United States. One of my first classes in the City University of New York Graduate Center (CUNY-GC) was American dialectology while the Ebonics debate was raging. Professor Walt Wolfram authored our textbook *Dialects and American English* (1991). This class was transformative to my understanding on language difference versus language disorders.

Figure P-1. Neurodiversity continuum.

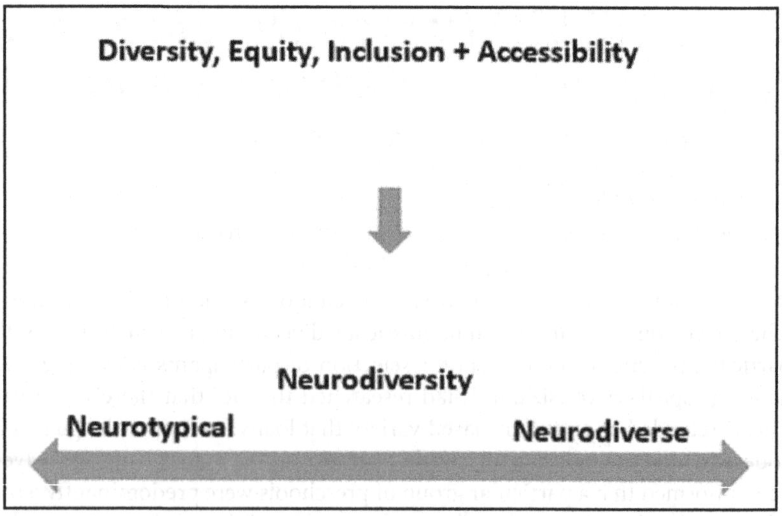

My passion for my profession and the need for culturally and linguistically diverse materials has taken me all over the world. It is somehow fitting that I now work at St. John's University, Queens Campus. St. John's is a global, Vincentian Catholic University that espouses the mission of St. Vincent De Paul, i.e., .. "we devote our intellectual and physical resources to search out the causes of poverty and social injustice and to encourage solutions that are adaptable, effective and concrete" (Mission of St. John's Global Engagement). Being located in Queens, New York, I encounter an ongoing need for culturally and linguistically diverse language assessment materials in my community, which is the most linguistically diverse area in the world with over 160 languages (Lubin, 2017).

Terminology of Diversity, Equity, Inclusion, and Accessibility Used in This Book

Every effort has been made to ensure that the terminology related to diversity, equity, inclusion, and accessibility used in this book reflects current clinical practice and research as Figure P-1 describes. Neurodiversity, which is integrated with inclusion and accessibility, is the most current term used in speech-language therapy and is a transformation from the medical/ableist model, which discriminates against people with disability due to the belief that typical abilities are superior and the adoption of the neurodiversity that promotes the notion that there is a wide range of ways in which people function and all of these are acceptable. The term *neurodiversity* was coined in the 1990s by journalist Harvey Blume and an autism advocate and sociologist diagnosed with Asperger syndrome, Judy Singer (Eusebio, 2017). Neurodiversity implies neurologically diverse or neuroatypical. Therefore, in this book the term *speech-language therapist* is used interchangeably with *speech-language pathologist*.

The terminology we use when assessing our individual clients is important. Traditionally, in "ableist policies" people with disabilities are discriminated against and endure social prejudices, based on "the belief that abilities are culturally defined as typical are superior" (Yu et al., 2021). Ableist ideologies stifle neurodiversity (Manalili, 2021). This in turn can prevent inclusion. Prizant et al. (2017) recommend that as speech-language therapists we should attempt to understand an individual's experience and the reason for their behaviors instead of trying to eliminate these.

Table P-1
Terminology

TERM USED IN THIS BOOK	ALTERNATIVE FORMS
Speech-Language Therapist	Communication Specialist; Logopedist; Phoniatrician; Speech, Language, and Hearing Professionals; Speech-Language Pathologist
Majority-World Countries	Global South, Middle- and Low-Income Countries
Minority-World Countries	Global North, High-Income Countries, Developed
Assessment	Evaluation
Disorder	Disability, Impairment, Challenge
English as a New Language	Dual Language Learner (DLL), English as an Additional Language, English Language Learner (ELL), English Learner (EL), First Language is Not English (FLNE)
First Language and Additional Languages	L1 and L2, Native Language, Mother Tongue

Speech-language therapists are taught to use a person-first nomenclature, for example, a person with aphasia. The reason for this is that the person is named first and the disorder or disability is secondary. This helps eliminate stereotypes and bias (Dunn & Andrew, 2015).

However, *deaf* is the cultural/linguistic term used and preferred by groups of people who use American Sign Language. A study conducted by Kenny et al. (2016) found that the majority of adult autistic people, family, friends, and parents prefer to be known as autistic. The reason for this is that this name emphasizes the value of the person's humanity. As speech-language therapists we need to ask our clients how they prefer to be addressed.

The profession of speech-language therapy uses different terminology in different parts of the world. Therefore, for the reader's convenience, Table P-1 provides a list of terms used in this book.

How to Use This Book

Each chapter of this book is written by an expert in their particular content area. A summary of research is provided. The next section contains a guide to developing language assessments. The chapters conclude with case studies. Tables, figures, images, and charts are included in each chapter.

This book is divided into five sections. Part 1: Background focuses on foundational knowledge that speech-language pathologists need when assessing language with multilingual clients (i.e., linguistics and the World Health Organization *International Classification of Functioning, Disability and Health* [WHO-ICF]). Alternative forms of assessment such as dynamic assessments are described in Part II: Methods of Assessment. Examples of different forms of language assessment are provided in Part III: Specific Examples of Global Assessments. Part IV includes assessment of language disorders, and Part V describes adult language assessment. A Glossary is also included in the book. Instructors can access a Repository of Language Assessment Materials according to six WHO-ICF regions at www.efacultylounge.com.

References

Arias, G., & Friberg, J. (2017). Bilingual language assessment: Contemporary versus recommended practice in American schools. *Language, Speech, and Hearing Services in Schools, 48*(1), 1-15. https://doi.org/10.1044/2016_LSHSS-15-0090

Bortz, M. A. (1995). *A language assessment for preschool IsiZulu speaking children* [Unpublished master's thesis]. University of the Witwatersrand.

Bortz, M. (2023). Assessing language in South Africa: Use of the passive construction. *Handbook of Speech-Language Therapy in Sub-Saharan Africa*, 403–422. https://doi.org/10.1007/978-3-031-04504-2_18

Bortz, M. (2023). Methods for devising a standardized language assessment for isizulu preschoolers: Implications for sub-Saharan Africa. *Handbook of Speech-Language Therapy in Sub-Saharan Africa*, 423–440. https://doi.org/10.1007/978-3-031-04504-2_19

Dakwar, R. K., Ahmar, M., Farah, R., & Froud, K. (2018). Diglossic aphasia and the adaptation of the bilingual aphasia test to Palestinian arabic and Modern Standard Arabic. *Journal of Neurolinguistics, 47*, 131-144. https://doi.org/10.1016/j.jneuroling.2018.04.013

Erickson, J., & Iglesias, A. (1986). Assessment of communication disorders in non-English proficient children. In O. Taylor (Ed.), *Nature of communication disorders in culturally and linguistically diverse populations* (pp. 181-217). College-Hill Press.

Fei, Y., & Weekly, R. (2020). Examining the parameters of translanguaging in the context of Chinese bilinguals' discourse practices. *International Journal of Multilingualism*, 1-21.

Freeman, L. A., & Staley, B. (2018). The positioning of Aboriginal students and their languages within Australia's education system: A human rights perspective. *International Journal of Speech Language Pathology, 20*, 174-181.

Goral, M., & Lerman, A. (2020). Variables and mechanisms affecting response to language treatment in multilingual people with aphasia. *Behavioral Sciences, 10*(9), 144.

Goral, M., Rosas, J., Conner, P. S., Maul, K. K., & Obler, L. K. (2012). Effects of language proficiency and language of the environment on aphasia therapy in a multilingual. *Journal of Neurolinguistics, 25*(6), 538-551.

Grosjean, F. (2012). An attempt to isolate, and then differentiate, transfer and interference. *International Journal of Bilingualism, 16*(1), 11-21.

Hammer, C. S., Detwiler, J. S., Detwiler, J., Blood, G. W., & Dean Qualls, C. (2004). Speech–language pathologists' training and confidence in serving Spanish–English bilingual children. *Journal of Communication Disorders, 37*(2), 91–108. https://doi.org/10.1016/j.jcomdis.2003.07.002

Klinger, J. K., & Artiles, A. J. (2003). When should bilingual children be in special education? *Educational Leadership, 61*(2), 66-71.

Levey, S., & Cheng, L. L. (2021). The plight of unserved and underserved populations across the globe. In S. Levey & S. Moonsamy (Eds.), *Unserved and underserved populations. New approaches to inclusivity* (pp. 1-22). Peter Lang.

MacWhinney, B., Fromm, D., Forbes, M., & Holland, A. (2011). AphasiaBank: Methods for studying discourse. *Aphasiology, 25*(11), 1286-1307.

McLeod, S. (2014). Resourcing speech-language pathologists to work with multilingual children. *International Journal of Speech-Language Pathology, 16*(3), 208-218. https://doi.org/10.3109/17549507.2013.876666

Mdladlo, T., Flack, P. S., & Joubert, R. W. (2019). The cat on a hot tin roof? Critical considerations in multilingual language assessments. *South African Journal of Communication Disorders, 66*(1), 1-7. https://doi.org/10.4102/sajcd.v66i1.610

Taylor, O. L., & Payne, K. T. (1994). Language and communication differences. In G. H. Shames, E. H. Wiig, & W. A. Secord (Eds.), *Human communication disorders: An introduction* (4th ed., pp. 136-177).

Wiig, W., Semel, E., & Secord, W. (2013). *Clinical evaluation of language fundamentals* (5th ed.). Pearson Publications.

Williams, C., & McLeod, S. (2012). Speech-langauge pathologists' assessment and intervention practices with multilingual children. *International Journal of Speech Language Pathology, 14*, 292-305.

World Bank. (2022). Poverty and share prosperity. https://www.worldbank.org/en/publication/poverty-and-shared-prosperity

FOREWORD

The writings of Egyptian economist Samir Amin equated globalization (commonly defined as the blurred national boundaries and interdependence among nations) with colonialism and imperialism. Amin's argument was that a *minority* of the world's countries (i.e., the United States and countries in Europe, as well as Israel and Australia) have a monopoly on the majority of the world's natural resources, machines used to create war, media content, money for investing in infrastructure, and access to healthy food, health care, and medicines (Amin, 2000, 2019; Hyter, 2022, p. 2; Maxman, 2021; McGrath, 2021). This global context makes it particularly important for speech, language, and hearing clinicians, educators, and scholars to engage in culturally and linguistically responsive and globally sustainable practices, teaching, and research (Hyter, 2022). Important aspects of approaching our work includes acknowledging and comprehending the history from which our discipline comes, employing an equity mindset in all aspects of our work, and incorporating principles of social justice—all of which are essential for creating and using culturally and linguistically responsive assessment processes and materials globally.

Coloniality—the continued existence of colonization in speech, language, and hearing sciences—has been fortified in the discipline by the foundation of positivist science and a medical model of disability (Abrahams et al., 2019; Pillay & Kathard, 2015, 2018). These models still influence the way speech, language, and hearing processes and materials (including assessment) are conceptualized and practiced (Hyter, 2022; Pillay & Kathard, 2015; St. Pierre & St. Pierre, 2018). These models may work well for a minority of the world's populations, but certainly do not work for most. Understanding this history is important for dismantling the inequities inherent in our discipline. This history underscores the need for effective global assessment materials. An equity mindset "requires explicit attention to structural inequality, and institutionalized forms of" *-isms* (e.g., ableism, classism, genderism, racism, sexism; Liu et al., 2021) and "demands system-changing responses" (Bensimon, 2018, p. 97). To activate equity, however, a shift to social justice is necessary. Social justice is the elimination of all forms of systemic exclusion, oppression, repression, and domination resulting in transformative remedies, such as those that dismantle "systemic barriers," "cultural and linguistic hierarchies" (Hyter & Salas-Provance, 2023), and "eliminates injustice at the root" (Heidelberg, 2019, p. 393). Efforts to develop and/or identify and implement global assessment processes and materials is a move in this direction toward equity and justice in speech, language, and hearing sciences.

One of the most important aspects of the work of speech-language hearing scholars, educators, and clinicians is to employ meaningful assessments that effectively measure the communication strengths and difficulties faced by the people with whom we work daily. This text, *A Guide to Global Language Assessment: A Lifespan Approach*, is a refreshing review of the importance of effective assessments for all, and shares remedies to the challenges we face when assessing language and communication abilities of multilingual speakers from varied cultural and country backgrounds and world views. Most language assessments in the world have been developed and standardized based on White, middle class linguistic standards (Abrahams et al., 2019), a population that does not match most of the people in the world, or many of the people with whom we work. As a culturally and linguistically responsive and globally engaged scholar, clinician, and educator in speech, language, and hearing sciences with 38 years in the discipline, I am thrilled about this text!

Dr. Mellissa Bortz has spent her career addressing the development of language assessment materials that would be culturally and linguistically responsive and effective around the globe. This work has been done through her research projects, student assignments, as well as networking and collaborating with other like-minded speech, language, and hearing scientists, researchers, educators, and clinicians. In 2018, Dr. Bortz reached out to me, and others, about joining a team of people to develop the Global Language Assessment Task Team (GLATT), which was launched during that year's convention of the American Speech-Language-Hearing Association. This text evolved out of that meeting.

All of your questions about global assessment are answered in this text, and its content will be a welcome and much needed addition to our discipline. It answers questions about challenges, as well as successes, of assessing language skills of individuals from a range of backgrounds, abilities levels, and world views. Each chapter is designed to encourage collaboration in the development of language assessment materials that will be effective for all of individuals and families with whom we work. Moreover, the chapters include information about existing culturally and linguistically responsive processes, such as dynamic assessment and ethnographic interviewing, and in addition includes information on how to assess individuals who have autism, aphasia, and dementia. This is an indispensable text to have on your shelf. You will not be disappointed!

—Yvette D. Hyter, PhD, CCC-SLP, ASHA Honors

References

Abrahams, K., Kathard, H., Harty, M., & Pillay, M. (2019). Inequity and the professionalization of speech-language pathology. *Professions & Professionalism, 9*(3), w3285. http://doi.org/10.7577/pp.3285

Altman, C., Burstein-Feldman, Z., Fichman, S., Armon-Lotem, S., Joffe, S., & Walters, J. (2021). Perceptions of identity, language abilities and language preferences among Russian-Hebrew and English-Hebrew bilingual children and their parents. *Journal of Multilingual and Multicultural Development.* https://doi.org/10.1080/01434632.2021.1974462

Amin, S. (2000). The political economy of the twentieth century. *Monthly Review,* 52, https://monthlyreview.org/2000/06/01/the-political-economy-of-the-twentieth-century doi:10.14452/MR-052-02-2000-06_1

Amin, S. (2019, July 1). The new imperial structure. *Monthly Review, 7,* 32-45. https://monthlyreview.org/2019/07/01/thenew-imperialist-structure/doi:10.14452/MR-071-03-2019-07_3

Bensimon, E. M. (2018). Reclaiming racial justice in equity. *Change: The Magazine of Higher Learning, 50*(3-4), 95-98. https://doi.org/10.1080/00091383.2018.1509623

Heidelberg, B. M. (2019). Evaluating equity: Assessing diversity efforts through a social justice lens. *Cultural Trends, 28*(5), 391-403. https://doi.org/10.1080/09548963.2019.1680002

Hyter, Y. D. (2022). Engaging in culturally responsive and globally sustainable practices. *International Journal of Speech-Language Pathology.* Early Online 1-9. http://doi.org/10.1080/17549501.2022.2070280

Hyter, Y. D., & Salas-Provance, M. B. (2023). *Culturally responsive practices in speech, language, and hearing sciences* (2nd Ed.). Plural Publishing.

Liu, D., Burston, B., Stewart, S. C., & Mulligan, H. H. (2021). *Isms in health care human resources: A concise guide to workplace diversity, equity, and inclusion.* Jones & Bartlett.

Maxmen, A. (2021, September 16). The fight to manufacture COVID vaccines in lower-income countries. *Nature, 597,* 455-457. https://www.nature.com/articles/d41586-021-0283-z. http://doi.org/10.1038/d41586-021-02383-z

McGrath, M. (2021, October 6). Climate change: Voices from global south muted by climate science. *BBC News,* https://www.bbc.com/news/science-enviornment-58808509

Pillay, M., & Kathard, H. (2015). Decolonizing health professionals' education: Audiology & speech therapy in South Africa. *African Journal of Rhetoric, 7,* 193-227.

Pillay, M., & Kathard, H. (2018). Renewing our cultural borderlands: Equitable population innovations for communication (EPIC). *Topics in Language Disorders, 38*(2), 143-160.

St. Pierre, J., & St. Pierre, C. (2018). Governing the voice: A critical history of speech-language pathology. *Foucault Studies, 24,* 151-184. https://doi.org/10.22439/fs.v0i24.5530

Part I

BACKGROUND

Chapter 1

Introduction

Mellissa Bortz, PhD, CCC-SLP

Failure to acquire language, or a disruption of the language acquisition process, is one of the most devastating and isolating events which can occur to a human being (O'Malley & Tikofsky, 1972, p. 3).

As speech-language therapists, one of our most important roles is to evaluate our clients' language to ameliorate the catastrophic effects of language impairment. The most important aspect of clinical management is assessment (Weiss et al., 1987). The challenge of language assessment is that "language is complicated and does not lend itself to easy assessments" (McCartney, 1993, p. 17).

Definition of Assessment

The aims of language assessment are to establish the presence or absence of a disorder and to plan and determine the appropriateness of a therapy plan. Assessments should have "foundational integrity" according to Shipley and McAfee (2021, p. 4). This integrity requires that assessments are thorough, include a variety of assessment modalities such as case history information and formal and informal testing, and should be valid and reliable. Most importantly we need to ensure that our assessments focus on the individual client. We need to devise "assessment materials that are appropriate for the client's gender, skill levels, and ethnocultural background" (Shipley & McAfee, 2021, p. 4). Assessment also requires the "integration and interpretation of results to make a judgement or a decision, i.e., the outcome of an assessment is usually a diagnosis ..." (Shipley & McAfee, 2021, p. 4).

Bortz, M. (Ed.). *A Guide to Global Language Assessment: A Lifespan Approach* (pp. 3-24).
DOI: 10.4324/9781003524472-2

Dia—gnosis

"apart"—"to know" (Greek)

Assessments allow us, speech-language therapists, to distinguish "a person's problem from the large field of potential disabilities" (i.e., to diagnose a challenge with language; Hedge & Pomaville, 2017; Pindzola et al., 2015).

Prevention of Language Disorders

Early detection prevents the more serious and long-term repercussions of language delay such as challenges with education, social, or vocational opportunities (Wetherby et al., 1989). There are significant long-term benefits to the early provision of children's language and literacy development. These benefits include maximizing their developmental potential (i.e., cognitive, linguistic, social-emotional), particularly when children are experiencing a critical period of development (i.e., early childhood to 9 years of age; McIntyre et al., 2017, abstract). Infancy and early childhood are critical times to engage in prevention and improvement of challenges that play a role in development and could later affect children's neurological development across the lifespan (de Koning et al., 2004 as cited in Fernandes et al., 2021). Late diagnosis of language disorders can be stressful for both family members and children (Fernandes et al., 2021) and affects the family's quality of life (Cardoso, 2019; Jones et al., 2016 as cited in Fernandes et al., 2021). In majority-world countries the time period from a family's first concern about their child's development and the definitive diagnosis could be as long as 5 years (Zanon et al., 2017 as cited in Fernandes et al., 2021).

The World Health Organization (WHO) 67th World Congress addresses these issues in relation to autism spectrum disorders. They recommend the mainstreaming of primary health care services in the promotion of child and adolescent development to ensure "timely detection" and management according to national circumstance of member countries (WHO, 2014). At the WHA 73 they reiterated the importance of addressing the current significant gaps in early detection, care treatment, and rehabilitation for metal and neurodevelopmental conditions including autism (WHO, n.d.).

Figure 1-1 depicts the three levels of prevention that speech-language therapists engage in. Primary prevention can be seen at the bottom and broadest part of the triangle where services can be provided to the most clients. Prevention of a language disorder is achieved through the use of primary prevention in the form of public education programs such as Early Intervention. Early Intervention targets an entire population in order to provide support and education before problems occur.

The American Speech-Language-Hearing Association's (ASHA's) position statement on prevention defines secondary prevention as the early detection and treatment of communication disorders (1988). As Figure 1-1 indicates, early detection (screening and language assessments) is achieved by secondary prevention (Eastern Mediterranean Region World Health Organization, n.d.) by speech-language therapists. Figure 1-1 shows that therapy or rehabilitation occurs at the tertiary level of prevention.

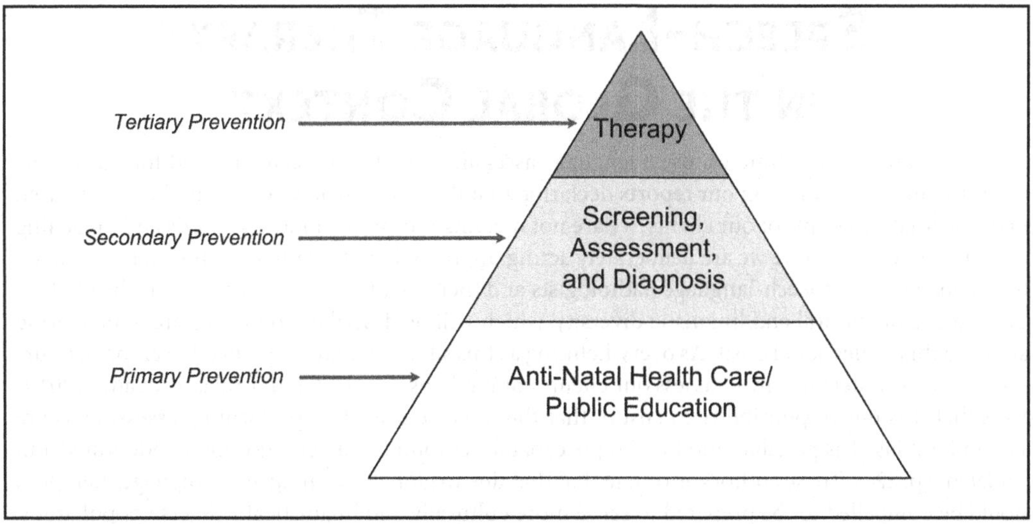

Figure 1-1. Primary health care model. (Adapted from American Speech-Language-Hearing Association [1994], Gerber [1990], and Marge [1991].)

Speech-Language Professional Role in Assessment

It is my belief that currently we are not fulfilling our professional roles as speech-language therapists in terms of assessment. Our professional associations clearly state that assessment of communication disorders is one of our professional and ethical responsibilities. Assessing communication and swallowing needs are one of the standards for speech-language pathologists in Australia (Speech Pathology Australia, n.d.; speechpathologyaustralia.org.au). ASHA's *Scope of Practice* (2016) states that "speech-language pathologists have expertise in the differential diagnosis of disorders or communication and swallowing; ... (should) administer standardized and/or criterion-referenced tools to compare individuals with their peers and ... (must) utilize culturally and linguistically appropriate assessment materials." As clinicians, ethically we are duty bound to our clients by ensuring their autonomy, beneficence, nonmaleficence, and justice.

Verdon et al. (2016) indicate that speech therapy associations are beginning to recognize the need for increased research with cultural and linguistically diverse populations to ensure that recommendations for practice are based upon the best available evidence. The proof of this is the establishment of significant interest groups (SIG) and panels in different countries' associations. These include the International Expert Panel on Multilingual Children's Speech, Royal College of Specific Interest Group in Bilingualism, and ASHA SIG 14 Cultural and Linguistic Diversity. ASHA's *Code of Ethics* requires the provision of competent services to all populations and the recognition of the cultural and linguistic experiences, or life experiences, of both the professional and those they serve. Caution must be taken not to attribute stereotypical characteristics to individuals (Issues in Ethics: Cultural and Linguistic Competence—ASHA). We also need to ensure that we are not committing linguistic racism or linguicism by not being able to assess our clients in all the languages that they speak.

Speech-Language Therapy in the Global Context

Dear readers, every time we use a language assessment that is not standardized for our clients or must write a disclaimer on our reports declaring that the assessment we performed was not based on the normative sample of our clients, we are not meeting our professional standards and breaching our ethics. I do not believe we are deliberately acting unprofessionally. Rather, the mismatch between the homogeneity of speech-language pathologists and their clients (Table 1-1) as well as the complicated nature of cultural and linguistic diversity, which will be described following, are contributing factors to this professional crisis. As overwhelming as this situation may be, we need to empower ourselves to work systematically to assess our clients comprehensively. Hyter and Salas-Provance (2019) stress that it is our responsibility to ensure that the tests we use when performing assessments are "fair and unbiased as possible, and the unique capabilities found in diverse groups are identified and validated" (p. 224). These authors also state that that due to globalization, speech-language therapists should be compelled to "be prepared to serve more culturally and linguistically diverse populations, and to make connections linking local and global concerns" (Hyter & Salas-Provance, 2023, p. 26).

Global Context

This section describes the global context in which this cultural and linguistic diversity occurs. This book uses the terms *majority-world countries* and *minority-world countries* and *majority-world contexts within minority-world countries.*

Majority-World Countries

"The chances that a disabled child in Africa receives the quality of care that children are all over the rest of the world receives are similar to the chances that an Antarctic penguin is fed a mackerel by a physiatrist" (Wylie et al., 2013, p. 3).

Majority-world countries, previously called colonial countries (Emmanuel, 2009), are now where most of the world's population live (e.g., India and African countries). These countries are rich in resources. However, the people in these countries do not have access to or benefit from these resources.

Minority-World Countries

Minority-world countries are where the minority of the world's populations live. These countries are rich and hold a monopoly on the world's resources (Hyter, personal communication, November 14, 2021; e.g., United States, Canada, France). WHO reports that health care systems in high-income countries provide multiple opportunities for prevention, early identification, and management of developmental difficulties in young children (Fernandes et al., 2021, p. 107).

Table 1-1
Ratio of Speech-Language Therapists to Clients

COUNTRY	NUMBER OF THERAPISTS	POPULATION TOTAL	RACE/ ETHNICITY	SPOKEN LANGUAGES IN COUNTRY	GENDER	MONO MULTILINGUAL	RATIO
Sub Saharan Africa (Angola, Benin, Botswana, Burkina Faso, Burundi, Cabo Verde, Cameroon, Central African Republic, Chad, Comoros)	33	1,136,046.77	POC 80%	Language Families	Female	Multilingual	1:2-4 million people
Taiwan	594	23,895,594	98% Han Chinese	Mandarin Chinese	NA	NA	1:40228
South Africa	1024	59.31 million (2020)	Black POC 80%	11	Female	Bilingual: English and Afrikaans	1:57919
United States	207,913	329.5 million (2020)	White People of color (POC) 8.5% Hispanic 6.1%	350	Female	Mono 92%	1:350 1:2500–470
English first language countries (Antigua, Barbuda, Australia, Bahamas, Barbados, Belize, Canada, Dominica, Grenada, Guyana, Ireland, Jamaica, Saint Lucia, Saint Vincent, United Kingdom)	213,115	335 million	White POC Hispanic	English	Female	Monolingual	1:2500 – 4700 (Wylie et al., 2013)

(continued)

Table 1-1 (continued)

Ratio of Speech-Language Therapists to Clients

COUNTRY	NUMBER OF THERAPISTS	POPULATION TOTAL	RACE/ ETHNICITY	SPOKEN LANGUAGES IN COUNTRY	GENDER	MONO MULTILINGUAL	RATIO
Vietnam	16	88 million	Kinh, Muong, Tho, Chut	Vietnamese, English	NA	Monolingual	70:88 million
New Zealand	838	5.084 million	European, Māori, Pacific peoples, Asian, MELAA (Middle Eastern/ Latin American/ African)	English, Māori NZ Sign Language, Samoan, Northern Chinese (including Mandarin), and Hindi	Female	NA	942 and the then population (4,699,755) there are 20 SLTs per 100,000 population

Majority-World Contexts in Minority-World Countries

It is very important to consider that majority-world contexts often exist in minority-world countries such as Aboriginal people in Australia (Hyter & Staley, personal communication, November 14, 2021). Clients may live in rural or remote areas rather than urban areas (Wylie et al., 2013). In addition, marginalized groups such as African American, First Nations, and Latinx people living in the United States have limited access to services (Copeland, 2005; Hyter & Salas-Provance, 2023).

Refugees, Migrants, and Asylum Seekers

The current global situation requires speech-language therapists to assess increasing numbers of refugees, migrants, and asylum seekers from majority- and minority-world contexts. Levey and Cheng (2021) describe refugees as people who are forced to leave a country due to war, poverty, persecution, and political instability. Refugees fear persecution due to race, religion, nationality, politics, or being a member of a particular group (worldpopulationsreview.com).

There are 25.9 million refugees around the world, and half of these refugees are children. This is the highest number ever recorded (UN Refugee Agency, n.d.). However, the number could be closer to 30 million due to the events in Ukraine resulting in over 4 million refugees having to flee their country. To exacerbate the refugee situation, approximately 80% of refugees resettle in majority-world countries who already have limited resources. Refugee populations are "confronted by numerous difficulties in assimilation and acculturation" (Westby & Levey, 2021, p. 42). A focus of assessment and treatment should be the use of narratives to describe the trauma that people, particularly children, have endured. McNeilly (2019) has written an important article regarding how speech-language therapists in the United States who work with migrant children should develop competence in distinguishing between language difference and language disability when learning English as a new language.

Underserved or Unserved Populations

Limited or unavailable health, educational, or other basic services results in increasing numbers of underserved or unserved populations (Levey & Cheng, 2021). Wylie et al. (2013, p. 2) cite the U.S. Department of Health and Human Services (2009) as defining medically underserved areas as those where there are not enough health workers to meet population needs, populations where there are barriers such as financial, cultural, or linguistic issues. Approximately 80% of the global populations who have health disabilities live in majority-world contexts. It is common that these clients will have more access to physical rehabilitation services than speech-language therapy (Wylie et al., 2013).

Linguistic Human Rights in Global Contexts

As speech-language therapists, we need to be aware that every human being has the right to their language, to be educated in their own language and have this respected, and to have the right to learn another language (Skutnuabb-Kangas & Phillipson, 1994 as cited in Hyter & Salas-Provance, 2019). Linguistic racism or *linguicism* is defined as "discrimination (or racism) based on the language of person or a group of speakers" (Baker-Bell, 2020; Phillipson, 1992 as cited in Hyter & Salas-Provance, 2023, p. 35). In all global contexts, linguistic imperialism occurs when "a language dominates internationally and includes exploitation, injustice and unequal rights" (Philipson, 2018 as cited in Hyter & Salas-Provance, 2023, p. 35). Colleagues, we need to take note of the fact that in language education the standard form of a language is used (Otheguy et al., 2015).

> Standard languages ... make room only for those features that index social prestige, that is only those idiolectal features found in the speech of those who share a superior class membership, political power, and in many cases ethnic identity. The linguistic canon that rules the teaching of what schools call native language arts, second languages, additional languages, foreign languages, and bilingual education has been shaped by acts of selective legitimation that license only linguistic features associated with powerful speakers and states. This means that schools everywhere seek to limit translanguaging in all students. (Otheguy et al., 2015, p. 301)

An example of linguicism is that African American English (AAE) has been stigmatized as being an inferior language when compared to Standard American English (SAE; Baugh & Labov, 1999; Wolfram, 2013). Further, Wolfram asserts that normative views of SAE attribute an inferior status to immigrants or refugees who speak other Englishes, such as Maay or Lebanese (Wolfram, 2013 as cited in Song et al., 2021). This description indicates that our majority-world clients (refugees, migrants, asylum seekers, and underserved or unserved clients) are at great risk of linguistic racism.

Challenge: Ratio of Clients to Speech-Language Therapists in the Global Context

One of the biggest challenges that we as speech-language therapists face in providing professional assessments to our clients in the global context is the lack of appropriate assessments and trained professionals to administer these assessments (Maulik & Darmstadt, 2007), as can be seen in Table 1-1. There is very limited information available on the number of speech-language therapists in the world. International speech-language therapy associations were surveyed, based on the ASHA list of associations, to determine the number of speech-language therapists compared to the populations of the particular countries. From the results, it can be seen that there is a global shortage of speech-language therapists.

Cultural and Linguistic Diversity Barriers in Majority- and Minority-World Countries

Wylie et al. (2013) provide a list of cultural and linguistic barriers to access speech-language pathology services as described in the following text. When considering devising culturally and linguistically diverse language assessments, we should apply our minds to ensuring that we eliminate these barriers. Therefore, we should ensure that the assessment matches or incorporates the client's cultural traditions and beliefs. We also need to consider that the language differences between provider and client need to be dealt with effectively to prevent challenges in communicating effectively. A challenge is that in minority-world countries, speech-language therapists may not be representative of minority groups. Speech-language therapists should educate themselves about culturally relevant information applying to their countries. In majority-world countries, the speech-language therapist usually only speaks English and a limited amount of the local language. There could be a cultural mismatch between the therapist and community in terms of child-rearing practicing, languages, beliefs about disability, and limiting engagement of the community.

Cultural and Linguistic Diversity in Assessment

Historical, Cultural Perspective of Assessment

To empower ourselves to conduct culturally and linguistically diverse assessments we need to consider the historic, scientific background of our profession. Speech-language therapy has conducted research and treated clients for the last century. The American Academy of Speech Correction was established in 1926. Speech-language therapy, like most allied health professions, originates from Western Eurocentric ideology or coloniality. This Eurocentric ideal supports "hegemonic control of how professions came to be or professionalization" (Mupawosa et al., 2021, p. 68). Abraham (2020) focuses on the fact that the profession defines and controls what is considered the truths of disciplinary knowledge. Colonialism includes power and knowledge and how these dimensions interact to oppress, marginalize, and dehumanize groups of people who are considered inferior by the dominant group (Mupawosa et al., 2021).

A similar view is that historically most of the research in our profession has been conducted in English for Western middle-class populations (Kathard et al., 2007). Currently, Verdon et al. (2016) state that research evidence indicates that speech-language pathology practice remains based on Western, educated, industrialized, rich, and democratic (WEIRD) societies. Henrich et al. (2010) describes researchers as being in a precarious position if they are trying to construct universal theories from a narrow and unusual slice of the population. The challenge with this assumption is "that these data are generalizable to all human populations without considerations of the vast diversity that exists between societies" (Heine et al., as cited in American Psychological Association, 2010, p. 11).

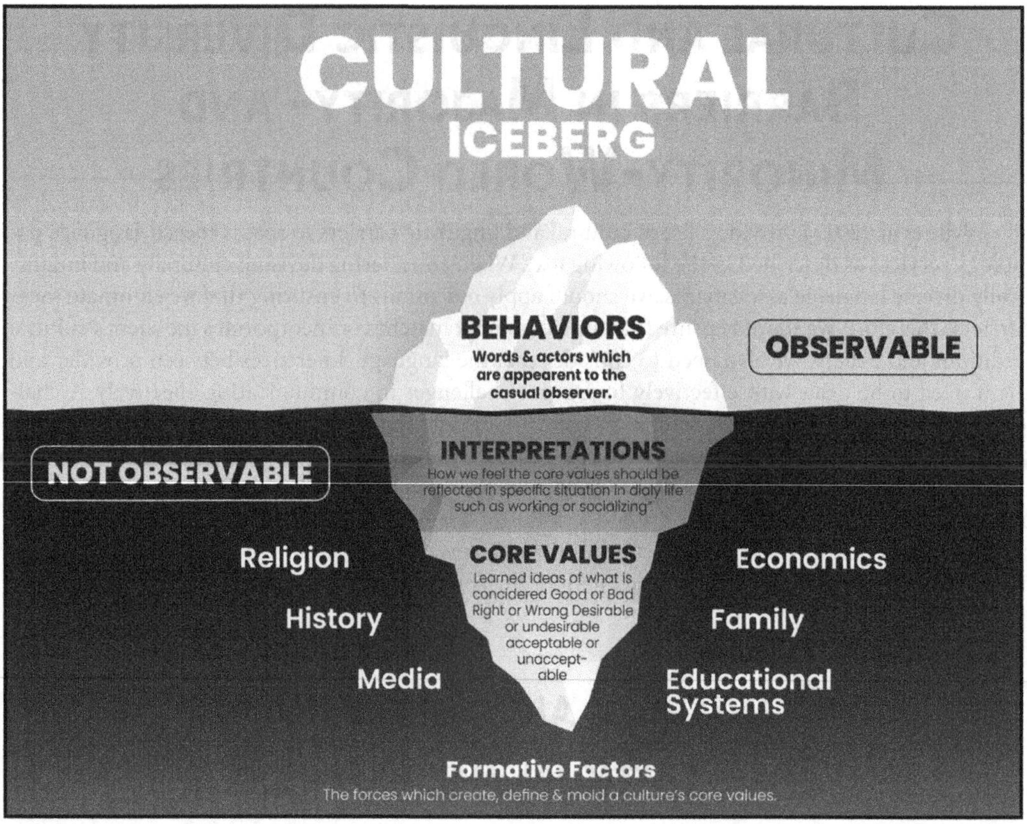

Figure 1-2. Iceberg Model of Culture. (iStock)

Similarly, Blum (2017) finds that "the unseen assumptions" of WEIRD people and what is thought to be "natural" or "optimal" is found to be narrow when there is cross-cultural evidence that relates to the "assumed proper way" to socialize children into language.

For speech-language therapists, the challenge of using language assessments normed on predominantly English-speaking British or American populations in their current form can present the speech-language therapist with inaccurate findings that may be used to determine the future of the children assessed (Arias & Friberg, 2017; Williams & McLeod, 2012). Mdladlo et al. (2019) contend that in fact "speech-language therapists could be guilty of what critical theorists would describe as 'social oppression' by ignoring more culturally and linguistically appropriate resources for assessment" (p. 6).

Deconstructing Cultural Diversity

Culture is a set of beliefs made up of many dimensions that describe how an individual or a group of people experience life and engage in daily practices (Hyter & Salas-Provance, 2023). As Figure 1-2 shows, the Iceberg Model of Culture consists of surface layers such as race, gender, and language. Deep culture includes age, religion, physical ability, and sexual orientation. Hyter and Salas-Provance (2023) contend that it is these invisible or internal aspects of culture are "what truly makes up culture" (p. 23).

Culture is like an iceberg; the deep layers are hidden from our view. We tend to see and hear only the uppermost layers of cultural artifacts. We can also witness the exchange of overt verbal and nonverbal symbols. However, to understand a culture—or a person in a cultural community—with any depth, "we must match their underlying values coherently with their respective norms, meanings, and symbols" (Ting-Toomey & Chung, 2012).

According to the Iceberg Model, when performing an assessment, the speech-language therapist will first observe the surface culture (i.e., the language that our clients speak, communication styles, and rules such as eye contact; facial expression are examples of deep culture). Speech-language therapists have to consider this interaction carefully, as when assessing a child who does not make eye contact we may assume that they have autism spectrum disorder. However, in many cultures such as Japanese, South-Eastern Zone Bantu, Middle Eastern, Latinx, and Native American cultures eye contact is regarded as disrespectful (Uono & Hietanen, 2015).

ASHA (2023) defines multicultural diversity as including, but not limited to, age, disability, ethnicity, gender identity (encompasses gender expression), national origin (encompasses related aspects [e.g., ancestry, culture, language, dialect, citizenship, and immigration status]), race, religion, sexual orientation, and veteran status.

When developing assessments, it is essential to consider our client's religion and beliefs, for example, the use of traditional and faith healers when developing culturally fair assessments. Semela (2001) reports that particularly in rural areas parents seek assistance from traditional healers. "Traditional healers are readily accepted and understood by Black communities as they have the same or similar cultural and African background" (Semela, 2001, p. 133). Further, Semela (2001) reports that "these healers are successful in providing support systems for families who have brain damaged children who have difficulty in language acquisitions" (p. 33).

Developing Cultural Competence, Responsiveness, and Humility

In order to assess the cultural diversity of our majority and minority clients, we need to ensure that we are providing equitable, diverse, inclusive, and accessible assessments. Beginning the lifelong quest for cultural competence, responsiveness, and humility will assist us in this challenge. Developing cultural competence has been found to reduce health disparities (Selig et al., 2006). We need to be aware of performing microaggressions and how to deal with these (e.g., using the term *illegal alien*).

Cultural Competence

ASHA's *Code of Ethics* (2023) requires the provision of competent services to all populations and the recognition of the cultural and linguistic experiences, or life experiences of both the professional and those they serve. Caution must be taken not to attribute stereotypical characteristics to individuals. Mophosho et al. (2021) cite Campinha-Bacote (2002) that when a speech-language therapist becomes culturally competent this requires the consideration of the following cultural factors—"desire, awareness, knowledge, cultural encounters and most importantly skills conducting culturally sensitive assessments" (p. 86). Cultural competence requires a "practical, concrete demonstration of the ethical principles of beneficence, nonmaleficence and justice," according to Hoop et al. (2008).

A very useful model describing how to become culturally competent is the VISION Model (Bellon-Harn & Garrett, 2008 as cited in Hyter & Salas-Provance, 2023, p. 67). This model provides information about cultural and linguistic differences between clients and professionals as Table 1-2 indicates.

TABLE 1-2
VISION MODEL

V	Values and belief systems of the family and professional
I	Interaction style refers to the style of communication that is preferred by the family and by the clinician
S	Structuring the relationship between the professional and family
I	Interaction style is the style of communication preferred by the family and clinicians
O	Operational strategies refer to the manner in which selecting and addressing goals carried out
N	Need (perceived) focuses on the outcomes agreed upon by the family members and the professional

Cultural Responsiveness

Cultural responsiveness requires global speech-language therapists assessing cultural and diverse cultures to adapt our interactions and be responsive to our clients (Mophosho et al., 2021, p. 88). Hyter and Salas-Provance (2023) consider that cultural responsiveness is a broader term than cultural competence because it provides a broader perspective from "which to view our behaviors as they relate to our actions with individuals across a variety of cultures that are different from our own" (p. 7). Figure 1-3 shows that these circles are dynamic, and we need to "move within and among them in a circular way rather than linearly" (Hyter & Salas-Provance, 2023, p. 9) with each client we encounter. This means that we speech-language therapists need to undertake a lifelong commitment to self-evaluation and self-critique and remedying the power imbalances that can occur in clinical interactions such as assessments (Tervalon & Murray-Garcia, 1998).

Cultural Humility

Mophosho et al. (2021) defines cultural humility as being the development of a "lifelong learning process that incorporates openness, power-balancing, and critical self-reflection when interacting with mutually beneficial partnerships" (p. 87). Hughes et al. (2020) state that cultural humility occurs at the intrapersonal and interpersonal levels. Cultural humility requires us to utilize knowledge, sensitivity, and competence skills (Papadopoulas et al., 2016). We need to use cultural humility when parents ask us why we are asking them what level of education they have.

Materials to Assess and Develop Cultural Competence, Responsiveness and Humility

There are several measures of assessing and developing cultural competence, responsiveness, and humility (e.g., ASHA's Cultural Competence quiz).

Another useful resource to determine clinicians' cultural competence for majority-world cultures in the United States has been devised by Shipley and McAfee (2021). They have devised multicultural case history forms for children and adults. Hyter and Salas-Provance (2023) describe a series of questions to obtain the cultural and linguistic background English as a second language speaker. Important questions include "what the acculturation pattern of the family has been?"(p. 250).

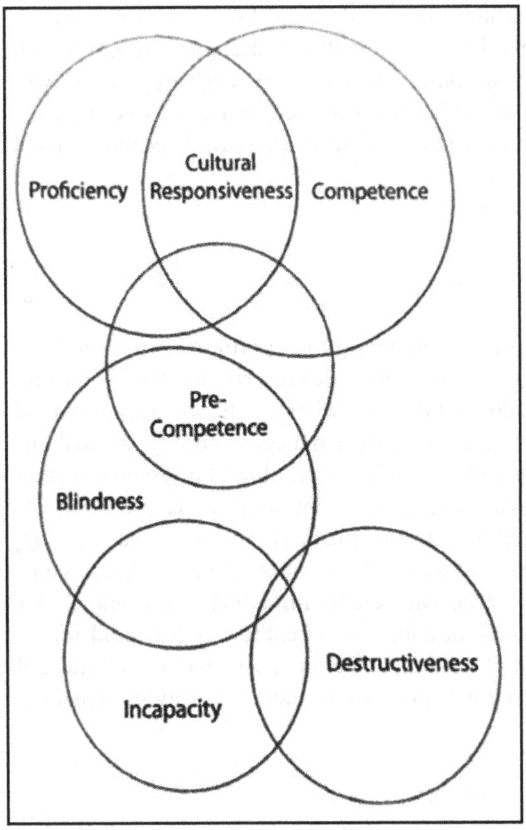

Figure 1-3. Cultural responsiveness. (From *Culturally Responsive Practices in Speech, Language, and Hearing Sciences, Second Edition* [pp. 1-448] by Hyter, Y. D., & Salas-Provance, M. Copyright © 2023. Plural Publishing, Inc. All rights reserved. Used with permission.)

Linguistic Diversity

One of the most important reasons that speech-language therapists have challenges in fulfilling our professional responsibility of assessing our clients in the languages that they speak is due to linguistic diversity in the majority- and minority-world contexts. The actual number of languages spoken in the world is difficult to determine and are more matters of opinion rather than facts according to Anderson (2010) and the Linguistics Society of America. The reasons for this are because languages are constantly changing. New languages develop while other languages die out. In 2022, it was estimated that there are 7,151 languages spoken in the world (Ethnologue, n.d.).

Multilingualism

The majority of the world's population speaks more than one language (Grosjean, 2012). Multilingualism[1] presents differently in different majority- and minority-world countries. In India, a majority-world country, there are 19 to 500 languages and dialects spoken. English and Hindi are the official languages spoken in India. There are 23 constitutionally recognized languages. Hindi and English are spoken by more than 50% of the population. The most diverse language group is the Tibeto-Burmese group with 66 languages. Twenty-six percent of the population is multilingual, and approximately 7% of the population are trilingual. There are large differences between urban and rural India (*The Times of India–Delhi* eEdition, November 7, 2018).

[1]In this book multilingualism incorporates bilingualism.

Minority-world countries such as the United States have a different linguistic reality. In the United States English is the only official language. Yet there are more than 350 languages spoken, with one out of every five children in the United States speaking a language other than English (Hyter & Salas-Provance, 2023). The Individuals with Disabilities Education Act ensures services to assist these children learn English by having English as a New Language teachers assist these multilingual children.

Translanguaging

Translanguaging occurs when a multilingual person's full linguistic repertoire is used and honored. Otheguy et al. (2015) posit that "translanguaging is the deployment of a speaker's full repertoire without regard for watchful adherence to the socially and politically defined boundaries of named (and usually national and state) languages." Therefore, a particular language cannot be defined linguistically in terms of lexical or structural grammar and is not a linguistic object but "something that a person speaks" (p. 286). The implications of translanguaging when devising language assessments for multilinguals *in a language* needs to be separated from testing proficiency *in language* (Otheguy et al., 2015, p. 299). As assessors we need to assess the size, development, flexibility, richness, complexity, and agility of deployment of an idiolect (i.e., true assessment of linguistic proficiency). This is different from and must be kept apart from assessing the ability of a client to recognize and adhere to politically defined boundaries in the deployment of an idiolect (i.e., an assessment of cultural and political proficiency). When assessing language-using narratives we would ask our multilingual clients to use all their languages.

Solution: World Health Organization Regions and Language Families

Language families are a group of languages related due to a common parental language or proto language (Greenberg, 1963; Gregersen, 1977; Wichmann et al., 2010). All language develops from a single ancestral family. Language families have common phonological, morphological, and syntactic features. Figure 1-4 illustrates the different South-Eastern Zone Bantu Languages spoken in South Africa. The Nguni and Sotho languages are mutually intelligible. In other words, a "family is a group of languages that can be shown to be genetically related to one another" (Anderson, 2010, paragraph 4). Chapter 3, Language and Language Families, provides more details of language families and shows maps of language families (Anderson, 2010).

An example of using language families is South Africa. There are 12 official languages spoken; nine of these are South-Eastern Zone Bantu languages, and two are Indo-European Languages: English and Afrikaans, and one is South African Sign Language. It is important to remember that the Nguni and Sotho languages are mutually intelligible. Figure 1-4 illustrates the nine South-Eastern Zone Bantu Languages used in South Africa.

Political and national borders do not correlate with where languages are spoken. An example is Bengali, an Indo-Aryan language with approximately 230 million speakers in the world. The Bengal region was part of India. However, after Partition in 1947 it became the Pakistani province of East Bengal (Van Schendel, 2020). In 1971, Bangladesh became an independent country after a war between India and Pakistan (Van Schendel, 2020). Bengal is now the official language of Bangladesh, but is also spoken by approximately 85 million people in India and 2 million speakers in Pakistan (AutoLingual, n.d.).

PHYLUM	Niger-Kordofanian
FAMILY	Benue-Congo
SUBDIVISION	Bantu
(LANGUAGE)	Setswana
BANTU SUBDIVISION: SOUTH-EASTERN BANTU ZONE	
SOTHO: Setswana, Southern Sesotho, Northern Sesotho NGUNI: isiZulu, isiXhosa, Seswati, isiNdebele Tshivenda Xitsonga/SHANGAAN	
Data sources: Greenberg (1963); Gregersen (1977).	

Figure 1-4. Classification of Setswana.

Therefore, according to Anderson (2010), what makes languages distinct from one another is related to social and political issues and not linguistic ones. Further, "what counts as a language rather than a 'mere' dialect typically involves issues of statehood, economics, literary traditions and writing systems and other trappings of power, authority, and cultures—with purely linguistic considerations playing a less significant role." In this global context, our clients are at risk for linguicism or linguistic racism (Phillipson, 1992). Otheguy et al. (2015) describe languages as "defined by the social, political or ethnic affiliation of its speakers" (p. 286). Linguicism often occurs when positive characteristics are assigned positive to a desired language such as English and negative characteristics to a dominated language such as Hmong (Hyter & Salas-Provance, 2023). When race in the form of "Whiteness" is combined with SAE, this forms language colonialism (Liggett, 2014; Flores & Rosa, 2015), in which Whiteness and SAE translates into social, cultural, and symbolic capital (Bourdieu, 2010 as cited in Song et al., p. 5).

I suggest that an organized way to deal effectively with all these variations of different languages is to make use of the six WHO regions of the world. The WHO regions are determined by the member states of the WHO. These regions are organizational groupings are based on geographical terms. It is important to note, however, that these are not necessarily synonymous with geographical regions (GreenFacts, 2001). The regions are the African Region (AFR = 46 countries), Region of the Americas (AMR = 35 countries), Southeast Region (SEAR = 11 countries), European Region (EUR = 53 countries), Eastern Mediterranean Region (EMR), and Western Pacific Region (WMR = 27 countries).

Practical Steps of Using Language Families

As speech-language therapists we need to familiarize ourselves with the language families and structures of the languages that our clients speak in order to assess their language effectively. A clinical example is that you are working in a busy National Health Service clinic in London and are asked to assess a 7-year-old multilingual child whose mother speaks isiZulu, father speaks Mandarin, and the child attends an English-speaking school. His teacher is concerned about his language development. This child will likely use translanguaging (i.e., use his individualized, integrated language system), as can be seen in the next example. Therefore, we need to familiarize ourselves with the different constructions used in the sentences such as the negative construction.

isiZulu is characterized by noun class systems, extensive agreement, and a suffixal system of verbal derivatives. It is also a tonal language (Doke, 1990). Mandarin is a Verb Object (VO) language. However, syntactically, Mandarin Chinese does have some word order patterns that are not seen in other VO languages. Mandarin is part of the Chinese family of languages, which are part of the Sino-Tibetan language family. English is an Indo-European language typified by inflections that have different endings in nouns. Adjectives and verbs represent the grammatical function of the word.

isiZulu: a-ngi-m-bon-anga

Neg-I-him-see-negative

"I didn't see him"

Mandarin: wo mei you kan jian ta / 我没有看见他。

I not see him (It can be "I do not see him" or "I did not see him").

We know the tense from the context. (Dr. Wendy Lee and Dr. Lucy Liu, personal communication, April 6, 2022).

English: **I didn't see him**

Possible translanguaged example: a-ngi **him** ta 他

"I didn't see him"

Historical Perspective of Language Assessment Translation

One who wishes to translate from one language to another, and tries to translate word by word and maintain the order of both the subject and the words, will find his work very difficult and will ultimately end up with a translation that is highly questionable and confusing. Rather, one who translates from one language to anther must first understand the concepts (Maimonides, 1135–1234; Letter to Shmuel ibn Tibbon, as cited in Kaplan, 1981).

Speech-language therapists have attempted to address the absence of a standardized test by translating existing standardized tests into one or more of the South-Eastern Zone Bantu languages. Masiloane (1983) performed a literal translation of the Reynell (1977) into Zulu. The results indicated that the test items were not culturally appropriate for Zulu children. An example was "Santa Claus" known as "Father Christmas" in South Africa.

Tests cannot simply be translated from English into the language in which the test is being devised. Literal translations ignore cultural and linguistic differences of the test population. These translations result in a structure that is different in syntactic complexity, semantic form, and pragmatic implications from the original (Paltiel, 1990). A specific example is that many concepts that are syntactically expressed in English are morphologically represented isiZulu. For example, verbs are expressed as part of a sentence that can be seen in the clinical example of past tense described previously. Bedore and Pena (2008) warn us that standardized measures should not be translated into another language for use as an informal measure. The reason for this is that there may be differences across languages regarding what would be important to convey meaning and what is developmentally appropriate, as well as cultural differences.

Table 1-3

Alternative Methods of Assessment

1. Use of criterion-referenced tests
2. Modification of norm-referenced tests by
   a. Varying prompting
   b. Completing test over several sessions
   c. Completing test under several conditions in different locations (office, classroom, playground, home, patient room)
   d. Using more than the allotted practice items
   e. Extending the time of the testing
   f. Allowing credit for a variety of responses beyond those accepted in test protocol
   g. Scoring test twice, once by examiner manual direction and one with nonstandard adjustments
3. Measure processing abilities rather than language knowledge
4. Use of portfolio assessment methods
5. Use of narrative assessment methods
6. Use of dynamic assessment methods
7. Include an interpreter in administration of test
8. Develop a new test

Although translation of assessments into other languages is problematic, back translation is a useful quality assessment tool (Brislin, 1970) that is available to us who are working cross-culturally in health research (Colina et al., 2017). In back translation an independent translator who has no knowledge of the original material translates it back into the original language literally so that the original meaning is shared.

Alternative Methods of Language Assessment

Hyter and Salas-Provance (2023, p. 254) provide an invaluable list of alternative methods of assessments, such as use of narrative assessments (Table 1-3). The later chapters of this book describe these methods in detail.

- Dynamic assessment is discussed by Dr. Washington and Dr. Núñez in Chapter 4.
- Ethnographic assessment is described by Dr. Davis-McFarland in Chapter 5.
- Narrative assessment is covered by Dr. Westerveld and Dr. Westby in Chapter 7.
- Chapter 12 details a new language test, as devised by Dr. Liu, Ms. Lee, Ms. Hutchings, Dr. de Villiers, and Dr. Rolfhus.

Utilizing Existing Structures to Devise Language Assessment

World Health Organization International Classification of Functioning, Disability and Health Model of Health and Disability

The World Health Organization *International Classification of Functioning, Disability and Health* (WHO-ICF) is a very useful model that we as global speech-language therapists can use to anchor all our assessments. The ICF is based on the integration of medical and social factors and represents functioning of the whole person. The ICF synthesizes the biological, individual, and social perspective of a client (WHO, 2001). Implementing the ICF allows us to assess our clients' challenges at the level of body—body functions and structures, level of the individual–activities of people and limitations that they may experience, functioning of a person as a member of society–participation and environmental factors, and whether these factors are facilitators or barriers (Centers for Disease Control and Prevention, n.d.). Dr. Carol Westby describes the use of the ICF Framework and Global Assessment in Chapter 2.

The diagnosis from the WHO-ICF can be coded using the *International Statistical Classification of Diseases and Related Health Problems* (ICD). ICD-11 would assign aphasia a code of R47.01. Due to the fact that functioning and disability associated with health conditions are classified using the ICF, the use of ICD-11 and the ICF together provides a more meaningful and complete picture of the individuals and populations (WHO, 2001).

In the context of language assessment, the main advantage of this system is that the method of assessing our clients and their environment is universal. Therefore, if a speech-language therapist in Haiti assesses a client with aphasia in French and Haitian Creole and the client moves to another part of the world, or the speech-language therapist requires assistance from a mentor working in China, the WHO-ICF template will be understood by both speech-language therapists. Other advantages of the WHO-ICF are that it can be used in interprofessional collaborative practice and for person centered care (ASHA, n.d.).

Collaboration

Collaboration requires teamwork, coordination, and networking (Reeves et al., 2017). One of the most effective methods of developing global language assessments is to collaborate.

Developing Interprofessional Teams for Developing Language Assessments

The development of a language assessment requires "buy in" from community members and many different professionals. Levey and Moonsamy (2021, p. 122) state that "no single practitioner possesses the knowledge to address the possible medical, communicative, sensory, and movement disabilities of an individual." Specific team members should include community members. This is essential as these are our clients who are going to be using the assessments. Researchers, statisticians, app developers, and linguists should also be included. In addition, we need to include Indigenous healers as part of our assessment teams (Mupawosa et al., 2021).

Networking

Networking is an invaluable tool available to speech-language therapists when devising language assessments. Countries that have speech-language therapy associations generally have committees or significant interest groups dedicated to clinical practice with culturally and linguistically diverse clients. If a group does not exist, the speech-language therapist can initiate one with local and global colleagues.

An example is the South African Speech Language Hearing Association (SASLHA) Collaboration with speech-language therapists and audiologists working in Africa. Our initial video conferencing meeting had eight participants. This meeting was followed by an introductory email to eight known African contacts and all SASLHA members in October 2016, explaining the projects and asking for emails contact details of other speech-language therapists. This had the snowball effect that within 4 months there were over 130 contacts in 20 countries. Currently there are 303 members of the African Connections project.

Cross-Linguistic Team Work

The COST ACTION A33 Cross-Linguistically Robust Stages of Children's Linguistic Performance was a comparative study of child language acquisition for the languages of the European Union (COST, n.d.). The main objective of this Action was "to discover methods that can be used for diagnosing language problems in children" in all European languages (cost.eu/actions/A33/). The proposed users of this action are speech-language therapists, education communities that work with children who might need language therapy, and doctors.

The findings of the COST ACTION A33 have resulted in COST ACTION ISO804 "Language Impairment in a Multilingual Society: Linguistic Patterns and the Road to Assessment" (LITMUS; 2019). LITMUS is a comprehensive set of tools designed and tested within the COST Action with the purpose of assessing the linguistic abilities of bilingual children. Examples of these tools include Sentence Repetition Tasks (Armon-Lotem & Grohmann, 2021).

The WHO resolution on autism spectrum disorders from the 67th World Health Assembly (WHA67.8; Rosanoff et al., 2015) stressed the need for comprehensive and coordinated management of autism spectrum disorders. This plan has been endorsed by over 60 countries. They recommend that part of this collaboration should be to develop clinical assessment tools.

University Repositories

Speech-language therapy master's and doctoral students have developed language assessments in fulfilment toward their degrees. These studies are freely available on university repositories all over the world.

Conclusion

In this chapter I have described the contexts and challenges that global speech-language therapists face when working with cultural and linguistic diverse multilingual children. We must ensure that we are providing the least biased and culturally responsive assessments. I have also attempted to share resources and methods of how we can meet these pressing challenges.

References

Abraham, G. Y. (2020). A post-colonial perspective on African education systems. *African Journal of Education and Practice, 6*(5), 40-54.

American Psychological Association (2010, May). Are your findings "WEIRD?" *Monitor on Psychology, 41*(5), 11. https://www.apa.org/monitor/2010/05/weird

American Speech-Language-Hearing Association. (1988). *Prevention of communication disorders* [Position Statement]. https://www.asha.org/policy/ps1988-00228/#:~:text=Secondary%20Prevention%E2%80%94the%20early%20detection,progress%2C%20thereby%20preventing%20further%20complications

American Speech-Language-Hearing Association. (1997). *American Speech-Language-Hearing Association.* https://www.asha.org/

American Speech-Language-Hearing Association. (2016). *Scope of practice in speech-language pathology* [Scope of Practice]. https://www.asha.org/policy/sp2016-00343/

American Speech-Language-Hearing Association. (2023). *Code of ethics.* https://www.asha.org/siteassets/publications/code-of-ethics-2023.pdf

American Speech-Language-Hearing Association. (n.d.). *International classification of functioning, disability and Health (ICF).* American Speech-Language-Hearing Association. https://www.asha.org/slp/icf/

Anderson, S. R. (2010). *How many languages are there in the world. Linguistic Society of America brochure series: Frequently asked questions.* Linguistic Society of America. https://www.linguisticsociety.org/content/how-many-languages-are-there-world

Arias, G., & Friberg, J. (2017). Bilingual language assessment: Contemporary versus recommended practice in American schools. *Language, Speech, and Hearing Services in Schools, 48*(1), 1-15. https://doi.org/10.1044/2016_LSHSS-15-0090

Armon-Lotem, S., & Grohmann, K. K. (2021). *Language impairment in multilingual settings: LITMUS in action across Europe.* John Benjamins Publishing Company.

AutoLingual. (n.d.). *Learn a foreign language by yourself.* https://autolingual.com/

Baker-Bell, A. (2020). Dismantling anti-black linguistic racism in English language arts classrooms: Toward an anti-racist Black language pedagogy. *Theory Into Practice, 59*(1), 8-21. https://doi.org/10.1080/00405841.2019.1665415

Baugh, J., & Labov, W. (1999). *Out of the mouths of slaves: African American language and educational malpractice.* University of Texas.

Bedore, L. M., & Peña, E. D. (2008). Assessment of bilingual children for identification of language impairment: Current findings and implications for practice. *International Journal of Bilingual Education and Bilingualism, 11*(1), 1-29.

Blum, S. (2017). Unseen WEIRD assumptions: The so-called language gap and ideologies of language, childhood, and learning. *International Multilingual Research Journal, 11*(1), 39-51.

Brislin, R. W. (1970). Back-translation for cross-cultural research. *Journal of Cross-Cultural Psychology, 1*(3), 185-216.

Centers for Disease Control and Prevention. (n.d.). *The ICF: An overview.* https://www.cdc.gov/nchs/data/icd/icfoverview_finalforwho10sept.pdf

Colina, S., Marrone, N., Ingram, M., & Sánchez, D. (2017). Translation quality assessment in health research: A functionalist alternative to back-translation. *Evaluation & The Health Professions, 40*(3), 267-293.

Copeland, V. C. (2005). African Americans: Disparities in health care access and utilization. *Health and Social Work, 30*(3), 265-270.

COST. (n.d.). *Cross-linguistically robust stages of children's linguistic performance.* COST. https://cost.eu/actions/A33/

Doke, C. M. (1990). *Textbook of Zulu grammar.* Maskew Miller.

Emmanuel. (2009). *"Majority world"—A new word for a new age.* https://masalai.wordpress.com/

Ethnologue. (n.d.). *How many languages are there in the world?* www.ethnologue.com

Fernandez, F. D. M., De La Higuera Amato, C. A., Molini-Avenjonas, D. R., Cardoso, C., Defense-Netral, D., & Garcia De Goulart, B. N. (2021). Children with communication disorders in Brazil: Rights and stigma of the unserved and underserved. In S. Levey & S. Moonsamy (Eds.), *Unserved and underserved populations. New approaches to inclusivity* (pp. 101-121). Peter Lang.

Flores, N., & Rosa, J. (2015). Undoing appropriateness: Raciolinguistic ideologies and language diversity in education. *Harvard Educational Review, 85*(2), 149-171. https://doi.org/10.17763/0017-8055.85.2.149

Gerber, S. E. (1990). *The etiology of communication disorders in children.* Prentice Hall.

Greenberg, J. H. (1963). *The languages of Africa.* Bloomington.

GreenFacts. (2001). *Facts on health and the environment.* https://www.greenfacts.org/en/index.htm

Gregersen, E. A. (1977). *Languages in Africa. An introductory survey.* Gordon and Breach.

Grosjean, F. (2012). An attempt to isolate, and then differentiate, transfer and interference. *International Journal of Bilingualism, 16*(1), 11-21. https://doi.org/10.1177/1367006911403210

Hedge, M. N., & Pomaville, F. (2017). *Assessment of communication disorders in children: Resources and protocols* (3rd ed.). Plural Publishing.

Henrich, J., Heine, S. J., & Norenzayan, A. (2010). The weirdest people in the world? *Behavioral and Brain Sciences, 33,* 61-83.

Hoop, J. G., DiPasquale, T., Hernandez, J. M., & Weiss Robers, L. (2008). Ethics and culture in mental health care. *Ethics Behavior, 18*(4), 353-372. https://doi.org/10.1.1080.105084270701713048

Hughes, V., Delva, S., Nkimbeng, M., Spaulding, E., Turkson-Ocran, R. A., Cudjoe, J., Ford, A., Rushton, C., D'Aoust, R., & Han, H.-R. (2020). Not missing the opportunity: Strategies to promote cultural humility among future nursing faculty. *Journal of Professional Nursing, 36*(1), 28-33. https://doi.org/10.1016/j.profnurs.2019.06.005

Hyter, Y. D., & Salas-Provance, M. B. (2019). *Culturally responsive practices in speech, language, and hearing sciences* (1st ed.). Plural Publishing.

Hyter, Y. D., & Salas-Provance, M. B. (2021). *Culturally responsive practices in speech, language, and hearing sciences* (2nd ed.). Plural Publishing.

Hyter, Y. D., & Salas-Provance, M. B. (2023). *Culturally responsive practices in speech, language and hearing sciences* (3rd ed.). Plural Publishing, Inc.

Kaplan, A. (1981). *The living Torah.* Maznaim Publishing Company.

Kathard, H., Naude, E., Pillay, M., & Ross, E. (2007). Improving the relevance of speech-language pathology and audiology research and practice. *South African Journal of Communication Disorders, 54,* 5-7.

Levey, S., & Cheng, L. L. (2021). The plight of unserved and underserved populations across the globe. In S. Levey & S. Moonsamy (Eds.), *Unserved and underserved populations. New approaches to inclusivity.* (pp. 1-22). Peter Lang.

Levey, S., & Moonsamy, S. (2021). The path forward. In S. Levey & S. Moonsamy (Eds.), *Unserved and underserved populations. New approaches to inclusivity* (pp. 121-128). Peter Lang.

Liggett, T. (2014). The mapping of a framework: Critical race theory and TESOL. *The Urban Review, 46*(1), 112-124.

LITMUS Sentence Repetition. (2019). *Home: Litmus sentence repetition tasks.* https://www.litmus-srep.info/

Marge, M. (1991). Introduction to the prevention and epidemiology of voice disorders. *Seminars in Speech and Language, 12*(1), 49-73.

Masiloane, M. (1983). *Performance of Zulu speaking children on a literal translation of the RDLS* (Doctoral dissertation).

Maulik, P. K., & Darmstadt, G. L. (2007). Childhood disability in low- and middle-income countries: Overview of screening, prevention, services, legislation, and epidemiology. *Pediatrics,* 120. https://doi.org/10.1542/peds.2007-0043b

McCartney, E. (1993). Assessment of expressive language. In J. R. Beech & L. Harding with D. Hilton-Jones (Eds.), *Assessment in speech and language therapy* (pp. 35-48). Routledge.

McIntyre, L. J., Hellsten, L. A. M., Bidonde, J., & Boden, C. (2017). Receptive and expressive English language assessments used for young children: A scoping review protocol. *Systematic Reviews, 6*(1), 1-7.

McNeilly, L. G. (2019). Strategies utilized by speech-language pathologists to effectively address the communication needs of migrant school-age children. *Folia Phoniatrica et Logopaedica, 71*(2-3), 127-134.

Mdladlo, T., Flack, P. S., & Joubert, R. W. (2019). The cat on a hot tin roof? Critical considerations in multilingual language assessments. *South African Journal of Communication Disorders, 66*(1), 1-7. https://doi.org/10.4102/sajcd.v66i1.610

Mophosho, M., Moonsamy, S., & Mupawosa, A. (2021). Cultural humility in interactions with different cultural identities: How do you see me? In S. Levey & S. Moonsamy (Eds.), *Unserved and underserved populations. New approaches to inclusivity* (pp. 83-100). Peter Lang.

Mupawosa, A., Mophosho, M., & Moonsamy, S. (2021). Critical reflections: A tool for intergroup relations for health-care services. In S. Levey & S. Moonsamy (Eds.), *Unserved and underserved populations. New approaches to inclusivity* (pp. 65-82). Peter Lang.

Otheguy, R., Garcia, O., & Reid, W. (2015). Clarifying translanguaging and deconstructing named languages: A perspective from linguistics. *Applied Linguistics Review, 6*(3), 281-307.

Paltiel, L. (1990). *The effects of translation on linguistic complexity and difficulty of development language tests: Evidence from three-subtests of Clinical Evaluation of Language Fundaments* [Unpublished master's thesis]. Department of Applied Linguistics, Bar Ilan University, Tel Aviv.

Papadopoulos, I., Shea, S., Taylor, G., Pezzella, A., & Foley, L. (2016). Developing tools to promote culturally competent compassion, courage, and intercultural communication in healthcare. *Journal of Compassionate Health Care, 3*, 2. https://doi.org/10.1186/s40639-016-0019-6

Phillipson, R. (1992). *Linguistic imperialism*. Oxford University Press.

Pindzola, R., Plexico, L. H., & Haynes, W. (2015). *Diagnosis and evaluation in speech pathology* (9th ed.). Pearson.

Reeves, S., Pelone, F., Harrison, R., Goldman, J., & Zwarenstein, M. (2017). Interprofessional collaboration to improve professional practice and healthcare outcomes. *Cochrane Database of Systematic Reviews*. https://doi.org/10.1002/14651858.cd000072.pub3

Reynell, J. R. (1977). *Reynell developmental language scales*. NFER Nelson Publishing Company.

Rosanoff, M. J., Daniels, A. M., & Shih, A. (2015). Autism: A (key) piece of the global mental health puzzle. *Global Mental Health, 2*, e2. https://doi.org/10.1017%2Fgmh.2014.7

Selig, S., Tropiano, E., & Greene-Moton, E. (2006). Teaching cultural competence to reduce health disparities. *Health Promotion Practice, 7*(3_suppl), 247S-255S.

Semela, J. J. (2001). Significance of cultural variables in assessment and therapy. *Folia Phoniatrica et Logopaedica, 53*(3), 128-134. https://doi.org/10.1159/000052667

Shipley, K. G., & McAfee, J. G. (2021). *Assessment in speech-language pathology: A resource manual* (6th ed.). Plural Publishing, Inc.

Speech Pathology Australia. (n.d.). *Home: Speech pathology australia*. Speech Pathology Australia. https://speechpathologyaustralia.org.au/

Song, K., Kim, S., & Preston, L. R. (2021). "No difference between African American, immigrant, or white children! They are all the same": Working toward developing teachers' raciolinguistic attitudes towards ELs. *International Journal of Multicultural Education, 23*(1), 47-66. https://doi.org/10.18251/ijme.v23i1.1995

Tervalon, M., & Murray-Garcia, J. M. (1998). Cultural humility versus cultural competence: A critical distinction in definition. *Journal of Health Care for the Poor and Underserved, 9*(2), 117.

Ting-Toomey, S., & Chung, L. C. (2012). What is intercultural communication flexibility? And what are the essential cultural value patterns? *Understanding Intercultural Communication, 29*(4), 22-63.

UN Refugee Agency. (n.d.). *Refugee statistics*. https://www.unrefugees.org/refugee-facts/statistics/#:~:text=In%20the%20first%20half%20of,remained%20at%20a%20record%20high

Uono, S., & Hietanen, J. K. (2015). Eye contact perception in the West and East: A cross-cultural Study. *Plos One 10*(2), E0118094. https://doi.org/10.1371/journal.pone.0118094

Van Schendel, W. (2020). *A history of Bangladesh*. Cambridge University Press.

Verdon, S., Blake, H. L., Hopf, S. C., Phạm, B., & McLeod, S. (2016). Cultural and linguistic diversity in speech-language pathology. *International Journal of Speech-Language Pathology, 18*(2), 109-110.

Weiss, C., Gordon, M., & Lillywhite, H. (1987). *Clinical management of articulatory and phonological disorders*. Williams & Williams.

Westby, C., & Levey, S. (2021). The mental health of migrants, refugees, and asylum seekers. In S. Levey & S. Moonsamy (Eds.), *Unserved and underserved populations. New approaches to inclusivity* (pp. 33-46). Peter Lang.

Wetherby, A. M., Yonclas, D. G., & Bryan, A. A. (1989). Communicative profiles of preschool children with handicaps: Implications for early identification. *Journal of Speech & Hearing Disorders, 54*(2), 148-158. https://doi.org/10.1044/jshd.5402.148

Wichmann, S., Muller, A., & Velupillai, V. (2010). Homelands of the world's language families: A quantitative approach. *Diachronica, 27*(2), 247-276.

Williams, C. J., & McLeod, S. (2012). Speech-language pathologists' assessment and intervention practices with multilingual children. *International Journal of Speech Language Pathology, 14*(3), 292-305. https://doi.org/10.3109/17549507.2011.636071

Wolfram, W. (2013). Challenging language prejudice in the classroom. *Education Digest, 79*(1). https://www.teachingtolerance.org

World Health Organization. (n.d.). *Fact sheets*. https://www.who.int/news-room/fact-sheets/details/autism-spectrum%20disorders

World Health Organization. (2014). *Comprehensive and coordinated efforts for the management of autism spectrum disorders*. https://apps.who.int/gb/ebwha/pdf_files/WHA67/A67_17-en.pdf

World Health Organization Eastern Mediterranean Region. (n.d.). *EMRO home page*. www.emro.who.int

Wylie, K., McAllister, L., Davidson, B., & Marshall, J. (2013). Changing practice: Implications of the World Report on Disability for responding to communication disability in under-served populations. *International Journal of Speech-Language Pathology, 15*(1), 1-13.

Chapter 2

The *International Classification of Functioning, Disability and Health* Framework and Global Assessment

Carol Westby, PhD, CCC-SLP

Introduction

This book addresses the challenges of assessing language abilities of multilingual speakers, or dual-language learners (DLLs), across the lifespan. Assessing multilingual speakers and DLLs is always a complex task, but is usually somewhat less difficult with adults who have acquired language impairments as the result of a stroke, traumatic brain injury, or degenerative neurological disease. In these cases, speech-language pathologists can gather information from the client or family members regarding the client's premorbid language skills. There is generally agreement that a language impairment is present. Assessment of language abilities of multilingual or DLL children is more challenging than language assessment of adults, because speech-language pathologists must differentiate the influences of the child's incomplete learning of a first language (L1) from the influences of the child's exposure to a second language (L2). With some children, such as those with autistic behaviors, obvious overall developmental delays, or unintelligible speech, adults readily acknowledge that a language impairment is present. But for DLL children who are referred because of concern of delayed or disordered language impairment alone, the assessment process is particularly challenging.

To understand the specific nature of language impairments in multilingual speakers/DLLs and to design an appropriate intervention program, speech-language pathologists must have an understanding of the characteristics of the languages that the client speaks, the client's comprehension and use of language in a range of contexts, and the influences of culture on the client's communication

Bortz, M. (Ed.). *A Guide to Global Language Assessment: A Lifespan Approach* (pp. 25-43).
DOI: 10.4324/9781003524472-3

style. This information cannot be gained from assessment of a client's comprehension and use of language on a formal measure of vocabulary and structural language in a clinical context. Clinicians need to see the "big picture" of the client's communication skills.

This chapter will provide a discussion of the nature of developmental language disorder (DLD) and the concerns regarding use of standardized language tests with DLL children. To provide appropriate assessment and intervention services for children and adults from culturally/linguistically diverse backgrounds requires that speech-language pathologists conduct a comprehensive assessment of a client's communication abilities. The World Health Organization's *International Classification of Functioning, Disability and Health* (WHO-ICF; 2001, 2007) provides a framework for a comprehensive language assessment, which enables clinicians to see the "big picture." The ICF components will be described with explanations of how these components can be addressed by speech-language pathologists conducting language evaluations. Because of the particular difficulties in diagnosing language impairment in DLL children, the majority of the examples of using the ICF in language assessment are child-based. The ICF framework, however, is intended to be used across the lifespan.

The Challenge of Language Assessment

Communication is a human right. Article 19 of the *Universal Declaration of Human Rights* (UDHR) states that everyone has a "right to freedom of opinion and expression," including the right "to seek, receive and impart information and ideas through any media and regardless of frontiers" (United Nations, 1948). This statement implies that all people have the right to be able to communicate. The WHO's *World Report on Disability* estimates that roughly one billion people around the world live with some form of disability (World Health Organization & World Bank, 2011). However, this same report acknowledges that people with communication disabilities may not be included in this estimate, even though they encounter significant difficulties in their daily lives.

Developmental Language Disorder

If communication is a right for all people, it is essential that those with communication impairments be identified and receive supportive services. In many countries, speech-language pathologists conduct assessments on children and adults for three reasons: (1) to diagnose a communication disorder, (2) to qualify a person for services, and (3) to develop a habilitation/rehabilitation program. Assessment of communication of multilingual speakers and DLLs is always more complex than assessment of monolingual speakers, but assessment of multilingual children is generally more difficult than assessment of multilingual adults because of the necessity to differentiate issues of language learning in two languages. Although persons of any age and disability usually benefit from interventions, children typically achieve optimal outcomes when their impairments are identified and treated as early as possible (Towle et al., 2020). Similarly, it is known that adults with acquired communication disorders can benefit from treatments received several years after the initial insult, but outcomes are usually best when interventions are received as soon as possible after the onset of the disability (Doogan et al., 2018).

Language impairments arising in childhood have had a variety of names: specific language impairment (SLI), primary language impairment (PLI), or DLD. DLD is becoming the preferred term around the world, being endorsed in a consensus study by an international panel of experts in child language (CATALISE Consortium; Bishop et al., 2017). Although the definition of SLI overlaps with

DLD, the CATALISE panel rejected the term SLI because it was viewed as overly restrictive in implying that the child had relatively pure problems with language in the absence of any other impairments. Yet children with SLI are also likely to exhibit executive function (EF) deficits in inhibition, sustained attention, auditory and visual working memory, and cognitive flexibility (i.e., shifting attention between tasks or mental sets; Tomas & Vissers, 2019). More children with SLI are late in reaching motor milestones than children without SLI (Diepeveen et al., 2018). Compared to typically developing children, they exhibit greater gross and fine motor difficulties. They stand on one leg for shorter periods of time, have their feet stray more often while walking in a straight line, and catch a bounced ball less frequently than typically developing children. Relative to children with typical development, children with SLI generally require more time to complete fine motor tasks such as drawing trails (drawing a line within the space of two lines), moving pegs, and threading lace (Sanjeevan & Mainela-Arnold, 2019). Children with true specific language problems are rare.

Diagnosis of Developmental Language Disorder

DLD is not well-recognized or well-understood. The amount of research conducted on DLD relative to other neurodevelopmental disorders remains low (McGregor, 2020). There is concern about potential overidentification of DLLs and culturally linguistically diverse (CLD) learners with DLD, yet overall the percentage of children who are deemed eligible for clinical services because of DLD falls well short of estimates based on the prevalence of DLD in community samples. A meta-analysis of research around the world indicates there is a disproportionality of overrepresentation of ethnic minority, immigrant, and Indigenous populations in special education in many countries (Cooc & Kiru, 2018). But this is not necessarily the case in all contexts or with students specifically diagnosed with language impairments. Disproportionalities may manifest differently at different grade levels. Nationally in the United States, linguistic minority children are underrepresented in special education services in kindergarten and first grade (Morgan et al., 2016; Samson & Lesaux, 2009). In fact, kindergarten Hispanic children were 46% less likely to receive speech-language services than non-Hispanic children; and children from non–English-speaking homes were 50% less likely than children from English-speaking homes to receive speech-language services (Morgan et al., 2016). Patterns of over- and underrepresentation vary at state and school district levels. In a California study (Artiles et al., 2005), second language (L2) learners in grades 6 to 12 were 3.5 times more likely to be identified as having a learning disability and placed in special education than their non–English learner (EL) counterparts. In contrast, EL disability placement rates reached underrepresentation levels in grades K-3, while placement odds were comparable for ELs and non-ELs in grades 4 and 5. It may be that teachers of young children are reluctant to refer L2 learners for special education services until they develop English proficiency. By later elementary, L2 learners are likely to have developed L2 conversational skills, but not the L2 academic language skills essential for classroom success.

The International Communication Project (ICP), conceived during the 2010 International Association of Logopedics and Phoniatrics (IALP) Congress in Athens, Greece, was founded because of concern that communication disabilities are largely ignored around the world (https://internationalcommunicationproject.com/; Mulcair et al., 2018). The ICP, with member agencies in 18 countries, was founded to raise awareness of communication disorders and their treatment. The current focus of the ICP is to influence international health and disability policy through interaction with world health policy bodies such as the United Nations and the WHO. Knowledge of current statements on and resources related to communication disabilities held by these international bodies is a critical underpinning to advocacy efforts. The ICP acknowledges that whether a person can communicate is influenced not only by their communication abilities (in one or more languages), but also by whether their communication abilities and preferences are accepted and supported in the environment, and whether they have access to the services they require to achieve their communication potential. Communication disabilities result from the interaction between individuals with impairments in multiple contexts and environmental barriers. Hence, an adequate language assessment must address factors beyond a person's performance on structured language assessment tasks.

Conducting assessments of children or adults with possible communication impairments, especially DLD, is a complex task under any circumstance; it is particularly challenging when a person to be assessed is multilingual and especially when the person is a child or adolescent. Speech-language pathologists are frequently charged with determining if students who are learning to speak a language in school that is different from their home language are exhibiting a language difference or a language disorder. This is a difficult task because the features of DLD overlap with the characteristic of L2 learning (Table 2-1).

In the United States, the majority of school districts and many health agencies require the use of standardized tests to determine eligibility for services. Speech-language pathologists readily acknowledge the multiple problems with using standardized tests to determine if students learning an L2 have a language impairment. CLD students may not be test-wise (i.e., they may not be familiar with the types of tasks and interactions required by standardized tests) or they may lack the motivation to attempt to perform their best. Similar issues are true for adults with acquired impairments such as aphasia or traumatic brain injury. Standardized assessments require that students are acculturated to the testing procedure, and any test in L2 is a measure of students' L2 proficiency. In the United States few standardized tests are available in languages other than English. Even using standardized Spanish language tests does little to reduce the difficulty in assessing L2 learners if they are unfamiliar with the testing process. There are multiple Spanish dialects and cultures around the world; children might not be familiar with the words and concepts on a particular test, and children might be in the process of losing their first language (L1) while learning their L2 so test scores in both languages are low. In the United States, ELs' rate of acquiring their L1 decreases as they begin to learn an L2; and in some instances, students begin to lose their L1 as they gain skills in L2.

Use of only structured, formal, standardized assessments of multilingual/multicultural persons is likely related to the fact that L2 learners are frequently disproportionally represented among students identified as having learning disabilities—that is, they may be identified as having a language impairment when none is present, or conversely they may not be identified, resulting in a situation where students are not provided with the services they need in order to access an optimal learning environment. For all students, there are two additional considerations when interpreting the significance of scores on standardized tests.

1. **Lack of eligibility for services does not mean lack of an impairment.** Typically, students must receive a score that is 1.5 to 2 standard deviations (SDs) below the population mean for a test. Frequently, it is also assumed that if students' scores are not below this predetermined level, they do not have an impairment. Sensitivity and specificity data for specific language tests differ however, indicating that tests differ markedly in their ability to diagnose language impairments. Sensitivity and specificity of a test are completely dependent on the cutoff point score that is used to determine a line between normal and impaired individuals. The cutoff score for one test can differ significantly from that of another test (Shahmahmood et al., 2016). Consequently, a single generic SD should not be used to diagnose a language impairment and qualify students for services. For example, based on specificity data for the Spanish Clinical Evaluation of Language Fundamentals (CELF-4), 48% of students who do indeed have a language impairment will not be identified as eligible for services if a cut score of -2 SD is required (Semel et al., 2006).
2. **Good scores on standardized tests do not guarantee effective communication in life activities.** Standardized language tests typically assess comprehension and production of components of language. They do not require simultaneous organized use of phonology, semantics, morphology, and syntax to generate complex discourse and to use that discourse in a variety

Table 2-1

Student Difficulties Explained Through Dual-Language Learners and Language Impairment Lenses

OBSERVED BEHAVIOR	REASONS FOR DIFFICULTY EXPERIENCED BY DUAL-LANGUAGE LEARNERS	POSSIBLE DEVELOPMENTAL LANGUAGE DISORDER EXPLANATION
Inappropriate word choice; morphological and syntactic errors when speaking	Has not yet learned the vocabulary, morphology, and syntax of the instructional L2	Difficulty with statistical learning, i.e., identifying the statistical regularities in word use, grammar, and syntax
Trouble retelling a story	Unfamiliar with the vocabulary and cultural schema and organization of story	Delays in developing micro- and macrostructures for narratives
Cannot remember information taught	Cognitive task load is high because child is attempting to process unfamiliar material in L2	Reduced working memory capacity and memory retrieval difficulties
Difficulty reading and spelling	Has not been taught or yet learned the L2 sound/grapheme relationships and orthography	Phonological processing and rapid automatic naming deficits
Difficulty comprehending texts	Insufficient English knowledge of vocabulary, syntax, pragmatics, and cultural schema/background knowledge	Difficulty recognizing and comprehending temporal and cause–effect relationships, understanding connectives, drawing inferences
Poor sustained attention; easily distracted	Does not understand the language of instruction sufficiently to sustain attention; fatigued because of cognitive load	Executive function deficits
Inappropriate or limited class participation with teacher and peers	Classroom cultural interaction expectations differ from home or previous educational experiences	Pragmatic or self-regulation deficits

of communicative interactions. This aspect of apparent adequate language comprehension and production on formal tests but not in life situations has been recognized in adults who have experienced a life-changing illness or trauma, but is less acknowledged as an issue with children.

Recent studies in the United States and Australia have explored the process that evaluation teams employ when assessing DLL or CLD students. These studies have revealed that the teams relied nearly exclusively on the use of standardized tests. They did not consistently specify children's language exposure/use, denote the language of the evaluation, prioritize appropriate assessment measures, conduct contextual or dynamic assessments, or indicate attention to cultural and linguistic differences when determining eligibility (Denman et al., 2021; Huerta et al., 2021). Because of the multiple issues with standardized tests, particularly when used to identify language impairments in DLLs, researchers recommend that speech-language pathologists employ a *converging evidence framework* to guide their diagnostic decision-making process (Castilla-Earls et al., 2020). A converging evidence framework involves the speech-language pathologist bringing together multiple pieces of assessment data to make a diagnostic decision. The WHO-ICF (WHO, 2001) provides a framework for the types of convergent evidence to gather.

International Classification of Functioning, Disability and Health

Traditionally, speech-language pathologists have used a medical model to guide assessment and treatment practices (Cunningham et al., 2017; Washington, 2007; Westby, 2007). However, in response to the 2001 publication of the ICF (WHO, 2001), there was a shift in practice beyond that of a medical model (Cunningham & Rosenbaum, 2015). The ICF is a biopsychosocial model of functioning and disability that integrates the medical and social models across the lifespan (WHO, 2001, 2007). According to a biopsychosocial model, the cause, manifestation, and outcomes of disease/disorder result from interactions between biological, psychological, and social factors. A purely medical model views disability as a feature of the person, directly caused by a trauma or health condition. A social model of disability sees disability as a socially created problem and not an attribute of an individual. Disability is a complex phenomenon that is both a problem at the level of a person's body and a complex social phenomenon. The impact of a disability is affected by the tasks persons must perform and the social context in which they must perform them. The ICF framework has been adopted by persons providing speech, language, and hearing services in many countries. The American Speech-Language-Hearing Association (ASHA) incorporated it into its scope of practice documents (2001, 2016), but it has not been widely used, particularly with children. The ICF is not an assessment tool per se, but rather a framework for assessment that speech-language pathologists can use to ensure they consider the multiple factors that influence persons' language skills.

Figure 2-1 depicts the ICF framework. Using the ICF framework, speech-language pathologists describe multiple components influencing persons' communicative functioning, including Body Functions and Structures (that are the bases of the *impairment*), the ways that the impairment may result in *limitations* of a person's ability to carry out Activities (the execution of tasks), and the ways that limitations in Activities may *restrict* a person's ability to perform activities so as to engage in Participation in daily life activities. The speech-language pathologist then considers the types and ways that Contextual Factors (Environmental and Personal) may serve as facilitators or barriers to a person's Activities and Participation. (*Note:* When words are used specifically to refer to the ICF components, they are capitalized.) When using the ICF framework, speech-language pathologists are collecting convergent evidence. They gather data on a client's performance in different types of tasks, such as decontextualized, contextualized, or activity-focused tasks; and on a client's performance across different contexts, including a clinical context, school context, or home/work/community context in order to best understand a child's language performance at a holistic level. These multiple perspectives on language use are important because persons may perform differently depending on the types of tasks targeted in an assessment.

The ICF has two primary parts: Functioning and Disability (Part 1) and Contextual Factors (Part 2), each of which has two components. The two components of Functioning and Disability are Body Functions/Structures and Activity/Participation:

1. Body Functions are defined as the physiological functions of a body system, including psychological functions. Body Structures are defined as the anatomical parts of the body such as brain, organs, limbs, and their components (WHO, 2007, p. 9).

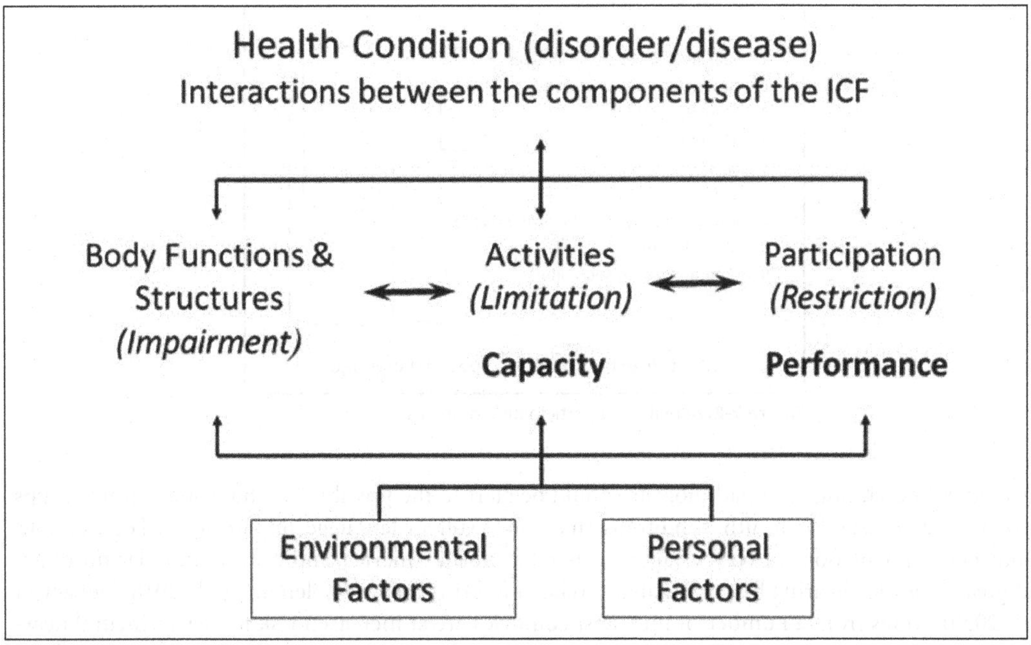

Figure 2-1. Interactions between the components of the ICF. (Reprinted from *How to use the ICF—A practical manual for using the* International Classification of Functioning, Disability and Health, World Health Organization, p. 7, © 2013.)

2. Activity represents an individual perspective and is defined as "the execution of a task or action by an individual" (WHO, 2007, p. 9) in a structured or standardized environment. Participation represents a societal perspective and is defined as "involvement in a life situation" (WHO, 2007, p. 9).

Body Functions/Body Structures

There are eight domains for Body Functions and eight related domains for Body Structures representing the major body systems. These Function/Structure domains comprise all body systems (e.g., cardiovascular/respiratory, digestive/metabolic, genitourinary, neuromuscular, skin). Three Body Functions and three Body Structures domains are most related to communication disorders: Mental Functions/Structures of the nervous system; Sensory Functions and Pain/Structures of the eye, ear, and related structures; and Voice and Speech Functions/Structures involved in voice and speech.

A problem in Body Function or Structure is termed an *impairment*. Impairments in body structures may be directly observable (e.g., a cleft lip and/or palate or ear atresia) or indirectly observable with x-rays or scans (e.g., brain hemorrhage); but for many impairments, particularly impairments in communication, structural impairments are not observable. Nor can one directly observe impairments in most mental functions that underlie speech and language disorders. One can only infer these structure/function impairments by observing how persons carry out activities (McCormack et al., 2012; WHO, 2013). One cannot directly observe the impairments in processing that underlie receptive and expressive language difficulties, only their manifestation in the use of phonology, morphology, semantics, pragmatics, and discourse in activities. Impairments in the Body Function, mental functions for language, lead to *limitations* in Activities that require comprehending or producing language. Limitations in Activities may result in *restrictions* in the ability to participate in life

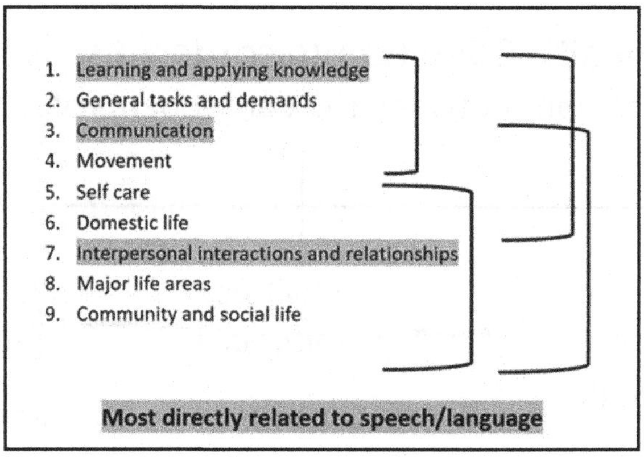

Figure 2-2. Activity and participation domains.

activities. Speech-language pathologists should be alert to the possibilities that some ethnic groups are at greater risks for health conditions that can result in language impairments. For example, Indigenous populations in New Zealand, Australia, North America, and the circumpolar north are at greater risk for hearing loss, particularly related to otitis media (Coleman et al., 2018; DeLacy et al., 2020). Arabs from a number of mid-East countries are at increased risk for sensorineural hearing loss (Sidenna et al., 2020). Persons of African descent are at increased risk for sickle cell disease. Children with sickle cell disease are likely to show language deficits even when they do not exhibit evident neurological events or brain damage (Arfé et al., 2018).

Activity/Participation

Activity

The Activity and Participation components of the ICF have a single list of nine domains that cover the range of life activities. Each domain can be coded for either Activity or Participation or both (Figure 2-2). The first four domains are primarily related to Activities; the last five are primarily related to Participation. Domains three through six can involve an overlap of Activity and Participation. Three of these domains are particularly applicable to communication disorders: Learning and Applying Knowledge, Communication, and Interpersonal Interactions and Relationships. The Activity component represents the *capacity* to carry out a behavior or skill in a situation in which the effect of the context is absent or made irrelevant (such as in a standardized evaluation setting). Participation requires *performance* of those behaviors or skills in naturalistic life contexts (WHO, 2007). Having capacity or skills is essential but not sufficient for Participation. For example, children may exhibit age-appropriate vocabulary and syntactic skills on a standardized test (demonstrating capacity), but not use these skills in conversation with peers or teachers (failing to demonstrate performance). Or a DLL student with some ability to comprehend and talk privately with a teacher in their L2 may be hesitant to participate in classroom discussions or social groups.

In most clinical practices around the world, the focus of language assessment is at the Activity level—what a person can or cannot do on a formal assessment in a specific situation with an evaluator. Speech-language pathologists typically use standardized formal assessments to assess persons' capacity at the Activity level. Such assessments provide norms that indicate the degree to which a person's score relates to the mean score of the test population. The ICF codes limitations in Activity in terms of the severity of the problem based on the amount of one's day that is affected or the percentage of the population with the impairment based on their standardized test scores. See Table 2-2.

Table 2-2
Qualifying Limitations in Activity

PROBLEM SEVERITY	PERCENTAGE OF DAY AFFECTED	SCORES ON STANDARDIZED TEST
0 = No problem	0% to 4%	<-1.0 SD (68%)
1 = Mild problem	5% to 24%	-1.0 to -1.5 SD (22%)
2 = Moderate problem	25% to 49%	-1.5 to -2.5 SD (6%)
3 = Severe problem	50% to 95%	-2.5 to -3.0 SD (3%)
4 = Complete problem	96% to 100%	-3+ SD (1%)

Although some school districts in the United States may require scores on standardized tests to qualify for services, the Individuals with Disabilities Education Act (IDEA), which guides services for children with disabilities in educational contexts, does not. Evaluation may include information regarding children's Activity and Participation gathered through informal assessments, observations of children in multiple contexts, and questionnaires and interviews completed by caregivers. Knowledge of children's development of skills in their L1 is important information in determining if a language impairment is present. If caregivers report language delays or disorders in L1, it is highly likely that children will have delays or disorders in L2. The Alberta Language Development Questionnaire (ALDeQ; Paradis et al., 2010) has proven to be a valid method of identifying DLLs in kindergarten and first grade who have a language impairment. The ALDeQ questions caregivers about both their child's L1 development and possible L1 attrition. L1 attrition characteristics pose complications for the bilingual assessment of DLLs, including overidentification. As children move through school, it becomes more difficult to have caregivers or teachers make judgments regarding students' academic language skills. Children who exhibit early delays and deficits in oral conversational language are highly likely to experience delays and deficits in academic language. But students who acquire oral conversational language may experience difficulty as language becomes more complex. Many DLLs develop academic language only in their L2, so comparison with L1 academic language is not possible. This increases the difficulty of determining if the L2 academic language difficulties are due to a true language impairment or insufficient exposure to academic language.

When persons are referred for evaluation of a possible language/learning disability, speech-language pathologists typically assess only the client's language skills. Yet because DLD is highly associated with deficits in EFs, speech-language pathologists should also consider evaluating clients' EFs at the Activity level. EF tasks assessing working memory, cognitive flexibility, and inhibition require minimal language. Ideally, the instructions for the EF tasks should be given in the client's dominant language; responses are nonverbal. Activity level EF deficits can provide convergent evidence for a language impairment. (*Note:* Persons may exhibit adequate Activity level EF skills but exhibit Participant level EF deficits. Activity level EF tasks involve basic processing, Participation EF requires higher-level mental states to initiate and monitor action. The type of EF required for participation is more dependent and interactive with language skills.)

Attempts are being made to develop language assessment tools for the Activity level that are appropriate and informational for DLLs. In response to increasing migration, the European Union established the COST Action IS0804 to address the challenges that multilingualism poses for the diagnosis and treatment of language-impaired bilingual children. This COST Action group has sought to disentangle bilingualism and language impairments by establishing the relative contribution of each by showing how LI can be identified in both of a child's languages and exploring the extent to which the manifestations of SLI/DLD are similar or different across languages in the same child. COST participants developed materials and assessment protocols to assess morphology, syntax, semantics, phonology, narrative discourse, and executive function skills in bilingual children, ages 4 to 9 years in a structured context. The Multilingual Assessment Instrument for Narratives (MAIN) has been extensively investigated (Gagarina et al., 2016). Picture sets are available for children to retell and to generate stories in two languages. These narrative materials have been recently updated for use with multiple languages (Bohnacker & Gagarino, 2020). A guide for use of the MAIN and the picture sets are available free by registering on the MAIN website (https://main.leibniz-zas.de/en/main-materials/main-materials/). Research on DLLs' language development indicates they achieve competency in their L2 first in narrative macrostructure, then vocabulary, and last morphology (Paradis, 2016).

Participation

Participation involves being actively engaged in tasks, activities, and routines at home, school, and the community that are typical for persons of that age. To participate in life situations, individuals need to integrate multiple pieces of information to comprehend subtleties in the situation or generate a complex response that considers others in the situation. Participation for adults can include engaging with others in work environments, socialization with family during meals or celebrations, or joining community activities (e.g., religious services, sporting events). For children, participation can include playing games with siblings, playing with peers on the playground, being a member of a sports team, collaborating with peers in a science experiment, offering meaningful comments in a classroom discussion, or going on a school trip. A restriction in Participation is identified by comparing an individual's participation to that which is expected of an individual without a disability in that culture or society.

Participation has two aspects: an objective aspect that can be observed—attendance, defined as "being there" and measured by frequency of attending and/or a range or diversity of situations; and a subjective aspect, involvement, which is the experience of participation while attending. Involvement is the idea of taking part or being included, accepted, or engaged. Involvement may include elements of motivation, persistence, social connections, and affect (Imms et al., 2017). Subjective aspects are related to the meaning and importance the individual may attach to particular life situations and the relative importance of participating in them. Worrell et al. (2011) asked persons with aphasia (PWA) about their experiences with therapy and if they received what they wanted. These PWA reported having goals across the ICF spectrum, but the majority of the goals they desired involved participation-level goals in everyday life activities. In contrast, the goals of speech-language pathologists at a rehabilitation center were aimed at the ICF levels of impairment and activity limitations with few explicit goals aimed at the level of participation (Leach et al., 2010). In a qualitative study of children with a variety of impairments (Heah et al., 2007), children defined successful participation as doing and being with others, having fun, feeling successful, and doing things by oneself (i.e., having autonomy or control). Parents identified successful participation as involving accomplishment, task completion, or something that increased the child's self-esteem. They also described good participation as a good fit between the child's interests and capabilities, the activity features and demands, and availability of resources in the environment. At present, the ICF does not include a qualifier for involvement or subjective satisfaction for the participation component.

Unless students exhibit autistic behaviors or social-communication difficulties, in the United States evaluation of children's participation is rarely conducted as part of an assessment to determine students' eligibility for special education services. School personnel in the United States often maintain that children can qualify for services only when their impairment in body structures and/or functions or limitations in Activities directly affects their academics tasks (under IDEA guidelines, this is not true); and they assume that only standardized test scores demonstrate that relationship. However, knowledge demonstrated on tests is not the only factor that influences students' performance in classrooms. Rather than determining service eligibility based on the diagnosis or severity of disorder at the Impairment/Activity levels alone, the ICF can be used to identify the gap between impairment/limitations in the components of Body Functions/Structures or Activity/ Capacity and restrictions in the component of Participation/Performance and use that information to set functional goals.

When evaluating persons' participation, speech-language pathologists should consider three components: (1) in what types of situations does the person participate, and to what degree; (2) does the person have the pragmatic knowledge and skills for participating; and (3) how might personal and environmental factors contribute to the person's participation or lack of participation. Evaluators can explore with clients the activities in which they want to participate or in which they participate and the degree to which they participate. For students in the United States, there are several scales that can be used to explore these factors (e.g., the Child & Adolescent Scale of Participation [CASP; Bedell, 2011], the Children's Assessment of Participation and Enjoyment [CAPE; King et al., 2004], and the Functional Abilities Classification Tool [FACT; Klein et al., 2018]). Students rate themselves on the CASP and CAPE; teachers rate students on the FACT. The Speech Participation and Activity Assessment of Children (SPAA-C; McLeod, 2004) was developed specifically for use with school-age children with identified speech and language disorders. (It has been used with children from a variety of cultural/linguistic backgrounds.) Some questions from the SPAA-C would be useful in language evaluations of DLLs (e.g., questions regarding who the children like to talk with and do not like to talk with, how they feel about talking with different people in different contexts, what they do when they encounter people who do not understand them or ask them to repeat).

Speech-language pathologists should observe clients' participation in multiple contexts. When observing DLL/CLD students in school settings, speech-language pathologists must exercise caution in their interpretations of students' pragmatic behaviors because these students may not share peers' or teachers' cultural expectations of behaviors. Books by Lynch and Hanson (2011) and Roseberry-McKibbon (2018) provide excellent discussions of childrearing practices across cultures that give speech-language pathologists insights into ways children's participation interactions may vary.

Guidelines for use of the ICF state that a person's participation in different contexts should always be observed because they reflect the actual functioning in real life settings. Since performance at the Participation level describes the interaction between the person and the context, it may change in different contexts (e.g., the functioning of an individual may change significantly when at home, school, community activity, or work). Consequently, it may be necessary to code separate profiles of performance for different environments. The combined coding of performance and capacity is a powerful technique to understand the effect of the environment on a person. The speech-language pathologist needs to note if there is a gap between a person's capacity and performance. Such a gap reflects the influence of current environments, and thus provides a useful guide as to what can be done to the environment to improve a person's performance (WHO, 2001). Persons may experience greater difficulties performing/participating in some situations because of increased cognitive load related to the intrinsic complexity of the activity, to the way the activity is presented, or to the type of response required. Cognitive load may be minimal with many Activity level tasks because isolated skills are assessed. Cognitive load can escalate in Participation events because students must process the language content, while simultaneously integrating social and academic knowledge and organizing a discourse response. If persons have limited working memory capacity (which is likely for persons with DLD or acquired communication impairments), cognitive load increases more quickly. Consequently, a task they may do easily at the Activity level becomes challenging at the Participation level. When evaluating students' participation in educational contexts, speech-language pathologists should consider how the cognitive load of tasks or routines might be altered to ensure participation in a given environment.

Activity and Participation can be qualified in terms of performance without assistance and capacity with assistance. Assistance might be a person who provides support or a variety of devices or technologies (e.g., wheelchairs, FM systems, medication, tablets). Dynamic assessment (DA) can be considered a type of assistance provided at the Activity and Participant levels. DA involves a structured test-teach-test framework. When apparent lack of skill or knowledge at the Activity level is observed, an evaluator can employ a variety of strategies to teach the skill or knowledge and then evaluate the person's learnability—how modifiable the person is, and how quickly and easily did the person acquire the skill or knowledge. Persons who learn more slowly, require more support, or who exhibit attentional, off-task behavior during the teaching are more likely to have a language/learning impairment (Petersen et al., 2017).

Contextual Factors

The knowledge and skills that persons exhibit at the Activity and Participation levels of the ICF are highly influenced by Contextual Factors. Contextual Factors (Part 2) "represent the complete background of an individual's life and living" (WHO, 2007, p. 15) and comprise two components:

1. *Environmental Factors* refer to all aspects of the external world of an individual's life that may have an impact on their functioning.
2. *Personal Factors* involve features of the individual that are not part of the health condition such as gender, age, temperament, other medical condition, culture/ethnicity.

The Contextual Factors interact with each other and with the health conditions and may serve as facilitators or barriers to a person's capacity to carry out activities or to participate in academic and social events. The personal and environment contextual factors can be qualified in terms of the degree to which they serve as a barrier (have a negative effect) or as a facilitator (have a positive effect) on functioning—or in this case, on the person's language use. They are coded as no barrier/facilitator, mild, moderate, severe, or complete barrier/facilitator.

The ICF does not provide a list of Personal Factors because of wide variability among cultures. In practice, common personal factors noted may include gender, temperament, family constellation, socioeconomic level, educational experiences, languages spoken, trauma history, health conditions, or other factors that could potentially influence a person's capacity and performance. The ICF lists five Environmental Factors: (1) products/technology, (2) natural environment and human-made changes to environment, (3) support and relationships, (4) attitudes, and (5) services, systems, and policies (Table 2-3). Environmental barriers might be no funding for hearing aids (products/technology), poor classroom acoustics (natural environment and human changes), a policy that allows assessment of DLLs only after 3 years of exposure to English, or a policy that permits language services for children only when they fall below two standard deviations on an approved standardized test (educational policies). Environmental facilitators might be involved grandparents (support and relationships), parent support groups, bilingual and heritage language programs (services, systems), or comfortable, child-sized furniture (human changes to environment).

Assessment of Contextual Factors is typically done by observation or by employing ethnographic interviewing of the client and significant persons in their environment. Speech-language pathologists can use ethnographic interviews of clients, caregivers, family members, and teachers to gather information regarding contextual factors that are serving as barriers or facilitators for a client's communication (see Chapter 5 on ethnographic assessment). If the client is an immigrant or refugee, speech-language pathologists may wish to incorporate elements from the Cultural Formulation Interview (CFI) for Immigrants and Refugees (Boehnlein et al., 2016) or the Refugee Services Toolkit (https://www.nctsn.org/resources/refugee-services-core-stressor-assessment-tool) when interviewing caregivers and adolescent/adult clients. The CFI can guide clinicians to efficiently recognize

Table 2-3
Environmental Factors With Examples

ENVIRONMENTAL FACTOR	EXAMPLES OF ENVIRONMENTAL FACTORS
Products/technology	• Augmentative devices, hearing aids, visual supports, therapy materials (books, games, toys) • Building construction/environmental design (curb cuts or wheelchair ramps)
Natural environment and human-made changes to environment	• Living density (number of persons in dwelling, community) • Weather (smoke, smog, sun, heat, cold) • Natural disasters (floods, fires, earthquakes) • Indoor environments (noise or acoustics, lighting, crowding)
Support and relationships	• Who is available at home, school, work for language, physical, emotional, or educational support (family, friends, teachers, religious leaders, health professionals, administrators) • Animals or pets
Attitudes	• About language/language impairments/disabilities, ethnicity/race, immigrants/refugees • Of family, friends, professionals, society
Services, systems, and policies	• Laws enabling access • Types of programs available/accessibility of programs • Qualification requirements for services (specific test scores, income levels, personal documents) • Transportation, health services or therapies

factors that may influence present functioning, such as premigration difficulties, exposure to violence and persecution, the historical time frame of migration, migration-related losses and challenges, continued ties to the country of origin, resettlement and life in the new country, and future expectations. The Refugee Services Toolkit provides users with information about four core stressors that refugees commonly face (e.g., pre-migration/migration trauma, resettlement, acculturation, isolation) and guides users through an assessment of a particular youth or family's needs.

When considering both capacity and performance in an assessment, speech-language pathologists can gain an understanding of the influences of the Contextual Factors on a student and consider ways to effect changes in the Contextual Factors to enhance the student's function. "The gap between capacity and performance reflects the difference between the impacts of current and uniform environments, and thus provides a useful guide as to what can be done to the environment of the individual to improve performance" (WHO, 2007, p. 14). By further evaluating capacity with assistance and performance without assistance, speech-language pathologists may gain better ideas of how to modify the Contextual Factors by using technology, personal support, or policies related to equitable access (WHO, 2013).

Case Study Application of the *International Classification of Functioning, Disability and Health*

Student Application of Language Disorders in the International Classification of Functioning, Disability and Health Framework

Isabella is a 14-year-old, ninth-grade, bilingual English-Spanish student who in elementary school should have had a comprehensive assessment as described in this chapter. Using the ICF framework, I have organized and summarized data regarding Isabella in Figure 2-3. From kindergarten through third grade, Isabella was in a bilingual classroom; since fourth grade, all her instruction has been in English. In third grade, Isabella was referred for evaluation because she was not making expected progress in math and reading. At that time, she was assessed with a nonverbal ability scale, a Spanish academic test battery, and an English academic test battery. On both the Spanish and English academic test batteries, her reading and math scores were considered borderline (-1.5 SD), but her lowest scores were in oral expression, listening comprehension, and working memory (-2 SD). Despite her low language scores, she was given a primary diagnosis of specific learning disabilities (SLD) and was not referred for a language evaluation. Since fourth grade, she has received supplemental instruction in math and reading.

In seventh grade, Isabella received a neuropsychological evaluation because of concerns of attentional problems and a depressed mood. She cried frequently during class. Isabella reportedly had experienced a significant trauma in her preschool years, which was believed to contribute to her depressed mood, but the specifics of this trauma were not shared with school staff. She was diagnosed with anxiety and a mood disorder, and her primary disability was changed to emotional disturbance. The school evaluation team believed that Isabella's emotional disturbance was the major contributor to her low academic performance. She began to receive mental health services at that time. A language assessment was not part of the neuropsychological evaluation.

Shortly after entering high school, Isabella's language arts teacher requested that Isabella be assessed for a language impairment. The teacher commented that Isabella struggled with retention and recall and that she required frequent step-by-step repetitions and rephrasing of instructions. The teacher noted that Isabella often appeared sad and was behind in all academic areas. However, she saw Isabella as a diligent, respectful student who tried everything, was aware of when she was confused, and appropriately asked for assistance. She had friendly interactions with her peers.

Isabella was assessed by a bilingual speech-language pathologist using Spanish and English versions of the Clinical Evaluation of Language Fundamentals (CELF; Semel et al., 2006; Wiig et al., 2013). Isabella's scores on the Spanish CELF were consistently higher (SS = 80) than her scores on the English CELF (SS = 65). Before high school, school staff had apparently not made the connection between Isabella's poor academic performance and possible language impairment, or they attributed her academic difficulties to her bilingualism and depression and possible dyslexia. There is no question that Isabella exhibits depression and anxiety, but it is not clear that the direction of the relationship is one way—that the depression is causing the low academic performance. It appears more likely that there is a two-way interaction between Isabella's depression and academic difficulties. Several

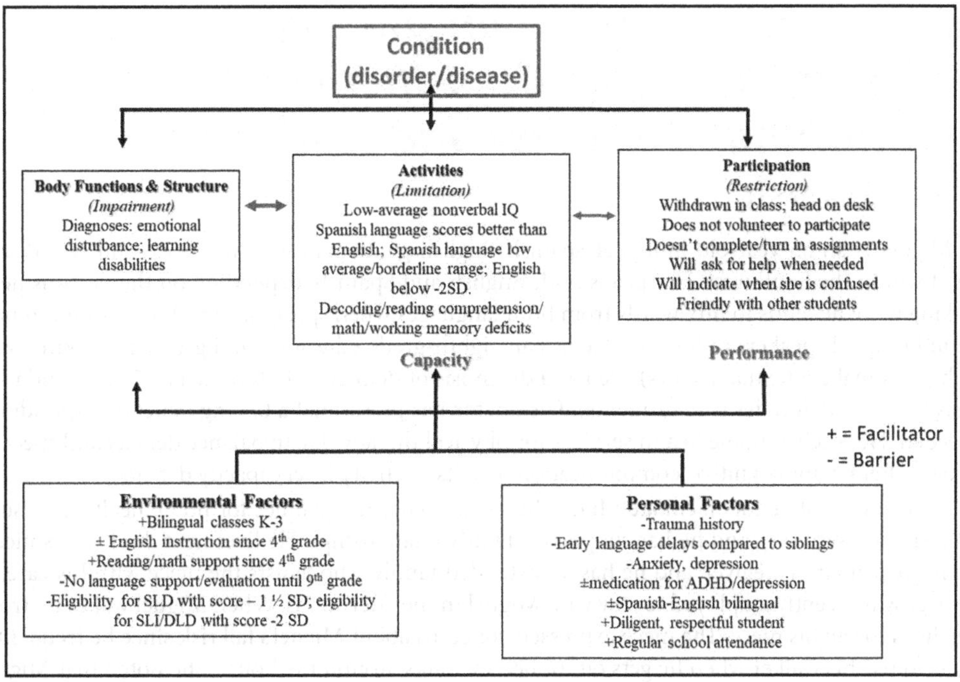

Figure 2-3. ICF case example.

teachers commented that Isabella tries to do the work that is presented and stays with tasks when she receives support. It is possible that the stress of doing academic work contributes to her anxiety and depression.

Because Isabella was bilingual and her CELF Spanish language score was not in the range to make her eligible for language services, the school diagnostic team initially wanted to deny language services, explaining that Isabella's Spanish scores indicated she did not have a language impairment and that her English scores were low because English was her L2. The speech-language pathologist noted, however, that since fourth grade all of Isabella's educational instruction has been in English. The high school she attends has a very large bilingual English-Spanish population. By high school, the majority of these students actually exhibit English dominance in testing. Isabella was learning English at a markedly slower rate than other students from similar backgrounds.

The speech-language pathologist concluded that Isabella did have DLD. Although Isabella was over the age for which the Alberta Language Development Questionnaire (ALDeQ) was designed, the speech-language pathologist used it to ask Isabella's mother about Isabella's language in Spanish compared to that of her siblings and cousins. Her mother reported that she had noticed that Isabella had always had more difficulty getting her ideas across than other children her age. On Activity level testing, Isabella's nonverbal intelligence was in a low average range, but she exhibited significant EF and language deficits, particularly in English. These deficits affected her performance on academic tasks at the Participation level. She tended to withdraw from classroom activities but would participate when given additional support, and it appeared that she did want to participate. Her EF deficits became more problematic at the Participation level. Due to her reduced working memory capacity, she could not maintain classroom instructions and she displayed limited reflective EF, which involves the use of language to plan and monitor one's work. As a result, she frequently did not complete assignments or remember to turn them in. Throughout most of Isabella's education, school personnel had not used convergent evidence to diagnose her language impairment. The ICF provides a framework for collecting and evaluating convergent evidence to make accurate diagnoses.

Adult Application of Language Disorders in the International Classification of Functioning, Disability and Health Framework

Miguel is an 85-year-old bilingual Spanish-English gentleman who was born and raised in a small town in the Southwest. He speaks both English and Spanish, depending on the persons he is speaking with; he tends to mix words from both languages when speaking, which is a common pattern in bilingual speakers in his area. He has an eighth-grade education and grew up working on a ranch (personal contextual factors). He has a diagnosis of dementia within the last 5 years and psychosis for several decades (Impairments). His doctor has prescribed a 0.5 mg tablet of risperidone, as needed. He receives home health services for physical therapy due to balance deficits and speech-language therapy for cognitive-communication deficits (Activity level capacity deficits).

Environmental factors facilitate Miguel living at home. He qualifies for home health care support (services, systems), and he has supportive family relationships. He lives next door to his niece, who is his primary caregiver, and he has an extended family who assists the niece with his care. A caregiver was recently employed to stay with Miguel in the afternoons. When Miguel wakes up from a nap he is to call his niece. The niece expressed concerns about Miguel's fall risk since he frequently forgets to use his walker when he gets out of bed or walks around the house. She noted that Miguel frequently perseverates on "nonreality" based events, talking about events that are not true. She tries to reason with him, but this increases the frustration for both of them. When the speech-language pathologist asked the niece what goal she would like for her uncle, she reported that she would like him to be able to cooperate in conversations. The niece also reported that Miguel has memory deficits that have led to him leaving the water running to overflow from the kitchen sink to the floor and leaving on the stove burner.

The speech-language pathologist developed goals and objectives targeting functional impairment-based goals at the Activity level and socially based goals at the Participation level. At the Impairment/Activity level, the speech-language pathologist used spaced retrieval to train Miguel's memory for using his walker in the house and then trained the niece and caregiver on using this technique to train behaviors such as turning off the faucet and stove. She reviewed with Miguel how to use his cell phone so he could call his niece when he wakes up from his nap.

Goals at the Participation level were particularly important for giving both Miguel and his niece a sense of well-being. The niece desired to have positive conversations with her uncle. Miguel appeared to have reasonably detailed memories from his early years and to enjoy talking about his life experiences. The speech-language pathologist asked Miguel if he would be interested in dictating stories from his life memories to his niece and helping her learn to write the stories down in Spanish. He agreed. Between therapy sessions the niece was instructed to spend time with Miguel daily as she wrote down personal narratives Miguel related from his autobiographical memory. These stories were reviewed in the following session with the speech-language pathologist, niece, and client. Additionally, the speech-language pathologist spoke with the niece about possible tasks that Miguel could do during the week to have him feel useful in contributing to the household. Both the niece and Miguel agreed that he could wash dishes, make the bed, water the plants outside (when accompanied), cook an egg, fold clothes, and separate kindling from bark in cardboard boxes on the porch. The speech-language pathologist suggested this last activity since he used to chop piles of wood for the winter and since he could actually help his niece prepare the kindling for a wood-burning stove. By using the ICF framework, the speech-language pathologist was able to develop goals for Miguel that facilitated his continued active involvement with his family.

References

American Speech-Language-Hearing Association. (2001, 2016). *Scope of Practice in speech-language pathology.* https://www.asha.org/policy/

Arfé, B., Montanaro, M., Mottura, E., Scaltritti, M., Manara, R., Basso, G., Sainati, L., & Colombatti, R. (2018). Selective difficulties in lexical retrieval and nonverbal executive functioning in children with HbSS sickle cell disease. *Journal of Pediatric Psychology, 43*(6), 666-677. https://doi.org/10.1093/jpepsy/jsy005

Artiles, A. J., Rueda, R., Salazar, J., & Higareda, I. (2005). Within-group diversity in minority disproportionate representation: English language learners in urban school districts. *Exceptional Children, 71*(3), 283-300. https://doi.org/10.1177/001440290507100305

Bedell, G. (2011). *Child and adolescent scale of participation.* Tufts University. http://sites.tufts.edu/garybedell/files/2012/07/CASP-Administration-Scoring-Guidelines-8-19-11.pdf

Bishop, D. V. M., Snowling, M., Thompson, P. A., Greenhalgh, T., and the CATALISE-2 consortium. (2017). Phase 2 of CATALISE: A multinational and multidisciplinary Delphi consensus study of problems with language development: Terminology. *Journal of Child Psychology and Psychiatry, 58*(10), 1068-1080. https://doi.org/10.1111/jcpp.12721

Boehnlein, J., Westermeyer, J., & Scalco, M. (2016). Immigrants and refugees. In R. Lewis-Fernández, N. K. Aggarwal, L. Hinton, L. C. Hinton, & L. J. Kirmayer (Eds.), *DSM-5® handbook on the cultural formulation interview* (pp. 173-181, 312). American Psychiatric Publishing, Inc.

Bohnacker, U., & Gagarino, N. (2020). Introduction to MAIN—Revised, how to use the instrument and adapt it to further languages. *ZAS Papers in Linguistics, 64,* xiii-xxi. https://doi.org/10.21248/zaspil.64.2020.549

Castilla-Earls, A., Bedore, L., Rojas, R., Fabiano-Smith, L., Pruitt-Lord, S., Restrepo, M. A., & Peña, E. (2020). Beyond scores: Using converging evidence to determine speech and language services eligibility for dual language learners. *American Journal of Speech-Language Pathology, 29*(3), 1116-1132. https://doi.org/10.1044/2020_AJSLP-19-00179

Coleman, A., Wood, A., Bialasiewicz, S., Ware, R. S., Marsh, R. L., & Cervin, A. (2018). The unsolved problem of otitis media in indigenous populations: A systematic review of upper respiratory and middle ear microbiology in indigenous children with otitis media. *Microbiome, 6*(1), 199. https://doi.org/10.1186/s40168-018-0577-2

Cooc, N., & Kiru, E. W. (2018). Disproportionality in special education: A synthesis of international research and trends. *Journal of Special Education, 52*(3), 163-173. https://doi.org/10.1177/0022466918772300

Cunningham, B. J., & Rosenbaum, P. L. (2015). A bioecological framework to evaluate communicative participation outcomes for preschoolers receiving speech-language therapy interventions in Ontario, Canada. *International Journal of Language and Communication Disorders, 50*(4), 405-415. https://doi.org/10.1111/1460-6984.12145

Cunningham, B., Washington, K. N., Binns, A., Rolfe, K., Robertson, B., & Rosenbaum, P. (2017). Current methods of evaluating speech-language outcomes for pre-schoolers with communication disorders: A scoping review using the ICF-CY. *Journal of Speech, Language, and Hearing Research, 60,* 447-464. https://doi.org/10.1044/2016_JSLHR-L-15-0329

DeLacy, J., Dune, T., & Macdonald, J. J. (2020). The social determinants of otitis media in Aboriginal children in Australia: Are we addressing the primary causes? A systematic content review. *BMC Public Health, 20,* 492. https://doi.org/10.1186/s12889-020-08570-3

Denman, D., Cordier, R., Kim, J.-H., Munro, N., & Speyera, R. (2021). What influences speech-language pathologists' use of different types of language assessments for elementary school-age children? *Language, Speech, and Hearing Services in Schools, 52*(3), 776-793. https://doi.org/10.1044/2021_LSHSS-20-00053

Diepeveen, F. B., van Dommelen, P., & Oudesluys-Murphy, A. M. (2018). Children with specific language impairment are more likely to reach motor milestones late. *Child: Care, Health and Development, 44,* 857-862. https://doi.org/pdf/10.1111/cch.12614

Doogan, C., Dignam, J., Copland, D., & Leff, A. (2018). Aphasia recovery: When, how and who to treat? *Current Neurology and Neuroscience Reports, 18*(12), 90. https://doi.org/10.1007/s11910-018-0891-x

Gagarina, N., Klop, D., Tsimpli, I. M., & Walters J. (2016). Narrative abilities in bilingual children. *Applied Psycholinguistics, 37*(1), 11-17. https://doi.org/10.1017/S0142716415000399

Heah, T., Case, T., McGuire, B., & Law, M. (2007). Successful participation: The lived experience among children with disabilities. *Canadian Journal of Occupational Therapy, 74*(1), 38-47. https://doi.org/10.2182/cjot.06.10

Huerta, L., Cycyk, L. M., Sanford-Keller, H., Busch, A., Dolata, J., Moore, H., De Anda, S., & Zuckerman, K. (2021). A retrospective review of communication evaluation practices of young Latinx children. *Journal of Early Intervention, 43*(4), 295-313. https://doi.org/abs/10.1177/10538151211012703

Imms, C., Granlund, M., Wilson, P. H., Steenbergen, B., Rosenbaum, P., & Gordon, A. M. (2017). Participation, both a means and an end: A conceptual analysis of processes and outcomes in childhood disability. *Developmental Medicine & Child Neurology, 59*, 16-25. https://doi.org/10.1111/dmcn.132337.

King, G., Law, M., King, S., Hurley, P., Hanna, S., Kertoy, M., Rosenbaum, P., & Young, N. (2004). *Children's assessment of participation and enjoyment (CAPE) and Preferences for activities of children (PAC)*. Pearson.

Klein, B., & Kraus de Camargo, O. (2018). A proposed functional abilities classification tool for developmental disorders affecting learning and behavior. *Frontiers in Education, 3*. https://doi.org/10.3389/feduc.2018.00002

Leach, E., Cornwell, P., Fleming, J., & Haines, T. (2010). Patient-centred goal setting in a sub-acute rehabilitation setting. *Disability and Rehabilitation, 32*(2), 159-172.

Lynch, E. W., & Hanson, M. (2011). *Developing cross-cultural competence: A guide for working with children and their families* (5th ed.). Brookes.

McCormack, J., Jacobs, D., & Washington, K. (2012). Specific mental functions: Language (B167). In A. Majnemer (Ed.), *Measures for children with developmental disabilities: An ICF approach* (pp. 129-153). Wiley.

McGregor, K. K. (2020). How we fail children with developmental language disorder. *Language, Speech, and Hearing Services in Schools, 51*, 981-992. https://doi.org/10.1044/2020_LSHSS-20-00003

McLeod, S. (2004). Speech pathologists' application of the ICF to children with speech impairment. *International Journal of Speech-Language Pathology, 6*(1), 75-81. https://doi.org/10.1080/14417040410001669516

Morgan, P. L., Hammer, C. S., Farkes, G., Hillemeier, M. M., Maxzuga, S., Cook, M., & Morano, S. (2016). Who receives speech/language services by 5 years of age in the United States? *American Journal of Speech-Language Pathology, 25*(2), 183-199. https://doi.org/10.1044/2015_AJSLP-14-0201

Mulcair, G., Pietranton, A. A., & Williams, C. (2018). The International Communication Project: Raising global awareness of communication as a human right. *International Journal of Speech-Language Pathology, 20*, 34-38. https://doi.org/10.1080/17549507.2018.1422023

Paradis, J. (2016). The development of English as a second language with and without specific language impairment. *Journal of Speech, Language, & Hearing Research, 59*, 171-182. https://doi.org/10.1044/2015_JSLHR-L-15-0008

Paradis, J., Emmerzael, K., & Sorenson Duncan, T. (2010). Assessment of English language learners: Using parent report on first language development. *Journal of Communication Disorders, 43*, 474-497. https://doi.org/10.1016/j.jcomdis.2010.01.002

Petersen, D. B., Chanthonqthip, H., Ukrainetz, T., Spencer, T. D., & Street, R. W. (2017). Dynamic assessment of narratives: Efficient, accurate identification of language impairment in bilingual students. *Journal of Speech, Language, and Hearing Research, 60*, 983-998. https://doi.org/10.1044/2016_JSLHR-L-15-0426

Roseberry-McKibbon, C. (2018). *Multicultural students with special language needs: Practical strategies for assessment and intervention* (5th ed.). Academic Communication Associated.

Samson, J. F., & Lesaux, N. K. (2009). Language-minority learners in special education: Rates and predictors of identification for services. *Journal of Learning Disabilities, 42*(2), 148-162. https://doi.org/10.1177/0022219408326221

Sanjeevan, T., & Mainela-Arnold, E. (2019). Characterizing the motor skills in children with specific language impairment. *Folia Phoniatrica et Logopedica, 71*(1), 42-55. https://doi.org/10.1159/000493262

Semel, E., Wiig, E. H., & Secord, W. A. (2006). *Clinical Evaluation of Language Fundamentals* (4th ed., Spanish Version [CELF-4 Spanish]). Pearson.

Shahmahmood, T. M., Jalie, S., Soleymani, Z., Haresabadi, F., & Nemati, P. (2016). A systematic review on diagnostic procedures for specific language impairment: The sensitivity and specificity issues. *Journal of Research in Medical Sciences, 21*(1), 67. https://doi.org/10.4103/1735-1995.189648

Sidenna, M., Fadl, T., & Zayed, H. (2020). Genetic epidemiology of hearing loss in the 22 Arab countries: A systematic review. *Otology & Neurotology, 41*(2), e152-e162. https://doi.org/10.1097/MAO.0000000000002489

Tomas, E., & Vissers, C. (2019). Behind the scenes of developmental language disorder: Time to call neuropsychology back on stage. *Frontiers in Human Neuroscience, 12*(517). https://doi.org/10.3389/fnhum.2018.00517

Towle, P. O., Patrick, P. A., Ridgard, T., Pham, S., & Marrus, J. (2020). Is earlier better? The relationship between age when starting early intervention and outcomes for children with autism spectrum disorder: A selective review. *Autism Research and Treatment, 2020*, 7605876. https://doi.org/10.1155/2020/7605876

United Nations. (1948). *UN Universal declaration of human rights*. https://www.un.org/en/about-us/universal-declaration-of-human-rights

Washington, K. N. (2007). Using the ICF within speech-language pathology: Application to developmental language impairment. *International Journal of Speech-Language Pathology, 9*(3), 242-255. https://doi.org/full/10.1080/14417040701261525

Westby, C. (2007). Application of the ICF in children with language impairments. *Seminars in Speech and Language, 28*(4), 265-272. https://doi.org/10.1055/s-2007-986523

Wiig, E. H., Semel, E., & Secord, W. A. (2013). *Clinical Evaluation of Language Fundamentals* (5th ed.; CELF-5). Pearson.

World Health Organization. (2001). *International classification of functioning, disability and health (ICF).* Author.

World Health Organization (WHO Workgroup for development of version of ICF for Children & Youth). (2007). *International classification of functioning disability and health—Children and youth version (ICF-CY).* Author.

World Health Organization. (2013). *How to use the ICF: A practical manual for using the international classification of functioning, disability and health (ICF).* Exposure draft for comment. Author.

World Health Organization & World Bank. (2011). *World report on disability.* Author.

Worrall, L., Sherratt, S., Rogers, P., Howe, T., Hersh, D., Ferguson, A., & Davidson, B. (2011). What people with aphasia want: Their goals according to the ICF. *Aphasiology, 25*(3), 309-322. https://doi.org/10.1080/02687038.2010.508530

Chapter 3

Language and Language Families

Tobias A. Kroll, PhD, CCC-SLP
and Dr. phil. Jan Wohlgemuth, MA

Introduction

Language is a foundational human capacity. Without language, humans would not have evolved as a species, and we most certainly would not have built cities, written books, or gone to the moon. Even our archaic cousins the Neanderthals probably had language (Dediu & Levinson, 2013), which means humans have been chatting away for at least 500,000 years (Barham & Everett, 2021; Everett, 2017).

No wonder, then, that humans have been thinking about this marvelous faculty for much of recorded history. In doing so, we have tried to answer the following questions: (1) What is language? (2) Is there a common logic underlying the world's different language systems? and (3) How and why did language evolve? While these questions may sound philosophical—and they are, even though they are also asked in anthropology—the answers do, surprisingly, shape the clinical work of speech-language therapists.

With regard to question 1, it is widely accepted that language has elements of both declarative and procedural knowledge. Put otherwise, it can be viewed as a networked inventory of mental representations—what we *know*—but also as a combination of cognitive and motor skills—what we can *do* with our knowledge. And like with other areas of knowledge, the quantity and quality of our mental network, and the efficacy with which we use our skills, depends on a host of factors: our exposure to relevant input, our ability to learn, our opportunity to practice our skills, and so forth.

Bortz, M. (Ed.). *A Guide to Global Language Assessment: A Lifespan Approach* (pp. 45-66).
DOI: 10.4324/9781003524472-4

For speech-language therapists working with clients and patients from an array of different linguistic backgrounds, it is therefore important to keep in mind that individual differences in linguistic functioning can have a host of reasons that may have nothing to do with a diagnosable problem—especially in the case of individuals whose first language is different from our own. If such speakers lack knowledge clinicians would otherwise expect from them, is it because they have a language problem, or simply because they have not yet had a chance to learn what we are looking for? This is not only a matter of time—how long they have been learning English—but also of culture and context. As an example, someone from a tropical country is less likely to have an in-depth concept of *snow*, and someone from a less complicated health care system may not be aware of the subtle difference between *primary care provider* and *family doctor.*

The same is true for skills. The ability to produce certain phoneme sequences or grammatical structure develops over time and depends not only on the person's capacity (or lack thereof) for learning, but also on exposure, practice opportunities, and even factors such as fatigue or emotionality. Clinical and anecdotal observation suggest that even proficient non-native speakers may produce more accented speech when they are tired (Dalhousie Accent Clinic, n. d.), or that their ability to accurately produce complex grammatical constructions decreases when they are emotional.

The challenge for speech-language therapists is to find their way through the thicket of factors contributing to the momentary performance of the person in front of them, and to arrive at a conclusion as to whether they are due to a clinical problem or simply to the fact that English is a new language for the speaker. Supporting clinicians in this challenge is, of course, the focus of this book, and this chapter will lay the foundations. It will provide an overview of the vast variety of languages of the world and present several ways of organizing this diversity. In the process, it will investigate cultures that routinely use more than one language, and how this affects speakers' functioning when compared to habitual monolinguals. It will then proceed to what is, in many ways, its central part: an outline—necessarily incomplete—of how speakers of English as a new language may differ from native speakers of English along each of the five components of language, as well as in their nonverbal and extralinguistic behaviors. Along the way, it will also consider speakers whose native idiom[1] is a variety of English other than the dialect dominant in professional contexts, i.e., Standard American English (SAE). In other words, it will attempt to give clinicians an overview of the *types* of productions and behaviors that should be treated as potentially indicative of a language *difference*, rather than a disorder.

Given the sheer number of languages spoken around the world, their structural variety (affecting speakers' procedural skills) and the multitude of cultural and environmental contexts they are spoken in (affecting speakers' communicative behaviors and their knowledge base), this is a daunting task, and so is the clinician's. In the conclusion the we will, therefore, return to questions 2 and 3 to illustrate how the answers to them can help speech-language therapists navigate this challenge.

Languages Around the World

In this section, the reader will be introduced to some of the major differences found among languages around the world. More precisely, it should be said, the focus will be on *communication* differences. As clinicians are well aware, language never happens outside of communication, and communication includes more than language—for example, nonverbal and paralinguistic behaviors. These, in turn, are part of the broader culture in which the language is spoken: How speakers deploy their body and voice while talking is shaped, not so much by the language itself but by the community that uses it.

[1]Note: in this chapter, the term *idiom* is used as a synonym for language to make for better readability.

This brings up an important point that will be reiterated throughout this chapter: most of the relations discussed—between culture and communication, first language structure and English productions, and so forth—are not simple and linear but multifaceted. This is especially true for a global language like English. To take the example of body language, White American Anglo speakers typically use gestures sparsely while African American or South Asian speakers of English typically use more emphatic gestures. These differences reflect cultural communication styles; however, this does not mean that every Black or Indian speaker of English will use emphatic gestures in every situation, nor will White Anglo speakers always be subdued in this regard. The actual communication behaviors of a person depend not only on their culture but also on their individual personality, mental-emotional state, the situation in which they communicate, and so on.

Thus, while the chapter will include general statements like "African American communication is characterized by expressive body language," such statements are always to be read as a statistical likelihood, not a general rule of the one-size-fits-all kind. The same is true for the cultural differences addressed in the following section, and for the patterns of interference and transfer discussed further within.

Cultural Communication Differences

Aside from full-on language barriers, the most obvious cultural communication differences occur in nonverbal and paralinguistic aspects of communication. Speakers from different cultures vary in how they use eye gaze, facial expressions, gestures and touch, and proxemics, as well as in their rate of speech, pitch range and intonation contours, and volume. For example, White (Anglo) American convention for eye gaze during conversation is that the speaker looks at the listener most of the time, while the listener alternates between having their gaze on versus away from the speaker, with about the same frequency and duration for each. In stark contrast to this, African and Native American as well as East Asian cultures require the listener to refrain from gazing directly at the speaker. Particularly in situations where the speaker has a higher social status (e.g., a teacher talking to a student), a direct gaze would be a sign of disrespect (Elliott et al., 2016). However, in White (Anglo) conversation, looking away from the speaker is a communication of lack of interest (or respect).

It is easy to see, from this brief contrast, how differences in nonverbal or paralinguistic conventions can contribute to serious miscommunication. A Native American child communicating respect to her White teacher by averting her gaze may well be seen as disrespectful by the teacher, and reprimanded (Elliott et al., 2016). The same pitfalls loom in all aspects of nonverbal and paralinguistic communication. Examples will be given in the discussion of interference and transfer in the next sections.

Language and Culture

Language and cultures are interrelated in many ways. Most obviously, this is relevant on the level of pragmatics and of semantics. What speakers say when greeting and parting, what counts as appropriate topics for conversation (and, just as importantly, as inappropriate ones), how directly or indirectly requests are made and so forth—all of these pragmatic rules are cultural as much as they are linguistic. Similarly, the concepts expressible in any given language are dependent on the shared cultural knowledge in which they are contained. Put simply, a culture with no experience with some real-world phenomenon will not have a word for it; for example, many Indigenous cultures in tropical regions do not have (Indigenous) words for *snow*.

On a subtler level, lexica may be organized differently across cultures. What gets classified as *domestic animal* or *food* depends on what is consumed in any given culture: in South Louisiana, for example, a client may list *alligator* among food items. Similarly, schematic association of concepts depends on the culturally prevalent status and uses of a referent. A *knife* may be associated with *food*, *hunting*, or *fighting* depending on which of these associations is most salient in a speaker's lexicon.

It may come as a surprise that aspects of linguistic form can also be tied to the culture in which it is used. For example, many languages encode social relationships using grammar. Examples are French and German, where social distance or closeness between interlocutors are expressed in the pronoun used to address each other: second person singular *(tu/du)* if speaker and listener are close, second (French) or third (German) person plural *(vous/Sie)* if they are not. Verb morphology is also adjusted based on the pronoun used. Japanese goes a step further and distinguishes three levels of politeness in its system of honorifics; they apply across all pronouns, as well as to verb morphology and phrasal formulation. In all three cases, these grammatical distinctions follow a traditionally complex and hierarchical culture.[2] English-speaking cultures, traditionally more egalitarian, do not encode hierarchy in grammar; in fact, even the distance/closeness distinction as encoded in first-name versus honorific-plus-last-name address (i.e., Jeff versus Mr. Bridges) has in many contexts been replaced by first-name only address.

For the clinician, the import is that ways of talking are intertwined with clients' cultures. And they should be honored as such, even if they show up in unexpected ways in the client's EL communication. Examples of what that might look like will be provided following, in the discussion of interference and transfer.

Structural Differences Unrelated to Culture

There are, of course, differences of form between languages that are not directly tied to culture. To get a handle on those, it is worth reminding the reader of the relevant characteristics of English. In the realm of *syntax*, for example, native speakers of English are used to the following:

- Sentences are analyzable into recognizable parts (e.g., subject and predicate), and even lay speakers may be able to provide such analysis
- Word order is relatively fixed, with SVO (subject-verb-object) as the "default"
- To count as a sentence, a sequence of language must minimally have a subject (noun or pronoun) and a verb or verb group
- Nouns are commonly (but not always) preceded by a determiner *(a* or *the)*
- In descriptive utterances where no action is expressed, and hence a full verb form is not needed, a sentence must have a form of to be as a copula to serve as a "logical connector" between subject and descriptor (e.g., *Paul is a doctor)*

None of these features are present in every language. In some Native American idioms, for example, utterances come as holistic "sentence-words" that follow a fixed form and whose parts are not altered (Marianne Mithun, personal communication). Some languages such as Italian or Russian are rather flexible in word order; many others do recognize a "default" order, but one that differs from English (e.g., SOV in Japanese, VSO in Filipino and Irish). Various idioms accept subject-less utterances as grammatical, e.g., Spanish, where *está durmiendo* ("he/she is sleeping," literally reads *is sleeping)* would make a perfectly acceptable statement. Others, such as Ukrainian, do not use determiners or copulas, resulting in utterances such as *trava zelena* (meaning the "the grass is green," literally reads *grass green)*.

---

[2]The authors' own, informal observation suggests that use of the closeness-signaling *du* is increasing in Germany, in tandem with the emergence of a more egalitarian culture.

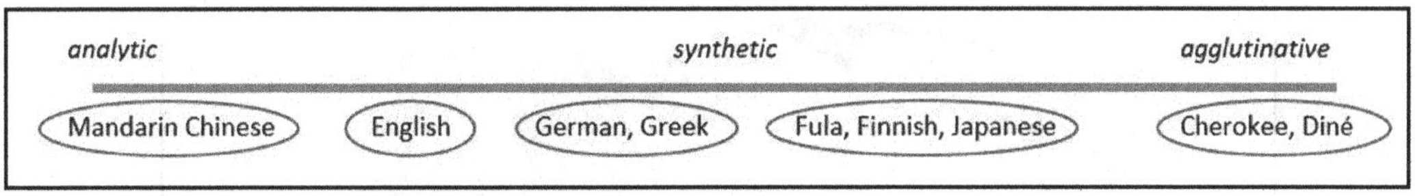

Figure 3-1. A continuum of morphological complexity (with example languages).

Similar variation is found in *morphology*. English has a morphological system of low complexity, meaning it does have prefixes and suffixes but not very many compared to other languages. In global comparison, English is thus placed towards the lower end of a wide continuum. Some idioms do not have any bound morphemes at all (e.g., Mandarin Chinese or Vietnamese); others have rich affix systems of various kinds (e.g., German or Greek); yet others have an comparative abundance of affixes, many of which serve functions fulfilled, in English, by prepositions (e.g., Fula, Finnish, or Japanese); yet others treat entire utterances as word-like constructions with a rich morphology, e.g., the Native American languages Cherokee and Diné,[3] alluded to previously in the mention of "sentence-words." Figure 3-1 shows the spectrum of the world's languages in terms of their morphological complexity, with the idioms discussed here placed on a continuum for illustration. *Analytic* refers to languages without any bound morphemes, *synthetic* to relatively rich bound morpheme inventories, and *agglutinative* to languages in which entire utterances, which would be analyzed into sentences in English or German, are formed from single word bases with affixes.

As the reader may expect by now, the same is true for *phonology*: variety is the norm. This applies both to the number of phonemes in any given idiom, and to the kinds of phonemes they have. As to the former, inventories can have anywhere between 11 and 141 phonemic segments, although few have more than 48. The two least phoneme-rich idioms, Pirahã (Native South American) and Rotokas (Papua New Guinean), share only 7 of their 11 sounds; the vastest inventory is found in !Xu, a South African language, which uses a large amount of click sounds in addition to the more frequent pulmonary ones. English is one of the more phoneme-rich languages, with around 42 sounds (and variations depending on the dialect); most languages have fewer sounds than English, in particular fewer vowels (Crystal, 1995; Leitung der Abteilung Phonetik der Goethe-Universität, 2018). To an extent, the sound substitutions and omissions clinicians can expect in speakers of English as an additional language are thus predictable (more detail on this will be provided later).

Language Families

There are around 6,000 to 8,000 languages in the world; counts differ depending on the criteria used to distinguish languages from dialects. Most of these belong to a *language family*, a group of languages descended from a common ancestor. The best-known example for the latter is the Romance language (sub)family, which contains idioms such as French, Italian, Spanish, and Portuguese; all of these are descendants of the Latin spoken in the Roman Empire. The Romance family, in turn, is a member of the larger Indo-European family, which has historically been spoken from Iceland in the west to India in the east, and contains languages such as English, Russian, Persian (Farsi), and Hindi, each of which is part of a subfamily within the Indo-European lineage. In the same way, most languages around the world are grouped into families and subfamilies. Some, however, are isolates, with no known other members in their family; examples are Korean and Basque.

[3] More commonly known under its Spanish name, Navajo.

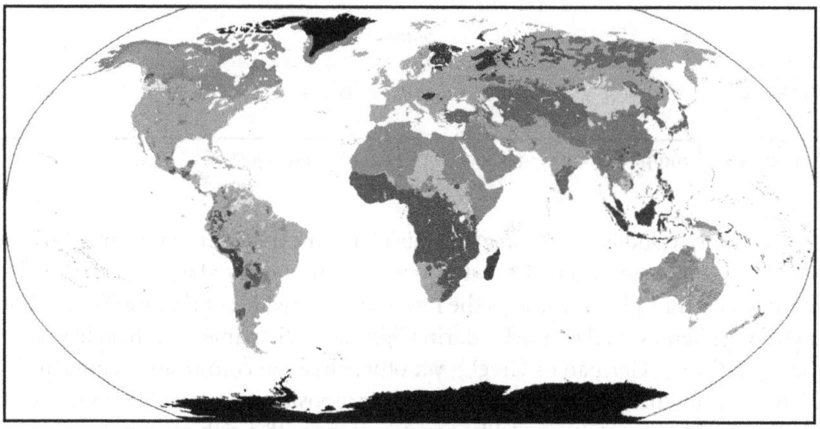

Figure 3-2. The world's language families. A full-color image (including the countries' names) can be viewed at https://upload.wikimedia.org/wikipedia/commons/e/ed/Primary_Human_Language_Families_Map.png (© Wikipedia contributor Alumnum, 2019).

Figure 3-2 shows the contemporary distribution of language families. Note that the Indo-European family covers the largest surface area by far; this is due to the past few centuries' history of colonization, which has led to the dominance of English, as well as Spanish and Portuguese, throughout the Americas and in Australia. Also because of colonization, Indo-European languages serve as linguas francas in much of Africa as well as South and Southeast Asia.

Known and presumed language families number in the dozens; most of these, however, comprise only a minute number of languages. According to the Glottolog 4.5 (Hammarström et al., 2021), the standard reference for linguistic genealogy, there are 16 families that each include at least one percent of the world's languages. Table 3-1 lists these families together with the geographical area as well as World Health Organization region in which they are spoken, and the most widely spoken members of the family.

As evident from this brief overview, language families and their relationship to geographical and World Health Organization regions are mainly useful for heuristic and overview purposes. Families and regions are only loosely associated with each other; also, regional linguistic contexts are characterized by considerable cultural and structural diversity, as we will see. And all of these factors impact a speaker's performance in a target language (e.g., English).

Bi-/Multilingual Cultures and Translanguaging

To make matters more complicated, many speakers whom clinicians encounter habitually speak more than one language. It has been estimated that the majority of the world's population is at least partly bi- or multilingual, that is, used to navigating more than one language at a time. While some of this linguistic richness stems from the legacy of colonialism, multilingualism has been the norm for most societies around the world throughout history. For example, Latin served as lingua franca for scholars in medieval Europe, and Sabir (the original "lingua franca") as shared idiom for traders around the Mediterranean. After the Mughal conquest, rulers of Northern India spoke Persian for a period and so did their administrations, while Hindustani served as the language of the street. Kiswahili was used for communication throughout vast stretches of Eastern Africa long before the advent of European tongues, and still has lingua franca status today (Genemo, 2021; Romaine, 2013).

Table 3-1

Prominent Language Families With Region and Example Idioms

FAMILY	AREA (WHO REGION)	MOST PROMINENT MEMBERS
Atlantic–Congo	West, Central, and Southeast Africa (AFR)	Yoruba, Igbo, Fula, Shona, Kiswahili, isiZulu, isiXhosa[a]
Austronesian	Southeast Asia, Pacific Ocean, Madagascar (SEAR, WPR, AFR)	Indonesian, Malay, Javanese, Tagalog, Hawaiian, Samoan, Maori, Malagasy
Sino-Tibetan	China, Myanmar (WPR)	Mandarin and other languages of mainland China; Burmese, Tibetan
Indo-European	All continents (all regions)	English, Hindustani, Spanish, Bengali
Pama-Nyungan	Australia (WPR)	Pitjantjatjara, Ngaanyatjarra, Arrernte, Warlpiri
Trans-New Guinea*	New Guinea (WPR)	Dani, Makasae, Enga
Afro-Asiatic	North and East Africa, Middle East (AFR, EMR)	Arabic, Hebrew, Hausa, Oromo, Amharic, Amazigh[b] languages
Nilo-Saharan*	Sahara Desert and Lower Nile area (AFR, EMR)	Luo, Kanuri, Songhay, Lugbara, Maasai
Oto-Manguean	Mexico (AMR)	Zapotecan, Mixtecan
Austroasiatic	Southeast Asia (SEAR, WPR)	Vietnamese, Khmer
Tai-Kadai	Southeast Asia (SEAR, WPR)	Thai, Lao
Dravidian	South Asia (SEAR)	Telugu, Tamil, Kannada, Malayalam
Tupian	South America (AMR)	Tupi, Guarani
Arawakan	South America (AMR)	Taino, Resigaro, Yucuna,
Mande	West Africa (AFR)	Mandinka, Yalunka, Kpelle, Soninke
Uto-Aztecan	North and Central America (AMR)	Luiseno, Hopi, Comanche, Nahuatl

*Note: the status of these families is disputed; they may actually be two or more separate families.
[a]The latter three are better known as Swahili, Zulu, and Xhosa; we use the Indigenous terms here.
[b]Better known as *Berber*; however, this term is now considered offensive.

With the advent of colonialism and globalization, multilingual societies became only more prevalent throughout the world. In many places, European languages became the idioms of administration; English serves as a de facto lingua franca for much of the world today and communities around the globe began adopting idioms of power. Sadly, many local languages became extinct in the process, and native tongues continue to disappear every day.

In a nutshell, practicing clinicians are likely to encounter persons for whom shifting between languages or blending them (a practice termed *codemixing* or, more recently, *translanguaging*) is a matter of habit. It is therefore important for the reader to be familiar with some of the basic dynamics in question. This includes the many facets of proficiency in bi- or multilingual individuals, a working understanding of the roles different languages may play in the lives of individuals and communities, and the resulting sociopsychological dynamics. We will discuss each of these in turn.

Proficiency in Bi-/Multilingual Speakers

It is a common misconception that only speakers who have "equal proficiency" in all their languages can properly be termed bi- or multilingual. This assumption relies on a twofold fallacy. The first aspect of it is the idea of "equal proficiency" itself. Even speakers who are fluent or native-like in both or all their languages are not typically equally proficient across all levels, domains, and modalities.

As regards to *levels*, someone may speak a second language proficiently and fluently but with an accent, or be pragmatically slightly "off" when compared with native speakers of English. Conversely, it is possible to speak with a heavy accent and grammatical mistakes but be pragmatically so proficient that conversation is not hindered. With regard to *domains*, speakers may be more comfortable talking about certain topics in one language and about others in another. As an example, the first author of this chapter is a native speaker of German but received his entire education in speech-language therapy in English; he would be hard-pressed to give a lecture about his field in his first language, as he lacks even the most basic vocabulary. Finally, speakers' proficiency may differ between *modalities*. Someone who has received intensive formal schooling in an additional language, but little interaction, may write it more proficiently than their own first language. This is the case for many speakers in India or African countries, where the language of instruction is commonly English.

The second aspect of the fallacy is the assumption that high levels of proficiency are needed for a language to have an impact on a speaker's communicative functioning or to play an important role in their life. In India, for example, English is woven so deeply into everyday discourse that even speakers with relatively low expressive proficiency understand it and intersperse English terms and phrases in their L1 utterances. Similarly, not everyone who speaks a form of Spanglish (a Spanish-English translanguage) is a fluent speaker of both languages (Bierly, 2019). Thus, proficient translanguaging should not result in an expectation of equal proficiency in all idioms involved. Conversely, codeswitching is one of the most common forms of adaptation used by members of minority or immigrant cultures, and regardless of the level of proficiency involved, it plays an outsized role in speakers' self-understanding and the ease, or lack thereof, with which they navigate the majority culture.

Translanguaging (Codemixing) and Codeswitching

In the field of speech-language therapy, the terms *codeswitching* and *codemixing* are often used interchangeably to refer to a wide range of very different behaviors—possibly because they sound so similar. Therefore, this chapter uses an alternative to codemixing that was coined by sociolinguists. *Translanguaging* (García & Wei, 2014) refers to the interwoven use of the repertoire of two (or more) languages in everyday conversation *within one speech community*. In other words, speakers of the same community, when translanguaging, draw from two or more languages to formulate their turns at talk or utterances.

Communities in which translanguaging is common include many Hispanic speakers in the United States, educated or middle-to-higher SES speakers in India, or bilingual speakers of Ukrainian and Russian in Ukraine (prior to the Russian attack on the country). In the first of these cases, the resulting idiom is often termed *Spanglish* (mentioned previously), and may take for example, the following form: "Alright because now we're gonna go to Los Tucanes de Tijuana con su tema La Chica Sexy" (Public Broadcasting System, 2005, minute 4:36). The speaker begins her utterance in English but switches to Spanish for the phrase *con su tema* (with their song). The song title features another example, i.e., the English word *sexy* used as an adjective to *chica* according to the syntactic rules of Spanish. Similarly, a native speaker of Tamil (a South Indian language) may utter *Amam Maa, inniku evening naan shopping panna poren* (yes, Mom, tonight we will go shopping; Anu Chandrasekaran, personal communication), inserting the English lexemes *evening* and *shopping* into the Tamil utterance. Other blends may occur at the sentence or discourse level, but the underlying principle is the same: speakers draw on two languages for communicative purposes so routinely that the resulting mix is the conventional idiom in their community.

The practice of *codeswitching* provides a stark contrast to this. Instead of one speech community drawing on two repertoires, codeswitching occurs when a speaker enters a speech community not their own and changes their communication to adapt to the conventions prevailing in that context (Kroll & Townsend, 2022). This can occur between languages, but also between dialects. Examples for the former are Spanish- or Vietnamese-speaking immigrants leaving their community (temporarily, if the community is within the United States; long-term with regard to their country of origin) to interact with native English speakers. Examples for the latter include African American persons switching from Black English to Standard American when interacting in majority-White spaces, or a White Southerner "losing" their accent when talking to Midwesterners.

It is clear that these two practices are very different in terms of both the resulting linguistic productions, and the sociopsychological dynamics involved. Regarding the former, codeswitching involves the change from one communication system to another. The systems are not mixed, except for remnants of the speaker's native system that are transferred into the target system. At least theoretically, it is possible to adopt an entirely different system without any such vestiges. By contrast, translanguaging involves the explicit blending of two systems at the word, phrase, sentence, or turn level. The resulting productions, while part of a unified repertoire from the speaker's viewpoint (García & Wei, 2014), can readily be analyzed into elements from both idioms involved, and typically are so even by lay listeners.

Regarding sociopsychological dynamics, change of communication systems does not happen in a vacuum but in within a complex web of culture(s), involving matters of group solidarity, intergroup relations, power, and historical injustices. All of these may complicate the act, already fraught, of adopting a way of communicating that is not one's own. Thus, when a client appears to reject the idea of codeswitching, clinicians are encouraged to think about the issue as a matter of identity, and of history shaping the present moment. As an example, an African American high schooler may be reluctant to adopt the standard dialect expected in academic work because they feel this would constitute a "selling out" of his identity at the behest of a dominating culture hostile to it (Kroll & Townsend, 2022). Similar dynamics may occur in immigrants, individuals with a strong working-class identity, or Indigenous people. In each of these cases, the clinician faces the challenging task of validating the client's linguistic and communicative identity while meeting the prescriptive expectations of their societal context.

Interference/Transfer

When speakers use a communication system (language or dialect) in which they do not have native-like proficiency, they are likely to produce communicative actions that do not fully conform to the target system because the speaker has introduced aspects of their own native system into their communication. This phenomenon is termed *interference* or *transfer*. It is distinctly different from translanguaging, discussed earlier, in that it does not involve a communally shared system of code-mixing, but rather reflects an individual speaker's struggles with a target system. As such, interference/transfer is a characteristic of codeswitching as defined previously.

The terms *interference* and *transfer* are largely used interchangeably, even though some attempts at differentiating them have been made. Grosjean (2011) suggests reserving *transfer* for patterned or stable productions (e.g., in cases where a non-native speaker of English consistently replaces the English liquid "r" with the globally more common tongue-tap "r"), and *interference* for one-off, idiosyncratic productions (e.g., when a speaker occasionally changes English word order to match that or their first language). Other authors use *transfer* when referring to similarities between first and target language that make acquisition of the latter easier, and *interference* for differences that make it harder (e.g., Hernandez et al., 2005). As for this chapter, these definitions are mentioned mainly for benefit of the reader. It is important to be aware that all these dynamics do occur in bilinguals; in order to avoid going into excessive detail, however, the terms will not be distinguished in the following discussion. The phenomena in question will be referred to jointly as I/T.

As suggested by the term *interference*, I/T can have detrimental impacts on communication. Listeners may *fail to understand* what the speaker is saying because their productions are too different from the listener's expectations, or—which is possibly more detrimental—they may *misunderstand* what the speaker is attempting to convey, up to and including a misreading of their intentions. Examples for these issues will be given below for each aspect of communication and language. Note that in order to keep the discussion succinct, it will be limited to examples of how I/T impact communicative actions in SAE contexts—not because the authors deem SAE intrinsically more important or interesting than other languages or varieties of English, but because it is the normative and reference dialect for speech-language therapists practicing in an Anglophone North American context.

Interference/Transfer in Communication

On the classic continuum of low- to high-context cultures (Hall, 1959), White North Americans fall decisively on the low-context end, meaning that nonverbal aspects of communication play a much smaller role for them in interaction than they do in Japanese or Apache culture, for example. In the latter, speakers routinely look for and produce minute clues that convey a wealth of information. By contrast, middle class Anglo North Americans will typically attempt to encode as much information as possible in verbal utterances. Thus, speakers from this background may be prone to missing vital signals when interacting with individuals from high-context communities. The following paragraphs will therefore go into some detail discussing communication differences of the nonverbal and extralinguistic kind.

There are two more reasons for giving extra attention to these aspects. First, nonverbal and extralinguistic differences are bound to shape the clinician's perceptions of the client, and vice versa. It is important for the clinician to keep in mind that initial impressions of others are formed quite quickly (Ambady & Rosenthal, 1992), tying an abundance of gestural communication to a perception of "aggression" or "intensity," or a gaze away from the speaker as lack of interest or respect, where in either case the speaker may simply be witnessing cultural communication differences. The same may be true for clients' perceptions of therapists, although their impression will often be mitigated by the power differential between experts and laypersons and by the fact that the client has likely been exposed to the dominant professional, middle class culture and knows what to expect in such a context.

The other reason is that in many instances, people interacting become more similar to one another in terms of communication behaviors; this is known as *accommodation* (Giles et al., 1991). Speech-language therapists trained to be sensitive to the minutiae of interaction may even (semi-) consciously attempt to accommodate clients in order to form a bond with them. There are, however, pitfalls associated with this when cross-cultural differences are involved; these will be touched on briefly here.

- *Eye gaze*, across cultures, can alternate from steady to shifting during conversation. As mentioned, in some cultures listeners communicates respect and attention by gazing at the speaker; in others, by averting gaze, typically downward. In cultures where gazing at the speaker is considered the default, variations exist along social hierarchies including gender and age. In Western culture, children may be admonished to "look at [the speaker]" while listening; by contrast, if an unflinching gaze were used by an adult male on another adult male, it could indicate aggression or contempt. The same variation holds for looking around along the horizontal axis: it may indicate discomfort or lack of interest, but it may also simply be prompted by other sources of information that the listener attempts to attend to simultaneously. As with all other communicative behaviors, intimacy with the (sub)culture in question and concurrent interpretation of the entirety of interlocutors' actions is needed to arrive at an accurate interpretation of this behavior. As for their own gaze, clinicians are best advised by sticking to what they are used to and comfortable with. Trying to match the client's gaze patterns may prove awkward and disruptive to the interaction.
- *Facial expressions* are vivid and ever-changing in some cultures, which may or may not vary by gender. In other cultures, faces are not used to convey direct information; instead, they are kept "stoic" (unmoved) or a smile is used for politeness regardless of the individual's emotional state. "Stoicism" is found in male communication styles in White Anglo and Hispanic cultures; smiles as default in several East Asian cultures regardless of speaker gender. In communicating with clients from diverse backgrounds, clinicians should use the amount of facial expressivity considered appropriate in their respective professional setting, while also considering the impact they may have on the client based on the best of their knowledge about them.
- *Gestures* can range from subtle and subdued to vivid, wide, and expressive. Examples for the former are found in Northern and Central Europe, as well as East Asia and among Native American groups; examples for the latter in Southern Europe, Southern India, and African American cultures (Elliott et al., 2016; Kendon, 1997, 2007). Potential for misunderstanding occurs based on listeners' cultural assumptions about gestures. In low-gesture cultures, expressive body language may be interpreted as an indicator of aggression or (excessive) excitement. In high-gesture cultures, lack of body movements may be read as a sign of subdued anger or, possibly, apathy. As with facial expressions, clinicians are advised to use their own gestures in line with the conventions of their workplace while keeping in mind the potential for intercultural misinterpretation.
- *Touch* is a special case of gesture that involves physical contact. In Western cultures, it may be initiated by speaker or listener and typically conveys an intention of caring in professional contexts. In other cultures, it may convey similar intents or be considered entirely inappropriate. As it involves the breach of each person's personal space, its use requires heightened sensitivity to the other person's mental-emotional state and cultural background, lest it be considered a transgression; this is true across cultures. Many cultures have specific conventions regarding touch. For example, in many Muslim and Orthodox Jewish cultures, touch should not occur between members of the opposite sex; in some Southeast Asian cultures, touching a child's head is seen as a bad omen, while in Hispanic culture it is considered a blessing. Given the extra sensibility surrounding touch, clinicians should refrain from touching clients unless they are confident it will be well-received; similarly, they should not be quick to make assumptions about a client's intent behind touching.
- *Proxemics* refers to cultural rules regarding the distance between interlocutors. As with all other aspects of communication, this too varies between cultures. Observed distances in nonintimate social interaction range from around one to several feet. If one interlocutor comes closer to the other than is culturally expected, discomfort arises as this is experienced as intrusive; conversely, if one interlocutor stays further away than expected, discomfort may arise from a perception of

distance and aloofness. Of note, White, middle-class North Americans are used to larger distances while interacting than most cultures (Hall, 1969). As with the other nonverbal behaviors discussed here, the clinician is advised to employ their own culture's rules for distance but to closely observe client interactions with members of their respective culture. If the clinician assumes their standard North American distance may come across as aloofness, they may intentionally use other means of connection to foster rapport.

This covers the *nonverbal* aspects of communication; next, cultural differences in *paralinguistic* features will be discussed, including prosody, rate, hearer feedback, and silence.

- *Prosody* refers to duration, intensity, and frequency aspects of verbal communication (Boutsen, 2003)—in other words, the speaker's intonation and volume. As the reader may suspect by now, these aspects vary widely between languages. Some do not distinguish between long and short syllables while others do. In some cultures, talk is considered conventional at a volume that would be considered shouting in others. Languages differ in their default intonation contours: in English or German, statements end with falling intonation,[4] in French, with same-level or rising intonation. Languages differ also in whether there *is* a default: tonal idioms such as Mandarin Chinese or Thai mark word meanings through intonation, so contours typically vary widely between utterances. Of note, this "melody" of language, the changes between lower and higher frequencies, is unique to every idiom and so deeply ingrained in everyday utterances that language defaults can be differentiated even in newborns' crying, as a result of exposure in the womb (Hardach, 2020). Like with other aspects covered in this section, the clinician is well-advised to use their own habitual prosody when interacting with clients and to interpret any unusual prosody in a client as a potential cultural difference.
- *Rate* is the speed at which verbal language is produced, usually measured as syllables per second or per minute. It is one of the most salient linguistic differences for untrained listeners, who frequently comment on the perceived speed with which speakers of a given language talk. However, actual average rate differences may be lower than they are perceived to be. English uses a strong contrast between long and short syllables; languages in which syllables are produced at about equal length may sound rapid to an untrained listener. As always, clinicians are called to investigate normative rate patterns in a client's L1 and to inquire with community members if there are rate concerns. Rate is a clinical issue only to the extent that it gets in the way of comprehensibility; in any idiom, clinical concern should not be about matching conventional rates but about ensuring that client does not talk too rapidly for hearers to understand them.
- *Hearer feedback.* Closely related to turn-taking rules (discussed later), norms regarding feedback while listening (such as head nods or fillers like mhm, ok, or yeah in English) not only differ between cultures but are a sensitive part of interpersonal communication. If listeners do not give the conventional type and amount of feedback, speakers may interpret this as lack of interest or attention; if they give too much of it, or not the expected kind, speakers may read it as interruption (particularly as hearer signals are also used to indicate assumption of speaker role; Sacks et al., 1974). Clinicians should not assume rudeness or pragmatic issues if a client's feedback behavior does not match SAE norms.
- *Silence.* This may be a surprising topic, but silence is an essential part of communication, and highly valued as such in an array of cultures. White North Americans are typically uncomfortable with silence, interpreting it as awkwardness or even a momentary interruption in relationship. Northern European cultures are used to pauses between interactions, by contrast, and Native American cultures have made silence a tool for relationship building (Basso, 1970). In many high-context cultures, silence is a normative part of communication (Hall, 1959). Children may not be willing to speak in front of unfamiliar adults; speakers of any age, faced with an unfamiliar

[4]A generational variation on this has emerged in American English: many younger speakers end statements with rising intonation these days.

and possibly incomprehensible situation—such as being asked assessment questions—may react with silence. Clinicians should always consider a client's cultural background when faced with an absence of verbal interaction.

Interference/Transfer in Language

In this section, I/T as they pertain to the traditional five aspects of language (pragmatics, semantics, syntax, morphology, and phonology) will be discussed. Note that this discussion will, of necessity, remain rather general. To assess whether a speaker's productions are due to a linguistic difference, clinicians have to familiarize themselves with the basic structure of the client's first language; recommendations as to how to do this will be given in Part V. In the present section, the focus will be on the most common patterns of I/T that can be found across a range of first languages.

- *Pragmatics* consists of the rules and conventions of language use. Pertinent rules may include appropriate or taboo topics during conversation, narrative structure, how to request or deny a request, rules for turn-taking, what counts as humorous versus offensive, and so forth. Thus, opportunities for pragmatic I/T and resulting miscommunications are virtually countless; we will confine our discussion to a few salient examples for illustration purposes.
    - *Appropriate versus taboo topics.* Some topics underlie broad restrictions across cultures, such as reference to sexual matters. Others are almost universally innocuous, such as the weather or food. On the continuum between these extremes, cultures vary widely as to what is considered acceptable talk. In some cultures, speaking about one's salary is considered normal; in others, offensive. The same is true for mentions of someone's looks. Other differences occur in *how* a topic is spoken about. In American culture, the tenor of conversation is expected to be positive, consisting largely of affirmations and appreciative appraisals. In Germany and other European cultures, conversations consisting of a large amount of merely factual and even critical remarks are perfectly acceptable.
    - *Narrative structure.* It has long been known that norms for storytelling differ widely (McCabe, 1997). Familiar "story grammar" elements such as "beginning, middle, end" or "characters, setting, problem, solution" reflect mostly middle-class, Anglo European norms. This *topic-centered* organization can be contrasted to *topic-associating* narratives as found in the African American tradition, where various episodes are told, sometimes in detail, to convey a common point frequently left implicit. Hispanic children place stories of personal experiences in a context that includes details about their family connections, locations, etc.; Japanese norms require the condensing of various experiences illustrative of the topic at hand into short, poetry-like accounts; similarly, Indigenous South African as well as Native American narratives may sound like poetry or verse meter. Of note, such structures show a considerable degree of overlap and similarity. Conversely, members of any given cultures may use "non-native" structures. For example, African American children may produce topic-centered stories, or mix topic-associating with topic-centered characteristics because they have been familiarized with the format by their families or during schooling.
    - *Requests and denials.* Across cultures, requesting and denying are structured by intricate cultural norms around directness versus indirectness, who can request what from whom, what are reasonable versus unreasonable requests, how to deny a request without causing the requester to lose face, and so forth. As the reader may expect, these rules differ considerably from each other; quite probably, the only cross-cultural commonality is that very young children generally request more directly than older children or adults because they have yet to learn the relevant cultural rules. Suffice to say, therefore, that the kinds of request common during speech therapy are not typically used outside of Western, professional contexts; this

includes asking for information using structured questionnaires, medical questions that may be considered intrusive, and those hallmarks of the field, requests to describe or repeat something. Refusal or uncertainty as a response to such requests should therefore be taken as indicators of a cultural difference if the clinician has reason to believe so, rather than of a disorder.

- *Turn-taking and overlap.* Speaker changes during conversation rely on intricate mechanisms of signaling and responding to signals (Sacks et al., 1974), the mastery of which requires intimate familiarity with pertinent conventions. In conjunction with nonverbal and paralinguistic differences, discussed previously, cultural gaps in turn-taking rules make for ample potential for cross-cultural misunderstanding. A notorious example in the United States is the divergence of White (Anglo) and African American conventions (Kochman, 1981). In the former culture, great care is exerted not to interrupt a speaker while in the latter, being expressive and assertive is valued. This often includes interrupting the current speaker to give feedback, or taking up the speaker role while the current speaker is finishing their turn. To White Anglo observers, this may appear rude or aggressive. Among Black speakers, Anglo reticence may be interpreted as lack of engagement, and may even come across as untrustworthy. This is an extreme example, but similar incompatibilities exist between many cultures. As clinicians, we are therefore called to vigorously check our "gut-level reactions" to speakers in order to make sure we are not falling into the common stereotypes of our larger culture.
- *Humor and its limits.* Speakers of all cultures value humor, tell jokes, and make jesting remarks. However, what counts as humorous and where the line between humor and offense is found varies widely and is also subject to personal differences and preferences. For example, in some cultures, humorous teasing is perceived as a characteristic of friendly relationships; in others, it is perceived as hostile. In addition, the interpretation of the speaker's intent may differ even between hearers from the same culture depending on their sense of self-confidence and security, perceived relationship to the speaker, or momentary mood. Conversely, in some cultures (e.g., in South East Asia) humor is often used to hide shame or insecurity or uneasiness about a topic, and its use by a speaker may be interpreted as such by the listener. That said, the authors do not wish to suggest that clinicians refrain from using (appropriate) humor in their work. Its tremendous value for rapport-building and motivation should be fully taken advantage of. Rather, their recommendation is for clinicians to be patient with themselves and their clients. Not everything clinicians say or do with a humorous intent will be received as such; also, an amount of adjustment and trial-and-error is to be expected before humor can be successfully incorporated into therapy, especially with clients from a different culture.

- *Semantics.* The way languages organize their lexica is a vast territory, too vast to comprehensively cover here. The following discussion will be confined to four important factors: categorization differences, connotative differences, false friends, and semantic confusions.
  - *Categorization differences.* It was mentioned previously that cultures differ in what is considered food; in a variety of cultures, for example, insects are considered a delicacy, while Americans typically shudder at that idea. Other differences pertain to societal organization and may be harder to detect, coming to the fore mainly when there is a misunderstanding. For example, this chapter's first author was asked during the first few months of his new life in the United States if he had come to America "to go to school." He was, in fact, pursuing his PhD. In his native German, however, the term *Schule* (school) strictly pertains to K to 12 education. An explicit clarification was needed to sort this confusion out. More pertinent to health care, the medical industry habitually uses a vast array of highly technical terms that are confusing even to members of this culture. Having a *primary care provider* is a requirement on most insurance plans in the United States; however, outside of the United States this term is likely unknown even to otherwise proficient speakers of English.

- *Connotative differences.* The term *connotation* refers to the emotional content of concepts, which is also reflected in a person's schematic associations. For example, some speakers may associate *dog* with feelings and terms such as *scary* or *repulsive*; others, with *cute* or *best friend.* There can be wide individual variability in connotations obviously, but some are culturally more or less stable. For example, *freedom* ranks high in positively appraised American values; while in more communal cultures, *family* or *harmony* occupy similar spaces. The number *four* is associated with death in East Asian cultures similarly to the unlucky properties American culture ascribes to the number *thirteen.* On a daily basis, the clinician will not have to navigate these subtle differences; they do come into play, typically, in moments of misunderstanding or unintentional (unexpected) offense. Like in any other situation of misunderstanding, culturally humble clinicians are called to investigate the client's reading of the situation, rather than dismissing it.
- *False friends.* This type of I/T happens especially between related languages that share cognates (i.e., words that are related to each other). In many cases, cognates facilitate learning (e.g., when a speaker of German uses their knowledge of *Haus,* or house, to acquire the English equivalent, or a Spanish speaker does the same for *carro,* or car). Cognate words do not always map neatly onto each other, however. In many instances, words of recognizably similar form differ in their semantic content. For example, German *Bank* can mean "bank" but also "bench"; Spanish *éxito* does not refer to an "exit" but to "success"; and French *blessé* means "hurt," not "blessed." Learners may use these "false friends" unawares of their actual meaning in English; this is indicative of efficient learning strategies, not of a learning problem (unless the learner is unable to acquire the difference).
- *Semantic confusion.* Conceptual meanings in every language are not distinct with clear-cut boundaries, but flow into each other and overlap. Thus, it is easy for learners to make nonconventional connections between a form and a meaning, particularly when there is a parallel form-meaning connection in their first language. As an example, speakers of Tamil may use the term *hand* to mean both "hand" and "arm," since the Tamil equivalent *kai* refers to both (Anuradha Chandrasekaran, personal communication).[5] Again, this is an indication of good associative skills needed for language learning, not of a problem unless there is reason to believe otherwise.

- *Syntax.* English sentence structure is deceptively straightforward at its simplest, uniformly requiring a subject and verb at minimum. The verb can be complemented by an adjunct and/or an object; the resulting word order is invariably SVA or SVO (subject-verb-adjunct/object). Yet even at this level, learners can run into difficulty because their first-language system differs from the English one. Default word orders are not uniform across languages, as seen previously; determiners, copulas and auxiliaries do not exist in every idiom and adjuncts can be challenging because they typically involve prepositions. English has an elaborate system of prepositions that do not always map on seemingly equivalent function words in other languages; in addition, many languages do not use prepositions in the first place but mark relationships through word order alone or with bound morphemes (discussed later). All of those obstacles become more salient the more complex the language involved: elaborate English sentences, especially written ones, are characterized by intricate rules around positioning of words, phrases, and clauses that are not easy to learn for non-native speakers. With this in mind, clinicians may find the following types of I/T at the syntax level:

---

[5]Depending on the level of subtlety in the concepts involved, native speakers of a language may run into similar issues. In the first author's experience, for example, many native speakers of English have trouble distinguishing the verbs to effect and to affect.

- *Word order errors.* As seen previously, languages differ in their default sentence order, with SOV and VSO being the most frequent alternatives to the SVO order to which English speakers are used. Particularly beginning learners may therefore produce English utterances that abide by their native syntax, such as *Daddy fire make* (SOV) or *Make Daddy fire* (VSO). Word order may also be altered within phrases; for example, beginning learners whose first language is Spanish may reverse adjective and noun according to their native system, resulting in *I see a truck big!* (Note that all these examples also feature other aspects of I/T, such as omission of morphological tense markers and of determiners.)
- *Non-use of copulas or auxiliaries.* As many languages do not feature these particular sentence parts, learners of English are likely to transfer their native patterns and leave out copulas and auxiliaries from their utterances. An additional difficulty is that these function words are frequently contracted in spoken English (e.g., *is* → *'s, have* → *'ve, or would* → *'d),* which turns them, effectively, into the equivalent of bound morphemes, both phonologically and semantically, and makes them easy to miss. (More details on this will be given in the morphology section.)
- *Non-use of determiners.* The English determiner system is simple enough to be acquired quickly by most learners. Its only elements, strictly speaking, are *a* and *the*, denoting newly introduced versus known referents, respectively. (In formal varieties, the indeterminate member of the pair is produced with a phonetic alteration if it precedes a vowel, as in *an apple*; however, this is not a uniform rule for informal registers.) That said, many languages do not use determiners, and speakers of those idioms may therefore omit them when beginning to learn English or deploy them inconsistently. Resulting constructions may take forms like *boy eating, the man going store,* or *car is in garage.* (In these examples, other elements such as copula, auxiliary, or preposition are also partially omitted; all of these omissions may occur jointly or independently.)
- *Substitution or non-use of prepositions.* English has an intricate inventory of prepositions to express subtle relational distinctions, many of which are somewhat idiosyncratic and do not easily translate into other languages that either have no prepositions, or their own idiosyncratic inventory. First-language speakers of an idiom that uses word order or affixes instead of prepositions may simply omit this part of speech, leading to utterances like *He go doctor* (He is going to the doctor). (In this example, copula, present progressive suffix, and determiner are also omitted; all of these omissions may occur jointly or independently.) Speakers of such languages may also use English prepositions erroneously; the same is true, of course, for individuals whose first language's inventory differs from English. As an example, this chapter's first author has been known to say *on the party* to mean "at the party," since the German equivalent *auf der Party* uses a preposition that translates into English as "on."
- *Nonconventional sentence formulation.* It is not only word order that differs between languages, but also arrangements of sentence elements (or their equivalents). Particularly in more complex utterances, learners of English may produce sentence elements that appear out of order to native speakers. As an example, consider this mini-narrative (describing a common experience for immigrant children): *When my brother was young, he spoke to the doctor for our mother.* A Chinese speaker may render this, according to the syntactic rules of Mandarin, as *My brother, he young, for mama he speak to doctor.* (Note that this example also features other aspects of Mandarin-English I/T, such as omission of the temporal conjunction *when*, of the copula, tense, as well as person markers; all of these may occur jointly or independently.)

- *Morphology.* As mentioned, English has a morphological system that is less complex than many other languages, but still complex enough to pose a challenge to learners whose L1 does not feature any bound morphemes at all. Learners from any language background (i.e., with or without affixes in their native inventory) may find it challenging to acquire a new system, of course, particularly since bound morphemes are, by definition, never encountered in isolation but have to be processed jointly with the lexeme base to which they are affixed. Phonological characteristics and systemic idiosyncrasies also pose obstacles. Bound morphemes typically occur at the end of words, which frequently results in a consonant cluster; thus, they are less phonologically salient than other sounds in a word, particularly as part of a cluster. With regard to idiosyncrasies, consider that the English suffix system looks deceptively simple (just add *-s* or *-ed* to a word base) but has, in fact, a variety of irregular past tense and plural forms (and of modal verbs that do not take a third-person singular -s, [e.g., *must, can,* or *would*]). With all this in mind, here are some common morphological differences exhibited by learners of English.
  - *Non-use of third-person singular -s.* English verb conjugation is fairly simple, with only one suffix (*-s*) used in the present tense (e.g., *she speaks, he swims*) while all other forms are equal to the word base. However, learners are more likely to encounter verbs in their present progressive form (e.g., *she is speaking, he is swimming*); also, -s is not very salient acoustically, hence it is easily missed in conversation. Thus, learners of English are likely to produce third-person singular verbs without the present tense *-s*, as in *he speak*. The same is true for many dialects of English, where unmarked third-person singular is often the rule.
  - *Non-use or overgeneralization of the past tense -ed.* In contrast to the comparably infrequent third-person singular *-s*, past tense *-ed* is the most commonly encountered past tense form, which would make it more learnable were it not for its similarly low acoustic salience. It either occurs in word-final consonant clusters (e.g., in *baked*) or voiced after a vowel (e.g., in *played*); both occurrences lack acoustic prominence and are easily missed. Also, we mentioned many languages do not have word-final consonant clusters, or even word-final consonants, thus both perception and production are fraught. (The same is true, of course, for most suffixes in varying degrees). As a result, learners may omit it or apply it erroneously to irregular verbs once acquired, much like children during development.
  - *Non-use or overgeneralization of plural -s.* Much like past tense *-ed*, and for the same reasons, plural *-s* may be missing in learners of English or be used on irregular plural nouns. Conversely, it may also be applied to mass nouns that do not take a plural form (e.g., when a speaker consistently says *stuffs* instead of *stuff*). This is an example of the intersection of semantics and morphology: since *stuff* typically refers to more than one object in the real world, the term may be conceptually plural to the speaker, who may then use the plural suffix on it.
- *Phonology.* English has a comparably rich sound system, making for three distinct difficulties for learners. One, it features several subtle vowel distinctions that are not found in most languages of the world, as well as two diphthongs for which the same is true. Two, it has a few consonants that are both rare and hard to produce, and its consonants occur at any position in syllables and words, which is not universal across languages. Three, English sports a variety of consonant clusters both the beginnings and at the ends of words and syllables, which poses another obstacle for speakers of other first languages. Here are some of the most common sound-level differences clinicians are likely to encounter.
  - *Vowel differences.* The sound systems of most languages include the *cardinal vowels* (the sounds represented, roughly, by "ah", "eh", "ee", "oh", and "oo"). Beyond that, inventories differ widely, and not many systems contain the same distinctions English does. For this reason, you may find the following productions in many learners of English:
    - Collapse of the vowels in *bed* and *bat* (both produced the same way, or inconsistently exchanged for each other)

- Collapse of the vowels in *beat* and *bit* (both produced the same way, or inconsistently exchanged for each other)
- Substitution of the vowel in *bus*, or the first vowel in *about*, with *"ah"*
- *"oo"* pronounced with the tongue all the way back towards the throat, in contrast to the more fronted version that is standard in many areas around the United States
- Diphthongs in *hose* and *hay* produced as single vowels *"oh"* and *"eh"*, respectively

In addition, clinicians need to be aware that many learners of English have acquired a British-based variety, and hence use the corresponding vowel qualities; speakers from India or Nigeria, for example, are likely to produce *fast* as *"fahst,"* or *got* as *"goht."*

- *Consonant differences.* The plosive and nasals of English are fairly widespread across languages and do not pose substantial problems to learners. The same is not true for some of its fricatives, affricates, and approximants, which are less widespread, as is the variety of consonant clusters it features. The following are some typical patterns of substitution you may encounter in learners of English:
  - The sounds spelled *"th"* → *"t, d"* or *"s, z"*
  - The sounds spelled *"f, v"* → *"p, b"*
  - The sound spelled *"j"* → *"ch"*
  - The sound spelled *"w"* → *"v"* (these may also be inconsistently interchanged, which may be a form of hypercorrection)
  - The English *"r"* sound →a tongue tap or tongue trill
- In addition, speakers may lack final consonants if their first language does not have this feature. For the same reason, they may simplify consonant clusters or insert a schwa-like vowel between the individual sounds of a cluster. This may hold even at word or syllable boundaries.

This concludes the discussion of interference and transfer. It will be closed with two final remarks. One, the authors wish to point out, once again, that I/T—speech and language differences—do not only occur in speakers whose first language is not English, but also in speakers whose first language is a *variety* of English other than the standard variety (SAE). In a context where speakers' communicative and linguistic functioning are assessed by comparing them to an SAE-based norm—which, it may be assumed, is implicitly or explicitly the case in most North American contexts—any variation from said norm is notable, whether it stems from a non-English system or from a dialect of English.

Two, recall that the differences listed here are not only *not* present in every speaker from a given linguistic background, but may also be inconsistently present in one and the same speaker. The reason for this is the cognitive effort it takes to produce structures or behaviors that are not present in one's first language or variety, and hence have not been entrenched in the person's system at a subintentional level. If the system is taxed by other processing demands, less effort can be put into the conscious production of non-native target structures, and native structures may take over, manifesting as differences in the speaker's English. Thus, individuals may or may not produce certain differences depending on whether they are distracted or focused, tense or relaxed, fatigued or alert, confident or insecure, emotional or serene, and so forth.

Sources of Linguistic Information

Clinicians who work with diverse populations may run into languages they are unfamiliar with at a moment's notice. Therefore, knowing where to find information about the properties of any given idiom is part of speech-language therapists' clinical competence. Unfortunately, it is also a rather exacting task. Linguistic information at the level of rules of form, content and use is not easily to come by. Parents, family, and community informants are typically adept at conveying whether a child is developing typically or whether an elder speaker's behavior has changed; they are less likely to be able to provide contrastive information about the syntax or the phonology of their first language. Where available, trained interpreters may be able to provide such information, but their training does not always include linguistics at this level of granularity. Thus, all too often the practicing clinician will find themselves scrambling for this information using whatever resources they have at hand.

A natural first step is to search the website of the American Speech-Language-Hearing Association (ASHA; 2022) for pertinent insights. Yet while ASHA's linguistic database is constantly expanding, it is still far from a comprehensive overview of the languages of the world. Take two important idioms mentioned in this chapter, Fula and Tamil, spoken in West-Central Africa and South India by around 40 million and 80 million people, respectively. A search of ASHA's website, conducted on May 16, 2022, yielded no results for *Fula* (or for the alternative forms of the name, *Fulah, Fulani, Fulfulde, Pular,* and *Pulaar*). A search for *Tamil* resulted in over 100 entries; however, these represented either brief mentions of the language or ASHA members who speak it.

What clinicians need for assessment and treatment is a concise yet comprehensive overview of the language system in question, ideally complemented by descriptions of nonverbal and extralinguistic conventions. Such descriptions do exist in book form (e.g., Kester, 2014; see also the summaries and boxes in the individual chapters of Battle, 2012), but obviously cannot cover all languages a clinician might encounter. They may also be found in academic journals, but practicing therapists do not typically have access to these. Thus, until ASHA issues a validated database for clinicians to utilize, clinicians are largely on their own in finding pertinent information.

There are several online sources that would seem useful for clinicians. One is the Ethnologue (Eberhard et al., 2022), the standard catalog of the world's languages. It requires subscription, however, and does not provide details about linguistic systems. Another is the Glottolog (Hammarström et al., 2021), which is freely accessible. While it does not provide structural information, it does include links to third-party sources. For sound-level only inquiries, PHOIBLE 2.0 (Moran & McCloy, 2019) offers a database of phonemic inventories. All of these have in common that they are meant for academic purposes, and require an amount of practice to become familiar with them.

The source the authors have found most widely useful is Wikipedia (Wikimedia Foundation, 2022). Most languages with a sizable number of speakers are featured in at least one dedicated entry, in which all aspects of form (syntax, morphology, phonology) are typically discussed (although information about pragmatics, semantics, or extralinguistic aspects is rare). Several entries may be found for more widely spoken languages, each dedicated to one particular aspect. Linguistic descriptions are concise yet detailed enough to provide clinicians with good insights into the respective structures.

The authors are aware that professionals and academics do not recommend using Wikipedia for clinical or scholarly purposes. They do, however, believe it is well-suited for the task in question here. The reticence toward Wikipedia stems from its nontraditional approach to knowledge dissemination. As is well-known, Wikipedia is an open-source encyclopedia to which anyone can contribute. In theory, this could lead to a poorly managed repository of inaccurate or biased entries. In practice, however, it results in a rapid editing process with quick remediation time for factual errors or biased content, leading to a level of reliability on par with academic standards (Mesgari et al., 2015; Michelucci & Dickinson, 2016). In particular with regard to language-related entries, the authors have consistently found them to be accurate, reliable, and concise enough to make for easy use by speech-language therapists.

Consider the entry for Fula (Wikipedia contributors, 2022a). A clinician who needs information about this idiom will find information about all aspects of its form there. To illustrate how this can be used for assessment, consider Table 3-2, where the information provided by the article and the conclusions for possible patterns of I/T the clinician can draw from it are summarized.

Table 3-2

Form Features of Fula and Clinical Inferences About Resulting Interference/Transfer

FEATURES OF FULA	POSSIBLE INTERFERENCE/TRANSFER
Rich morphology; suffixes serve grammatical purposes that prepositions do in English	Client may confuse English morphemes with each other; client may confuse or omit English prepositions
Rich system of noun classification via suffixes	Client may "gender" referents (using he or she) that would be neutral (it) in Standard English; client's conceptual categories for referents may differ from those of English
Plural marked by initial consonant mutation (e.g., /w/ ↔ /b/ ↔ /mb/ or /f/ ↔ /p/)	Client may produce mutations of word-initial English consonants along number lines (singular versus plural)
Does not distinguish grammatical gender → only one pronoun	Client may confuse he and she
Consonant system does not include /v/, /th/, /z/, /sh/, or English /r/	Client may substitute these with the closest sounds Fula does include, i.e. /w/, /t/, /d/, /s/, /ch/, /dj/, and a trilled /r/
Vowel system includes only /ah/, /eh/, /ee/, /oh/, /oo/	Client may substitute English vowels and diphthongs with the closest sound in their native system

The entry on Fula does not contain any information about pragmatic or nonverbal aspects of communication. In practice, this information can be obtained through clinical observation of the client's social environment, and through cultural informants. Of note, Wikipedia does offer some audiovisual material in its language entries; while none was found under *Fula*, it is provided in the entry on *Pular* (Wikipedia contributors, 2022b), a dialect of Fula. Videos of two speakers provide ample insight into typical pragmatic, prosodic and nonverbal behaviors, showing a prevalence of emphatic gesturing while speaking, a conventional greeting, and an amount of translanguaging between Pular and West African French. All of this information can be valuable for the practicing clinician assessing a client with a Fula background.

Conclusion

This chapter began with three philosophical and anthropological questions about language that, the authors hope, helped frame its discussion of linguistic diversity for the practicing clinician. And as promised, it is now time to return to them in order to provide a humanistic view that lends some coherence to the sheer diversity of cultural and structural differences the reader has encountered. Question 1 was answered in the introduction; questions 2 and 3 can be summarized as follows: Is there a common logic underlying the world's different language systems? And how and why did language evolve? The authors hope that the following answers to these give the clinician some guidance through the vast variety of linguistic productions they may encounter.

Question 2 has been answered decisively. While the cognitive skills of all humans are the same—that is, any human can, in theory, fully acquire any language if exposed to it early enough in life—the grammatical diversity of human languages cannot be collapsed into some shared underlying logic (Dabrowską, 2015). The takeaway for clinicians is that the syntax and morphology of clients' first languages cannot simply be mapped onto English. For example, teaching the copula to someone whose first language does not use this part of speech involves introducing the speaker to a syntactic structure that is entirely new to them. The therapist cannot rely on notions such as "deep structure," presuming that at some subconscious level the client's linguistic system does involve copulas because they are "logical" or "necessary." To the client, saying *Paul a doctor* to mean "Paul is a doctor" is entirely logical and natural.

That said, while there is no shared structure underlying the world's languages, there *is* a shared human need: the need for connection facilitated by communication. And this moves the discussion to question 3. While the "how" and "why" of language evolution may never be determined with absolute certainty, the more plausible of theorized scenarios place the need for socializing and for joint thinking at the heart of the dynamic. Language, the reasoning goes, may have evolved from primate vocalizations as a means of maintaining social bonds as hominid groups became larger and more complex (Barham & Everett, 2021; Trudgill, 2020). A second pathway may have been the increasing need for collaboration in early human species. Childrearing and adaptation to new environments required the development of shared or joint intentions, which in turn facilitated the use of abstract symbols such as nondeictic gestures or sound sequences (Tomasello, 2008). Taken together, this would suggest that the underlying communality of languages that linguists have been looking for is actually found at a level deeper than language: that of interacting, sharing, collaborating, and forming bonds.

For clinicians working across cultural, communicative, and linguistic barriers, the takeaway is that beneath the many outward differences in how humans interact and communicate there is a shared need for communication and collaboration. Barring issues of trauma, mistrust, or mental illness, people from any cultural context can thus be expected to react positively to someone who shows genuine interest in them, no matter how awkward or inadequate their interlocutor may feel while trying to communicate. This avenue—that of creating a genuine human bond in order to reach shared goals—is thus always available to clinicians working with cultural and linguistic diversity.

References

Ambady, N., & Rosenthal, R. (1992). Thin slices of expressive behavior as predictors of interpersonal consequences: A meta-analysis. *Psychological Bulletin, 111*(2), 256-274.

American Speech-Language-Hearing Association. (2022). https://www.asha.org

Barham, L., & Everett, D. (2021). Semiotics and the origin of language in the Lower Palaeolithic. *Journal of Archaeological Method and Theory, 28*, 535-579.

Basso, K. H. (1970). "To give up on words": Silence in Western Apache culture. *Southwestern Journal of Anthropology, 26*(3), 213-230.

Battle, D. E. (2012). *Communication disorders in multicultural and international populations* (4th ed.). Elsevier.

Bierly, R. (2019). *Spanglish: The validity of Spanglish as a language.* https://www.panoramas.pitt.edu/opinion-and-interviews/spanglish-validity-spanglish-language

Boutsen, F. (2003). *Prosody: The music of language and speech. The ASHA Leader, 8*(4). https://leader.pubs.asha.org/doi/10.1044/leader.ftr1.08042003.6

Crystal, D. (1995). *The Cambridge encyclopedia of the English language.* Cambridge University Press.

Dabrowską, E. (2015). What exactly is Universal Grammar, and has anyone seen it? *Frontiers in Psychology, 6*, 852.

Dalhousie Accent Clinic. (n. d.). *Frequently asked questions.* https://www.dal.ca/faculty/health/scsd/accent-clinic/frequently-asked-questions.html

Dediu, D., & Levinson, S. C. (2013). On the antiquity of language: The reinterpretation of Neandertal linguistic capacities and its consequences. *Frontiers in Psychology, 4,* 397.

Eberhard, D. M., Simons, G. F., & Fennig, C. D. (2022). *Ethnologue: Languages of the world* (25th ed.). SIL International. http://www.ethnologue.com

Elliott, C., Adams, R. J., & Sockalingam, S. (2016). *Communication patterns and assumptions of differing cultural groups in the United States.* https://www.awesomelibrary.org/multiculturaltoolkit-patterns.html

Everett, D. L. (2017). *How language began: The story of humanity's greatest invention.* Profile Books.

García, O., & Wei, L. (2014). *Translanguaging: Language, bilingualism and education.* Palgrave Macmillan.

Genemo, T. B. (2021). Multilingualism and language choice in domains. In X. Jiang (Ed.), *Multilingualism.* https://www.intechopen.com/chapters/79781

Giles, H., Coupland, J., & Coupland, N. (1991). *Contexts of accommodation: Developments in applied sociolinguistics.* Cambridge University Press.

Grosjean, F. (2011) An attempt to isolate, and then differentiate, transfer and interference. *International Journal of Bilingualism, 16*(1), 11-21.

Hall, E. T. (1959). *The silent language.* Anchor Books.

Hall, E. T. (1969). *The hidden dimension.* Anchor Books.

Hammarström, H., Forkel, R., Haspelmath, M., & Bank, S. (2021). *Glottolog 4.5.* Max Planck Institute for Evolutionary Anthropology. http://glottolog.org

Hardach, S. (2020). Do babies cry in different languages? *The New York Times.* https://www.nytimes.com/2020/04/15/parenting/baby/wermke-prespeech-development-wurzburg.html

Hernandez, A., Li, P., & MacWhinney, B. (2005). The emergence of competing modules in bilingualism. *TRENDS in Cognitive Sciences, 9*(5), 220-225.

Kendon, A. (1997). Gesture. *Annual Review of Anthropology, 26,* 109-128.

Kendon, A. (2007). Some topics in gesture studies. In A. Esposito, M. Bratanić, E. Keller, & M. Mariano (Eds.), *Fundamentals of verbal and nonverbal communication and the biometric issue. NATO Security through Science Series E: Human and Societal Dynamics* (Vol. 18, pp. 3-19). IOS Press.

Kester, E. S. (2014). *Difference or disorder: Understanding speech and language patterns in culturally and linguistically diverse students.* Bilinguistics.

Kochman, T. (1981). *Black and White styles in conflict: The hegemony of culture.* University of Chicago Press.

Kroll, T. A., & Townsend, C. (2022). The sociopsychological cost of AAE-to-SAE codeswitching: A symbolic interactionist account. *Journal of Interactional Research in Communication Disorders, 13*(1), 120-144.

Leitung der Abteilung Phonetik der Goethe-Universität. (2018). [*Interface to the UPSID database.*] http://www.phonetik.uni-frankfurt.de/upsid_nr_seg.html

McCabe, A. (1997). Cultural background and storytelling: A review and implications for schooling. *Elementary School Journal, 97*(5), 453-473.

Mesgari, M., Okoli, C., Mehdi, M., Nielsen, F. Å., & Lanamäki, A. (2015). "The sum of all human knowledge": A systematic review of scholarly research on the content of Wikipedia. *Journal of the Association for Information Science and Technology, 66*(2), 219-245.

Michelucci, P., & Dickinson, J. L. (2016). The power of crowds. *Science, 351*(6268), 32-33.

Moran, S., & McCloy, D. (2019). *PHOIBLE 2.0.* Max Planck Institute for the Science of Human History. http://phoible.org

Public Broadcasting System. (2005). *Do you speak American? Part 3* [Video]. https://www.youtube.com/watch?v=6PR34EJOZFs

Romaine, S. (2013). Keeping the promise of the Millennium Development Goals: Why language matters. *Applied Linguistics Review, 4*(1), 1-21.

Sacks, H., Schegloff, E. A., & Jefferson, G. (1974). A simplest systematics for the organization of turn-taking for conversation. *Linguistic Society of America, 50*(4), 696-735.

Tomasello, M. (2008). *Origins of human communication (Jean Nicod Lectures).* Massachusetts Institute of Technology.

Trudgill, P. (2020). *Millennia of language change: Sociolinguistic studies in deep historical linguistics.* Cambridge University Press.

Wikimedia Foundation. (2022). *Wikipedia: The free encyclopedia.* https://en.wikipedia.org/wiki/Main_Page

Wikipedia contributor Alumnum (2019). *Primary human language families map.* https://en.wikipedia.org/wiki/Language_family#/media/File:Primary_Human_Languages_Improved_Version.png

Wikipedia contributors (2022a, May 16). *Fula language.* https://en.wikipedia.org/wiki/Fula_language

Wikipedia contributors (2022b, March 22). *Pular language.* https://en.wikipedia.org/wiki/Pular_language

Part II

METHODS OF ASSESSMENT

Chapter 4

Conducting Dynamic Assessments in Culturally and Linguistically Diverse Individuals

Samantha Washington, EdD, CCC-SLP
and Giselle Núñez, PhD, CCC-SLP

Introduction

Individuals from culturally and linguistically diverse backgrounds can be misdiagnosed as having a language disorder based on their home and school language experiences, as their language experiences can impact their performance on standardized measures (Kapantzoglou et al., 2012, Peña et al., 2001). According to American Speech-Language-Hearing Association (1993), language disorders are defined as a disorder of spoken and written language skills which may impact an individual's vocabulary, grammar, sentence structure, pragmatic, and phonological skills. Researchers have expanded on this definition to indicate other characteristics for language impairment. These characteristics include the impairment is not associated with intellectual disabilities or other conditions (Rombouts et al., 2020), the cause is unknown (St. Clair et al., 2019), and the individual has typical sensory and motor capacity (Rudolph & Leonard, 2016).

Differentiating a language disorder from a language difference is imperative to educators, as the population of culturally and linguistically diverse students continues to rise in the United States. A language difference occurs when an individual's first language has some linguistic influence on their second language. According to Kohnert et al. (2021), an individual's cultural experiences also impacts all of their communicative interactions. Differences in communicative interactions can manifest in using or in understanding the second language. In other words, the speaker's language skills will

Bortz, M. (Ed.). *A Guide to Global Language Assessment: A Lifespan Approach* (pp. 69-90).
DOI: 10.4324/9781003524472-6

match that of their primary speaking community, but will differ from their second language (Prasad, 2015). Many culturally and linguistically diverse students are exposed to more than one language, and some with limited English skills before starting their academic journey.

Furthermore, there are a number of limitations that static assessments demonstrate. Hasson and Joffe (2007) reported that educational psychologists in the United Kingdom and speech-language therapists in the United States have found dynamic assessment more useful than static assessment measures. Static assessments are limited in being able to capture a client's multidimensional nature of language or provide information about how children approach a task (Hasson & Joffe, 2007). Static assessments are also based on a client's abilities from one moment in time. To fully understand a client's language skills, clinicians must be able to capture the various areas of language and understand the client's ability to grasp the concept or skill being assessed.

Currently, there is a global need for unbiased assessment options for culturally and linguistically diverse students that can differentiate language differences from language disorders. Research does not support assessing culturally and linguistically diverse students with standardized measures that are normed on monolingual students or exhibit a small representation of culturally and linguistically diverse individuals (Hasson et al., 2012; Kapantzoglou et al., 2012). Cultural biases in assessing students' language skills require careful consideration, as the administration of assessments normed on a dominant cultural group is not appropriate when used on a nonmainstream group. These biases may underestimate the student's language abilities (Kramer et al., 2009) or reveal cultural and linguistic differences. In addition, many speech-language pathologists in the United States are often trained during their studies to use Brown's (1973) morphemes to analyze the child's ability to mark morphological markers. However, Brown's stages of morpheme development are based on the acquisition of Standard American English. The stages do not consider obligatory versus nonobligatory morphological markers, which are used in children who use dialects outside of Standard American English or who are bilingual (e.g., Baron et al., 2018).

Based on the difficulties in accurately identifying students with language disorders there is both an underrepresentation and overrepresentation of culturally and linguistically diverse students in special education programs (Hasson et al., 2012; Kapantzoglou et al., 2012; Ukrainetz et al., 2000). Underrepresentation of culturally and linguistically diverse students in special education may result from educators attributing second language learning difficulties to the deficits they witness in language and literacy skills (Hasson et al., 2012; Kapantzoglou et al., 2012). Additionally, culturally and linguistically diverse students may also demonstrate difficulties with their language skills which may be underestimated as a language difference (Camilleri & Law, 2007). Conversely, culturally and linguistically diverse students may be overrepresented in special education programs in their later educational years if they present with decreased academic skills (Kapantzoglou et al., 2012).

To reduce cultural and linguistic assessment bias, the use of dynamic assessment has been suggested as an appropriate assessment tool to assess the language skills of culturally and linguistically diverse clients (Hasson et al., 2012). Dynamic assessment is a process in where the individual is assessed on a general domain, for example, a discourse analysis, instead of a specific skill, such as receptive vocabulary skills (Camilleri et al., 2014) and is evaluated on how they learn instead of how much they know while being provided with interventions and support within a short time (Gilliam & Peña, 2004; Kapantzoglou et al., 2012). During a dynamic assessment, the examiner and student interact extensively in structured clinical tasks (Peña et al., 2006, 2007). According to Grigorenko (2009), dynamic assessment is similar to a shortened response-to-intervention program. Additionally, Gustafson et al. (2014) agreed that the use of dynamic assessment in Sweden has shortened the response to intervention window and has allowed clinicians to meet the needs of learners through a systematic and dynamic approach.

Throughout the dynamic assessment process, clinicians analyze an individual's fast mapping skills and engage the learner in mediated learning through a fluid process within a short time. Fast mapping skills consist of one's ability to grasp and demonstrate an understanding of a new concept within a fairly short amount of time. This time frame will vary for each person, but generally clients will gain the skill given only a few examples and explicit instruction within a therapy session. On the other hand, mediated learning encourages the client to think and make inferences as the clinician uses strategic questioning. Mediated learning will be discussed further in later sections.

Theories Supporting Use of Dynamic Assessment

Dynamic assessments have been influenced by Vygotsky's theory of cognitive development and Feuerstein's mediated learning experience (e.g., Gutierrez-Clellen & Peña, 2001; Kramer et al., 2009).

Based on Vygotsky's theory, the student will learn and develop skills by socially interacting with others in their environment that are proficient in the student's language and culture (1978). Vygotsky (1978) presented the zone of proximal development as the level of performance a student can complete a task independently or with adult support and a comparison can be made on the student's pre- and post-teaching performance, as a competent learner would complete a task better after instruction. For example, an educator can present a child with an assessment that looks at the child's ability to use grammatical markers when speaking. If the child does poorly on this assessment, the educator would be able to determine what skills need to be addressed. A plan can then be created to address the errors that the child made, and teaching of these skills would occur. Based on this theory, if the child does well on a retake of the assessment, then a conclusion can be made that the child had not been taught that skill, but with the right support from an adult, the child learned the skill. If the child continues to demonstrate areas of need following the retake of the assessment, then it can be assumed that the child required more intensive and direct intervention from an adult to learn the skill.

Feuerstein's theory of mediated learning experience is focused on academic-based learning and carefully examines the student's learning characteristics, or the child's response to the adult instruction (Feuerstein et al., 1981). During this process, the focus is on the individual's response during tasks that the student cannot complete (Camilleri et al., 2014). Additionally, dynamic assessment provides information on the student's error patterns, their ability to self-correct, and their *modifiability* skills (Ukrainetz et al., 2000). Modifiability is defined as the strategies the students use when learning new skills, the amount and types of prompts (e.g., scaffolding) the students require in response to the interventions provided, and an analysis of the types of gains the students made during the interventions (e.g., Kapantzoglou et al., 2012; Peña et al., 2007; Ukrainetz et al., 2000). The benefit of this theory is that an educator can focus on how the child learns and applies learning tools with the goal of becoming an independent learner. For example, if a child has difficulty with story retelling, the adult can administer a pre-test to determine what the areas of need are. If the areas of need are in the ability to sequence a story, instead of comparing the pre-and post-test scores, the educator can focus on the amount of cues and support the child needed to complete the task, and other areas, such as the child's motivation or their ability to think about the task. The educator is then able to make a comparison about the child's learning skills. Case Study One, at the end of this chapter, provides an example of mediated learning.

The benefits of learning how to use dynamic assessments ensure that a child is being assessed holistically and there is thinking through the child's language strengths and abilities. This can be completed in collaboration with classroom teachers and the academic curriculum. This in turn can determine if the child actually presents with language learning difficulties or lack of exposure to a new task. The speech-language pathologist can then develop appropriate goals without the use of static or biased standardized assessments that compare them to their peers. In using this framework, speech-language pathologists can benefit from making informed decisions and ensuring that they are thinking of the child's cultural background and thinking of the child's own abilities.

Types of Dynamic Assessment

There are several types of dynamic assessment. However, the two most common types used in communication sciences and disorders are test-teach-retest and a graduated prompting format (Austin, 2010). These two types of dynamic assessments, as well as testing the limits, will be described in this chapter. When deciding to conduct a dynamic assessment, clinicians must first identify the specific and appropriate skill or task needing to be targeted. The skills can vary across several areas of language, such as vocabulary knowledge, grammar, phonological awareness, and narrative language skills. When deciding which skill to target through dynamic assessment, the clinician should be mindful of and consider developmentally appropriate skills for the client's age and increase their communication skills across settings.

Dynamic assessment is a means of assessing one's language abilities not only in the United States but in other countries as well. Dynamic assessment has been used as an assessment tool in South Africa due to their school-aged learners demonstrating educational handicaps secondary to historical segregationist policies (Skuy et al., 2002). Murphy and Maree (2006) conducted an analysis of the effectiveness of dynamic assessment in South Africa. These researchers concluded dynamic assessment had a small to medium effect across studies implicating its use is effective when using the test-teach-retest model. Mirzaei et al. (2017) conducted a study on the effectiveness of group dynamic assessment for a group of junior high school students in southwest Iran. Using the test-teach-retest dynamic assessment model, these researchers also concluded the implementation of dynamic assessment not only improved the participant's immediate post-test scores but also their delayed post-test scores when compared to the control group. Furthermore, Lebeer et al. (2012) expressed the continued use of standardized psychometric testing in Europe contributes to barriers for learning when used in a diagnostic way. Dynamic assessment has been consistently shown to be an effective means and accurate form of assessment for culturally and linguistically diverse persons.

Review of Research

Review of Dynamic Assessments

Six reviewed studies identified how the test-teach-retest dynamic assessment model differentiated stronger language learners from weaker language learners by comparing post-test scores from their pre-test scores. (See Table 4-1 for details on studies.) Dynamic assessments of vocabulary, categorization, and narrative skills were researched. All of the studies reviewed used school-aged students with culturally and linguistically diverse backgrounds.

Dynamic assessment of categorization skills. A study by Ukrainetz et al. (2000) investigated a dynamic assessment task of categorization in Native American kindergarten students. The authors used a categorization task to evaluate the students' ability to group words and examine their vocabulary skills. The students were assigned to a strong or weak language learning group based on classroom observation and teacher reports. Post-test scores on the categorization test were greater for stronger language learners than the weaker language learners.

Table 4-1
Dynamic Assessment: Test-Teach-Retest

AUTHOR	PARTICIPANTS	DESIGN	FOCUS	ASSESSMENT	PROCEDURE	OUTCOME
Camilleri & Law (2007)	• 14 typical language students aged 41 to 48 months • 40 referred students for speech and language services aged 41 to 50 months	Experimental design, two-group comparison using test-teach-retest design	Will a dynamic assessment of receptive vocabulary skills provide more information than standardized measure alone?	Standardized vocabulary testing and nonverbal cognitive testing	• Single session lasting 45 minutes • Used both dynamic and standardized measures • Intervention phrase carried out as game	Dynamic assessment provided more information than standardized measures Post-test scores were greater for stronger learners than weaker learner
Kapantzoglou et al. (2012)	• 4- to 5-year-old low SES Spanish-speaking students from Southwest • 15 typical developing students • 13 students with possible language impairment	Experimental design with two groups using a pre-test, teach, post-test design	Can dynamic assessment evaluating word learning skills identify bilingual students with a language impairment?	30- to 40-minute tasks, parent report, language sample, vocabulary test, story retelling task, modifiability checklist	• Dynamic assessment task presented in Spanish • Three sessions, sessions 1 day apart • Target words taught using scripted play	Students with typical language skills had better skills in phonological and semantic skills than students with a language impairment

(continued)

Table 4-1 (continued)
Dynamic Assessment: Test-Teach-Retest

AUTHOR	PARTICIPANTS	DESIGN	FOCUS	ASSESSMENT	PROCEDURE	OUTCOME
Kramer et al. (2009)	• Third-grade bilingual First Nations students from Canada • 12 students with normal language abilities • 5 students with possible language disorders	Experimental design with two groups with pre- and post-test score comparisons, grouped into typical language learning and possible language learning disorder	Would dynamic assessment of narrative identify students with language disorder from typical developing children?	Dynamic assessment used narration with wordless picture book, Dynamic assessment and intervention (DAI) record form	• Child seen individually • Student audio recorded • Test phase child's narrative scored using DAI • Teach phase: two mediation sessions 3 days after test phase • Retest phase: 10 days after test session using narrative and scored using DAI	Typical children demonstrated growth compared to children with possible delays DAI accurately classified children Post-test scores were greater for stronger learners than weaker learners
Peña et al. (2001)	• 79 bilingual children ages 3 to 5 from Northeastern city	Experimental design using test-teach-retest design with two comparison groups	Assessed students using a dynamic assessment of a word-learning task to determine validity of measure in differentiating a disorder from difference	Used *Expressive One Word Picture Vocabulary Test Preschool Language Scale, Stanford Binet Test of Intelligence for Children* (4th ed.)	• 12 weeks: 4-week pre-test with two 30-minute mediation session lasting 4 weeks and post-testing lasting 4 weeks	Typically developing students did better during the dynamic assessment compared to students with low language skills *(continued)*

Table 4-1 (continued)

Dynamic Assessment: Test-Teach-Retest

AUTHOR	PARTICIPANTS	DESIGN	FOCUS	ASSESSMENT	PROCEDURE	OUTCOME
Peña et al. (2014)	• 18 children with language impairment • 18 children with typical language skills	Experimental and quantitative measures	Access accuracy of dynamic assessment of narrative skills in children learning English	DAI testing narrative skills, observation, standardized testing	• DAI completed in kindergarten over three sessions in 7-to-14 day period • Wordless picture books pre-tested in pre-test and post-test story • Two mediated learning experience (MLE) sessions 30 minutes long using scripted interventions	High accuracy using DAI scores and narrative sample
Ukrainetz et al. (2000)	• Bilingual Native American kindergarten students • 15 stronger language learners • 8 weaker language learners	Experimental design using test-teach-retest test	Dynamic assessment examines categorization skills to identify stronger and weaker language learners	Categoriztion subtests from *Assessing Semantic Skills through Everyday Themes* (ASSET)	• 20-minute testing • Assessment lasted 3 weeks • ASSET administered once 1 to 5 days prior mediation session and 1 to 5 days after final mediation session	Test-teach-retest test reliably identified students as stronger or weaker learners Post-test scores were greater for stronger learners than weaker learners

Although the findings in this study demonstrated that using a categorization method of dynamic assessment was positive, the inter-reliability of the study was impacted, as the same rater was used for the classroom observations and to fill out the modifiability rating scales. Of concern in this study was that the authors did not use a group of students diagnosed with a language disorder; therefore, the students selected for either the weaker or stronger language group may have been biased in the way they were selected. Interobserver reliability could not be ruled out, as one graduate student observed two play sessions to determine the students who had communication concerns. The students in this study were selected after being in an academic setting for 6 months. There was no indication if the weaker language learners were receiving interventions or outside therapy in the study. As indicated by the authors, using the standardized measures during the study, the *Assessing Semantic Skills Through Everyday Themes*, was culturally biased as it was not normed on Native American persons. Additionally, the results of this study are unable to be generalized to a greater population and the sample size was small.

Dynamic assessment of vocabulary skills. Word-learning skills of culturally and linguistically diverse students were examined by three studies: Camilleri and Law (2007), Kapantzoglou et al. (2012), and Peña et al. (2001). Kapantzoglou et al. (2012) reported word-learning skills in culturally and linguistically diverse students reduced testing bias during a dynamic assessment model compared to examining the students' current vocabulary skills, as the students' previous experiences and cultures are not heavily considered.

Peña et al. (2001) compared word-learning skills of typical and bilingual preschool students suspected of having language delays. Standardized instruments were selected to examine pre- and post-test differences focusing on single-word vocabulary in the mediated sessions. Findings indicated that typically developing students performed better during the dynamic assessment than students with depressed language skills. Children with typical language skills with low pre-test scores demonstrated improvement on other language tests following mediated sessions compared to the students who had depressed language skills and those in the no-mediation group.

Word-learning skills of students were examined by Camilleri and Law (2007). The authors compared students with typical language monolingual English skills with students that were referred for a possible language disorder. Some of the students referred for possible language disorder were also English learners. Standardized measures were used to compare receptive vocabulary skills and nonverbal cognitive skills. Mediated sessions addressed the students' ability to match a word to a referent. The findings of the studies indicated that monolingual students did not score significantly different from the EL students on dynamic assessment measures of nonverbal scores. However, the students who were English learners did score lower on standardized vocabulary measures. Students with typically developing language skills were differentiated from students that were referred for language difficulties.

Kapantzoglou et al. (2012) examined if a dynamic assessment of word-learning skills that used verbal and visual support would identify bilingual students with a primary language disorder from their typically developing peers. The authors examined students with typical language skills and those with possible language disorders. Word production, identification, and modifiability were examined in predominantly Spanish-speaking students. Students with typical language skills demonstrated better phonological and semantic skills than students with language disorders. Of concern in this study was that 79% of students were correctly classified as with a language disorder, much below the desired classification of 90%.

All three studies determined positive findings in using a test-teach-retest model during word-learning tasks. However, caution with generalization to other populations needs to be considered, given that the participants used were with a specific population (e.g., Headstart) and in a particular part of the United States. None of the students were randomized in any of the studies. In all of the studies, the parental level of education or socioeconomic status was not defined, which may directly impact the child's vocabulary knowledge and skill level.

Dynamic assessments of narrative skills. The narrative language skills of culturally and linguistically diverse students were assessed by Kramer et al. (2009) and Peña et al. (2014). Evaluating the narrative language skills of culturally and linguistically diverse students may assist in differentiating students with a language disorder, as students with a language disorder may demonstrate difficulty with storytelling skills, such as story complexity (Kramer et al., 2009). In addition, assessing the narrative skills of culturally and linguistically diverse students may result in lower levels of testing bias (Peña et al., 2014) as this format allows an alternative venue for assessing students from various cultures (Kramer et al., 2009). Both studies used the dynamic assessment and intervention to assess narrative skills.

Kramer et al. (2009) examined third grade First Nations students. School personnel identified if the students had a possible language delay or were typical language learners, with examiners unaware of the students' language skills. The study found that the test and retest scores were more significant for the students with typical language skills than those with a possible language delay. After the students had received mediation, the students with a potential language disorder had difficulty learning and using new information in their narratives.

Narrative skills were studied by Peña et al. (2014) in kindergarten students learning English as a second language. The participants included students diagnosed with language disorders and those with typical language skills that were matched on various variables, such as age and intelligence quotient. The students selected for this study were English/Spanish speakers and were in the early stages of English language learning. The study results indicated that students who were language impaired scored lower than the students with typical language skills, with all students scoring higher on the post-test.

Although both studies showed positive findings, they both demonstrated that small sample sizes and findings could not be generalized to other populations. Both studies used a specific set of students; for example, Peña et al. (2014) used students that had a year of exposure to English. Based on the studies analyzed, dynamic assessments of narrative skills appear to be the most culturally nonbiased assessment tool for culturally and linguistically diverse students. Although categorization and word finding dynamic assessments also demonstrated promising results, narrative skills have an academic advantage in that the student's grammar, organization, higher-order thinking, and processing skills can be analyzed. Additionally, assessing a student's word learning and categorization skills are very specific aptitudes that may not be relevant or appropriate when diagnosing a language disorder.

Please refer to Chapters 7 and 8 in this book for additional resources on global narrative development.

Measures of Modifiability Characteristics

Nine studies reviewed identified how modifiability can assist in differentiating culturally and linguistically diverse students with typical language skills from culturally and linguistically diverse students with language disorders. An additional five studies examined the accuracy of determining if a culturally and linguistically diverse child had a language impairment by examining modifiability scores and changes in test scores. (See Table 4-2 for study details.) Modifiability is based on the examiner's ratings of the students' responses and the amount of support the students required during the mediated learning experience sessions (Patterson et al., 2013). The checklists used in the studies reviewed employ a Likert scale, where scores are obtained by combining scores from separate checklists (Ukrainetz et al., 2000). The scales measure several abilities, such as the students' ability to attend to tasks and transfer new skills (Gutierrez-Clellen & Peña, 2001). All studies indicated that modifiability ratings were the most substantial factor when determining if a student presented with a language disorder.

Table 4-2
Dynamic Assessment: Modifiability

AUTHOR	PARTICIPANTS	DESIGN	FOCUS	ASSESSMENT	PROCEDURE	OUTCOME
Gutierrez-Clellen & Peña (2001)	• Two bilingual 4-year-old students from Philadelphia	Case study	Case study: Two children had their modifiability profiles evaluated	Modifiability ratings: LSC and Modifiability Scale	• Rating scales used in MLE within and across each session	Modifiability scores are useful to determine difference from disorder
Kapantzoglou et al. (2012)	• 4- to 5-year-old low SES Spanish-speaking students from Southwest • 15 typical developing students • 13 students with possible language impairment	Experimental design with two groups using a pre-test, teach, post-test design	Can dynamic assessment evaluating word-learning skills identify bilingual students with a language impairment?	Modifiability ratings: LSC and the Modifiability Scale	• Scales used at the end of third session • Analyzed scales separately instead of together	Modifiability measurement was the best indicator of a language impairment

(continued)

Table 4-2 (continued)
Dynamic Assessment: Modifiability

AUTHOR	PARTICIPANTS	DESIGN	FOCUS	ASSESSMENT	PROCEDURE	OUTCOME
Kramer et al. (2009)	• Third grade bilingual First Nations students from Canada • 12 students with normal language abilities • 5 students with possible language disorders	Experimental design with two groups with pre- and post-test score comparisons, grouped into typical language learning and possible language learning disorder	Would dynamic assessment of narrative identify students with language disorder from typically developing children?	DAI used to obtain teacher effort and child modifiability during teach component	• Child seen individually with one examiner • Two mediation sessions with first session occurring 3 days after initial test phase • Student rated on scales	Students with possible language impairment required more effort to teach and were less responsive to mediation than student with typical language skills
Patterson et al. (2013)	• 32 bilingual typically developing 4-year-old preschoolers from Southwest	Experimental design that compared students' performance	Measured modifiability of students to determine of students' performance improves during dynamic assessment framework	Parent interview, dynamic assessment tasks completed in single session in Spanish/English: word-learning task, semantic task, and phonological awareness task	• Testing session video recorded • Dynamic assessment tasks presented	Performance improved on dynamic assessment tasks with adult support which indicate that dynamic assessment can provide information on modifiability
Peña et al. (2001)	• 79 bilingual children ages 3 to 5 from Northeastern city	Experimental design using test-teach-retest design with two comparison groups	Assessed students using a dynamic assessment of a word learning task to determine validity of measure in differentiating a disorder from difference	Used LSC and Modifiability Scale during MLE sessions	• MLE sessions presented in 30-minute sessions 1 to 2 weeks apart • Sessions were partially scripted • Scales used to measure modifiability	Highly modifiable students maintained focus, planned, self-regulated and were highly responsive compared to students with limited language abilities

(continued)

Table 4-2 (continued)
Dynamic Assessment: Modifiability

AUTHOR	PARTICIPANTS	DESIGN	FOCUS	ASSESSMENT	PROCEDURE	OUTCOME
Peña et al. (2006)	• 27 students with typical language skills • 14 children with language impairment • Control group of 30 students with no treatment • 1st and 2nd grade students from TX and CA	Experimental design using a test-teach-retest test control group design Mixed within and between participants design	What kind of measures differentiated students with language impairments than typically developing students?	Used DAI to measure examiner effort and child responsivity during MLE session using a 5-point rating scale	• Modifiability scores obtained at end of second MLE session • Sessions video and audiotaped	Modifiability measurement was the best indicator of a language impairment
Peña et al. (2007)	• 1st and 2nd grade students from TX and CA • 25 students with typical language skills • 15 students with language impairment	Experimental design comparing two groups	Examined modifiability when MLE sessions are scripted during a dynamic assessment of narrative skills	Sessions focused on stories using scripts Measured modifiability with mediated learning observation (MLO)	• Two 30-minute MLE sessions focused on narratives • MLO completed after each MLE session	Cognitive strategies were the strongest predictors of language skills
Peña et al. (2014)	• 18 children with language impairment • 18 children with typical language skills	Experimental and quantitative measures	Accessed accuracy of dynamic assessment of narrative skills in children learning English	Modifiability measured using MLO	• Examiners completed MLO after first session	High accuracy rate when modifiability measures used

(continued)

Table 4-2 (continued)
Dynamic Assessment: Modifiability

AUTHOR	PARTICIPANTS	DESIGN	FOCUS	ASSESSMENT	PROCEDURE	OUTCOME
Ukrainetz et al. (2000)	• Bilingual Native American kindergarten students • 15 stronger language learners • 8 weaker language learners	Experimental design using test-teach-retest test design	Dynamic assessment of categorization to identify stronger and weaker language learners	Calculated combination score from *Learning Strategies* checklist and *Response to Mediation* checklist	• Two mediation sessions 30 minutes each with participants seen in pairs • Examiner filled out checklists during sessions	Modifiability scores greater for stronger than for weaker language learners
Petersen et al. (2017)	• 42 Spanish-English bilingual kindergarten to third-grade students • 10 with language impairment • 10 without language impairment	Experimental design with two groups using a pre-test, teach, post-test design	Dynamic assessment of narrative language skills	Modifiability scores, post-test scores, and teaching duration	• Two 25-minute test-teach-retest sessions conducted in English	Sensitivity and specificity rates over 90% with a combined modifiability and teaching duration score

Modifiability factors. Peña et al. (2007) explored the modifiability factors of narrative skills of first- and second-grade students. The authors found that the combination of metacognition and flexibility differentiated students with and without a language disorder. The students' self-awareness of their errors and ability to change strategies during the mediated learning experience resulted in accurate language disorder diagnoses. Students that demonstrated motivation, persistence, flexibility, and awareness of mistakes had increased gains in their narrative skills. A follow-up case study by Peña et al. (2007) examined two second-grade African American students. The student with a language disorder had difficulty with arousal and elaboration. This student presented with higher anxiety levels and lower motivation compared to the student with typical language skills. This student also needed more verbal repetitions, prompting, redirection, and rewording of questions compared to the student with typical language skills. The student with typical language skills was described as engaged and demonstrated awareness of their errors.

Gutierrez-Clellen and Peña (2001) examined two 4-year-old bilingual students in case studies to evaluate the modifiability profiles of students during single word labeling tasks. The student with typical language skills demonstrated increased effort, transfer of skills, motivation, and focus compared to the child with a possible language disorder that had difficulty with planning and self-regulation skills. Patterson et al. (2013) examined whether typically developing preschool students with bilingual experience demonstrated evidence of learning within a brief dynamic assessment task of language skills. The authors did not use a specific form to evaluate modifiability, but offered a microscopic approach where they concluded that students with typical language skills demonstrate change when provided with support during tasks compared to students with a language disorder who would not make such gains.

Kramer et al. (2009) examined the learning characteristics of First Nations students during a dynamic assessment of narrative tasks. Findings indicated that the students who were typical language learners benefited from direct instruction during the mediated learning experience session and students with possible language disorders had increased difficulty learning and with the narrative task. Students with language disorders required more effort to teach, did not demonstrate transfer of skills, and were less responsive to mediation.

In all the studies presented, sample sizes were small, and results were unable to be generalized to other populations as they used a specific population (i.e., preschool). It is important to consider that although many of these studies have a small participant pool, many of these studies are qualitative in nature. However, dynamic assessments offer assessment practices that are less biased for populations that have historically little options when examining language strengths and areas of need. Given that each study used a different type of modifiability checklist, it was difficult to generalize the results. As a result, the fidelity of the studies was impacted. Based on the findings of the studies presented, using student learning characteristics appears to be beneficial when comparing strong language learners to weak language learners. Characteristics such as transfer of skills, frustrations levels, and flexibility seem to be unique skills to the students with possible language impairments.

Modifiability classification accuracy. Ukrainetz et al. (2000) examined modifiability in a categorization task of Native American students. The authors examined modifiability scores and changes in test scores classified students with a language disorder with 100% accuracy. On a word learning dynamic assessment task, Peña et al. (2001) examined the modifiability skills of bilingual preschool students. Students were classified with a language disorder with 92% accuracy when modifiability scores and changes in test scores were considered. Students who had decreased modifiability skills demonstrated frustrations with tasks requiring praise and encouragement. The students who were highly modifiable had characteristics such as motivation and focus.

Modifiability skills of first and second graders following a dynamic assessment of narrative skills by Peña et al. (2006) were examined. After mediated sessions, students with typical language skills had greater modifiability ratings than students with language impairments. Students were classified with a language disorder with 100% accuracy when modifiability scores and changes in test scores were considered. Word-learning skills during a mediation session were examined by Kapantzoglou et al. (2012), and students were correctly identified with a language disorder with 80% accuracy when modifiability scores were combined with scores in test changes. The modifiability of narrative skills was examined for students learning English by Peña et al. (2014). Students were classified as having a language disorder with 87% accuracy when modifiability scores and changes in test scores were considered. The authors determined that students with language disorders required more support in cognition, compliance, problem-solving, and flexibility.

Petersen et al. (2017) also assessed the classification accuracy of dynamic assessments. The study included 42 kindergarten to third-grade students who were Spanish-English bilingual speakers. The participants included 10 students diagnosed with language disorders and 32 students with typical language skills. In this study, the researchers utilized a test-teach-retest format for narrative language skills. Throughout the dynamic assessment process, the participants were taught story grammar elements and subordination. The study results indicated the use of modifiability ratings and teaching duration during dynamic assessment had sensitivity and specificity rates of more than 90%.

In the studies presented, sample sizes were small and results could not be generalized as they used specific populations. However, comparing post-test scores to pre-test scores and combining these scores with modifiability results appears promising. The results from all the studies had a high accuracy rate when differentiating whether a student has a language disorder from one that did not. Using a modifiability scale combined with the test score changes may also reduce inter-reliability, as the focus is not solely based on test score changes.

It is essential that all educators, including education administrators, be aware of the assessment processes of the culturally and linguistically diverse students in their district. With an increase of culturally and linguistically diverse students in the United States, it is imperative the availability of assessments differentiating a student with a language disorder from a language difference exists. Therefore, the purpose of this chapter is to report on the existing literature; addressing the use of a dynamic assessment with culturally and linguistically diverse students to differentiate strong language learners from students with weak language skills and how to conduct three types of dynamic assessment.

How to Do Dynamic Assessment

Test-Teach-Retest

Most dynamic assessments follow a test-teach-retest pattern (Kapantzoglou et al., 2012; Peña et al., 2007) focusing on the learning patterns to differentiate a student with a language disorder from a language difference (Guiterrez-Clellen & Peña, 2001; Peña et al., 2001). The procedures for test-teach-retest are outlined in Figure 4-1. During the initial test phase, the student may be assessed through standardized, static, or nonstandardized measures. When choosing a standardized measure, clinicians need to be aware of the specificity, sensitivity, dialect considerations, and the extent to which the individual's ethnicity is represented in the normative sample. If any of these factors are minimal, the clinician should consider an alternate assessment to administer. After administering the assessment, the clinician should choose which skill or skills the individual appeared to have difficulty with to target in the next phase. When selecting the skill or skills to target, consider the concerns of the individual and their caregiver, the academic needs if the person is school aged, and (more importantly) what will increase the person's communication abilities.

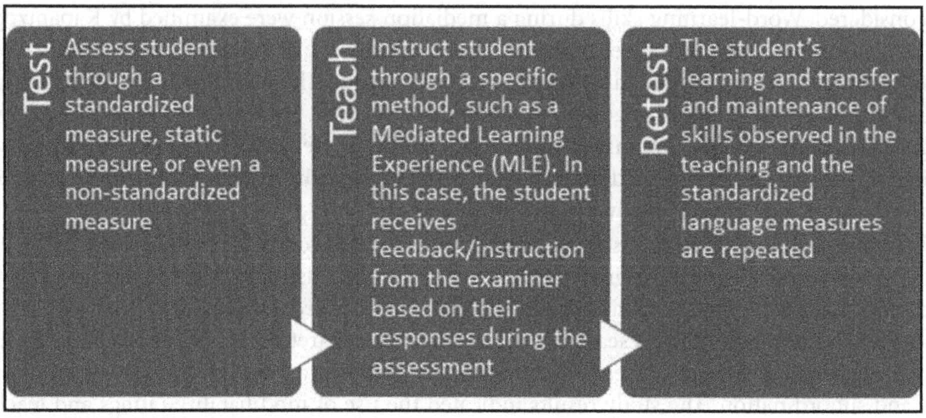

Figure 4-1. Test-teach-retest procedure.

Example: A student from Taiwan was administered the *Structured Photographic Expressive Language Test—Third Edition.* During the administration of the *Structured Photographic Expressive Language Test—Third Edition,* the student is presented with a photo and the examiner asks the student to state what they see in the picture or complete a sentence based on the picture. For instance, the clinician shows an image of one book and another of a stack of books. The examiner states, "Here is one book and here are ... " The student is expected to respond with a response with the plural form of book. During the assessment, the Taiwanese student demonstrated difficulty with forming verbs in past tense, as well as forming plurals. According to the classroom teacher, the student is demonstrating increased difficulty with English word order, although they are trying to form sentences the best they can. At home, the student only speaks Taiwanese Mandarin and the parents have not expressed much concern. To determine whether the student has the ability to learn or grasp plural forms in English, the speech-language pathologist decides to target these in small group sessions. The speech-language pathologist also takes into consideration that in Mandarin, words tend to only have one grammatical form, thus the student may be unaware of this grammatical change in English. This scenario will continue in each phase of test-teach-retest.

The second phase of the test-teach-retest dynamic assessment strategy is to teach. While in the teaching phase, the student may be instructed through various methods, such as a mediated learning experience in which the student receives feedback and instruction from the examiner based on their responses during the assessment (Kapantzoglou et al., 2012). The length of the teaching phase will depend on each situation. If the teaching phase is occurring during an evaluation, this is likely to happen within one session. If the teaching phase is a part of response-to-intervention, the phase may last over the course of 1 to 4 weeks.

Example: In this phase of the test-teach-retest model, the speech-language pathologist will explicitly teach English past tense and plural forms to the student. The speech-language pathologist begins by simply presenting two pictures: one of a single item (e.g., a dog) and a second with many pictures of that same item (e.g., dogs). When presented with the photo of the single item, the student named the item correctly with no difficulty. When presented with the photos of the plural form of the item, the student again stated the singular form of the word. Over the next 2 weeks, the speech-language pathologist conducted the same task while providing written visual and verbal cues for the needed grammatical change (adding the /s/) for regular plurals.

In the retest stage of the assessment, the student's learning and transfer and maintenance of skills observed in the teaching phase are evaluated (Kapantzoglou et al., 2012), and standardized language measures are repeated (Peña et al., 2014). To determine if a student presents with a language disorder, the changes between test scores are compared, and the student's response to instruction is evaluated.

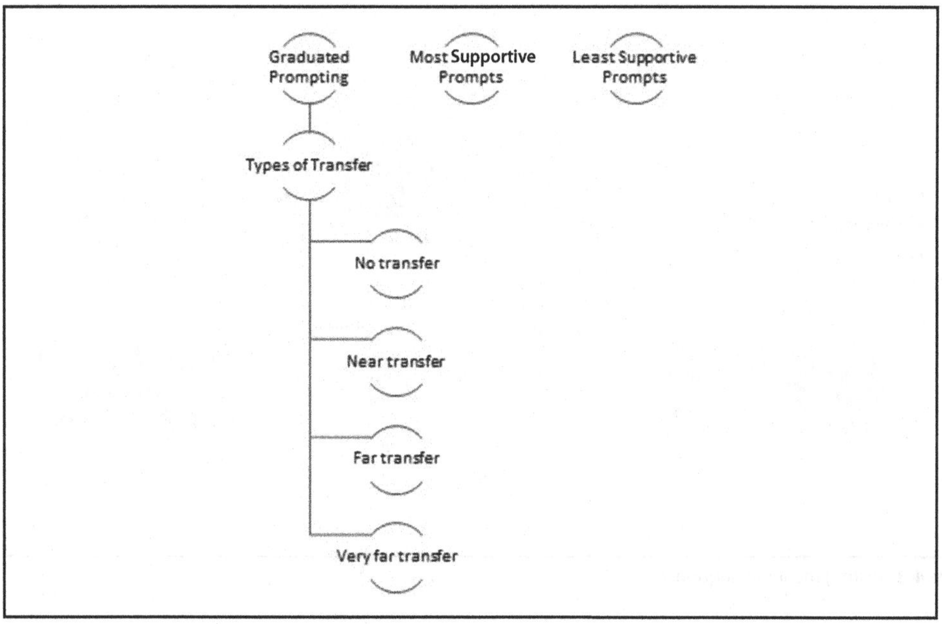

Figure 4-2. Graduated prompting sequence.

If the scores improve and cognitive strategies are used appropriately, an impairment could be ruled out; however, if there are minor improvements and the students demonstrate difficulty with cognitive strategies, then it is likely that the student presents with a language disorder (Peña et al., 2014).

Example: After 4 weeks of working on regular plurals, the speech-language pathologist readministers the items targeting plurals on the *Structured Photographic Expressive Language Test—Third Edition.* On the post-test trials, the student improved from 0% accuracy to 50% accuracy. These results indicate the student's difficulties with forming regular plurals in English were likely due to a language difference and not a language disorder. Case Study Two, at the end of the chapter, provides an example of the test-teach-retest approach.

Graduated Prompting

Graduated prompting is the second type of dynamic assessment to be discussed in this chapter. Graduated prompting entails the clinician going through a prompt hierarchy to determine how much prompting or how many prompts the client needs to be successful or grasp the desired skill. The prompts used should range from least supportive to most supportive (Austin, 2010). The prompts used can be, but are not limited to, questions, modeling from the clinician, or cueing. Once an individual appears to have grasped the skill or concept, it is important for the clinician to check whether the client is able to demonstrate the target skill or concept in a different setting, a similar task, or in other tasks. The extent a client is able to apply the learned concept in another task or concept is called transfer distance. The four types of transfer are no transfer, near transfer, far transfer, and very far transfer (Gutierrez-Clellen & Peña, 2001). The full sequence is outlined in Figure 4-2. No transfer would occur if the client was not able to grasp the concept or demonstrate it in a similar task after being taught. Whereas very far transfer would be the ability to demonstrate the skill across activities, contexts, and in unstructured settings without cues.

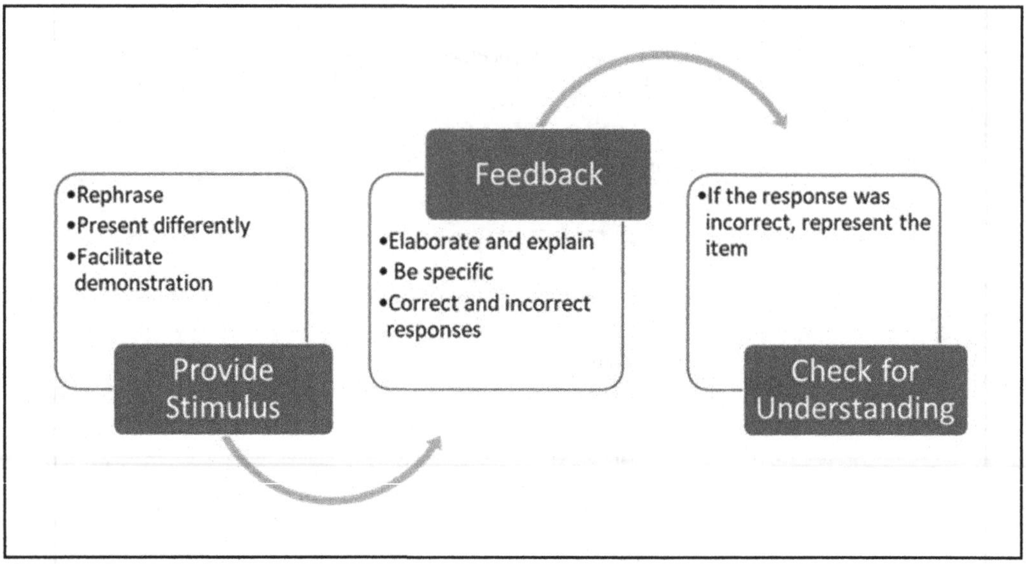

Figure 4-3. Testing the limits sequence.

To conduct a graduated prompting dynamic assessment, one needs first to identify the target skill or concept needing to be addressed. The next step is to determine the types of prompting appropriate for the skill you would like to teach. For instance, if you were targeting the plural grammar marker plural -s, a verbal cue or a visual prompt may be appropriate. The third step is to engage the individual in tasks eliciting plural -s. During elicitation of the task or trials, the clinician should provide the necessary prompting or cues needed to be successful for the client. During this process, the clinician will need to document the type and amount of cues required. The clinician then can begin teaching the client the target skill or concept while reducing the amount and types of cues over time. Suppose the individual continually requires the same amount and types of cues needed as the initial trial. In that case, this is indicative they may demonstrate a true deficit in that area and demonstrate no transfer. If the client can show mastery or make progress with fewer cues and prompts throughout the dynamic assessment, this is indicative that the person demonstrated a difference or had not previously been exposed to the concept and demonstrates some form of transfer.

Testing the Limits

Testing the limits is a third type of dynamic assessment. Testing the limits is a means of gauging a client's skills during the assessment or an intervention trial. Upon the client providing a response, the clinician first would rephrase the wording of the question, pose the item in a different way, or facilitate the client's ability to demonstrate what they know. The second step in testing the limits is to provide the client with elaborate feedback about their response. The elaborated feedback would explain or describe why the client's response was correct or incorrect rather than simply expressing whether their response was correct or incorrect. The explanation aspect of testing the limits is the aspect of this type of dynamic assessment that facilitates the client obtaining more depth in their understanding of the concept or target skill being targeted. If the clinician is providing feedback for an incorrect response provided by the client, the final step in testing the limits would be to check for understanding. If the clinician provided elaborated feedback on a correct response, checking for understanding is not needed. An example of testing the limits is presented in the next two paragraphs. See Figure 4-3 for an outline of the procedures.

Harper is an English-speaking third-grade student who is working on her English written expression skills. Her first language is Cantonese, and this is her second year attending an English-speaking school. Amiah is the speech-language pathologist in Harper's school and has been asked to assist with providing small group intervention for her. Amiah decides to have Harper work on creating and using different types of sentences. In a session, Harper is given a sentence and has to create a question that the sentence would answer. The sentence given to Harper reads: "The cat is on the chair." On her sheet of paper, she writes: "Where is the cat?" Amiah then explains to Harper how she used the correct question word and subject in her question. Amiah also expressed that the question word *where* is indicative of a location or a place. In this example, Amiah allowed Harper to demonstrate what she knew and provided elaborate feedback to her. In this scenario, Amiah does not need to check for understanding since Harper answered correctly. Let's look at another example in which the clinician would need to check for understanding.

Nelson, a Tagalog speaker, is 6 years old and attends primary school in the Philippines. Nelson has been in therapy for 3 years to increase his expressive language skill. Up until he was 5 years old, he generally spoke in one-word utterances. One of his goals in therapy is to describe people and objects. For this task, the clinician obtained pictures of some of Nelson's family members. The clinician presents Nelson with a photo of his aunt and he responds, *Tita si magandà* (Aunt is beautiful). The clinician provides an explanation of how sentences begin with descriptive words and verbs in Tagalog. She emphasizes to Nelson the words he used were correct but were out of order. The clinician then writes the word *magandà* on a green index card and explains the green words are describing words and they go first. The clinician then puts a red border around the photo to indicate it goes last in the sentence. The clinician then hands Nelson the word and the photo to make a sentence. Nelson lays the items out and states, *Magandà si tita*. The clinician provides positive reinforcement for use of the correct word order.

Conclusion

Dynamic assessment appears to show a positive alternative to standardized measures when examining the language skills of culturally and linguistically diverse students across various settings and countries. Using a test-teach-retest dynamic assessment model to assess a student's narration skills appears to be the most culturally sensitive way to examine a student's language skills. Assessing a student's narrative language skills may be the closest related to a student's academic achievement, as it considers cognitive processes, such as higher-order thinking, organization, and grammar. Also, based on the findings of the studies, it is not the checklist itself that differentiates the student's abilities; rather, it is the examination of the student's learning characteristics that determine if a client presents with a language disorder or not.

Based on the review of the studies in this chapter, there appears to be limited research in dynamic assessment with a culturally and linguistically diverse population in general. Limited studies were done using dynamic assessment with older culturally and linguistically diverse students (e.g., middle school) or adults. Most of the studies that were found in preparation for this chapter included participants that were preschool-aged or were in their early years of elementary school. Only a few studies examined specific language areas of categorization, vocabulary, and narrative skills. Other areas of language, such as phonological and phonemic awareness, require careful consideration as well.

Case Study One

Jenna, a monolingual speech-language pathologist, was asked to evaluate a new student in her school, Charlie. Charlie came from a monolingual home where French was spoken and was placed in a French-speaking classroom. The classroom teacher reported Charlie was struggling with language skills, but the speech-language pathologist did not have access to any appropriate standardized measures. She therefore decided to administer a nonword repetition task to examine his modifiability skills. Jenna asked Charlie to repeat a variety of single syllabic, and two- and three-syllable words. Jenna ensured the words contained sounds that were found in French and that were developmentally appropriate. During this task, she was able to examine Charlie's modifiability skills; specifically, his ability to attend to, retain, and process information. While he did not present with any speech sound errors, she noted that he had difficulty repeating several words back to her without the use of several repetitions and required several visual and tactile prompts. He appeared anxious that he was unable to complete the task, and began to avoid her questions by requesting water and snack breaks. She wanted to observe him in the classroom setting and noted that he struggled in this environment. For example, he was unable to answer questions without having information repeated or broken down into several steps. He also had demonstrated difficulty with retelling stories and writing his ideas on paper. He appeared anxious, upset, and at one point he erased his paper so hard he ripped it. She noted similar behaviors when she worked with him one-on-one, especially making a mental note that she had a high amount of examiner effort with the child having difficulty responding. While she was not there to assess other children, she was able to make a comparison to their behavior and noted that they did not demonstrate similar frustrations with the tasks as asked by the classroom teacher. Based on the results of her dynamic assessment, Jenna noted the difficulties Charlie was having in class and was confident in her decision to begin to provide services based on the child's modifiability in completing two tasks that were challenging for the student.

Case Study Two

Jorie works as a bilingual speech-language pathologist in a public school. She was asked to assess Jordan, a first-grade student, to determine if the child presented with a language difference or disorder. Jordan came from a home where Spanish was the primary language spoken; however, he was a student in a class where English was the primary language of instruction. The classroom teacher was not sure if Jordan was struggling in class due to a language difference or disorder and asked the school-based speech-language pathologist's professional opinion. Jorie was confident that standardized testing would not be an appropriate measure to determine eligibility for services, so she decided that she was going to administer a test-teach-retest dynamic assessment task. She felt that this would be an easy way to determine the child's growth in a specific skill, and so she picked vocabulary.

To complete this process, Jorie first administered an academic-based vocabulary test in both English and Spanish, and the results indicated that both test scores were low in both languages, which ruled out a language difference. She then decided to work on increasing the child's vocabulary skills in both English and Spanish. She developed a plan that addressed the child's receptive and expressive vocabulary skills and worked with the student and the classroom teacher to continue to develop the child's vocabulary. She pushed into the classroom and completed tasks with Jordan such as semantic word mapping and addressed tiers two and three vocabulary words.

After providing Jordan with explicit vocabulary instruction and taking data over the course of 10 weeks, Jorie readministered an academic-based vocabulary test to determine if Jordan made growth over the course of the intervention. The results of the pre- and post-assessment results revealed Jordan made growth across his vocabulary skills in both English and Spanish. While the results demonstrated more growth in English than in Spanish, Jorie was able to rule out that Jordan was struggling due to a difference and not a disorder.

References

American Speech-Language-Hearing Association. (1993). *Definitions of communication disorders and variations* [Relevant Paper]. www.asha.org/policy. https://doi.org/10.1044/policy.RP1993-00208

Austin, L. (2010). Dynamic assessment: Whys and how's. *Perspectives on School-Based Issues, 11*(3), 80–87. https://doi.org/10.1044/sbi11.3.80

Baron, A., Bedore, L. M., Peña, E. D., Lovgren-Uribe, S. D., López, A. A., & Villagran, E. (2018). Production of Spanish grammatical forms in U.S. bilingual children. *American Journal of Speech-Language Pathology. 27*(3), 975-987. https://doi.org/10.1044/2018_AJSLP-17-0074

Brown, R. (1973). *A first language: The early stages.* George Allen & Unwin.

Camilleri, B., Hasson, N., & Dodd, B. (2014). Dynamic assessment of bilingual children's language at the point of referral. *Educational & Child Psychology, 31*(2), 57-72. http://www.bps.org.uk

Camilleri, B., & Law, J. (2007). Assessing students referred to speech and language therapy: Static and dynamic assessment of receptive vocabulary. *Advanced Speech and Language Pathology, 9*(4), 312-322. https://doi.org/10.1080/14417040701624474

Feuerstein, R., Miller, R., Rand, Y., & Jensen, M. (1981). Can evolving techniques better measure cognitive change? *Journal of Special Education, 15*, 201-219.

Gillam, R. B., & Peña, E. D. (2004). Dynamic assessment of children from culturally diverse backgrounds. *Perspectives on Communication Disorders and Sciences in Culturally and Linguistically Diverse (CLD) Populations, 11*(2), 2-5. https://doi.org/10.1044/cds11.2.2

Grigorenko, E. L. (2009). Dynamic assessment and response to intervention: Two sides of one coin. *Journal of Learning Disabilities, 42*(2), 111-132.

Gustafson, S., Svensson, I., & Fälth, L. (2014). Response to intervention and dynamic assessment: Implementing systematic, dynamic and individualised interventions in primary school. *International Journal of Disability, Development and Education, 61*(1), 27-43. https://doi.org/10.1080/1034912X.2014.878538

Gutierrez-Clellen,V., & Peña,E., (2001). Dynamic assessment of diverse students: A tutorial. *Language, Speech, and Hearing Services in Schools, 32*(4), 212-224. http://dx.doi.org/10.1044/0161-1461(2001/019)

Hasson, N., Camilleri, B., Jones, C., Smith, J., & Dodd, B. (2012). Discriminating disorder from difference using dynamic assessment with bilingual students. *Child Language Teaching and Therapy, 29*(1), 57-75. https://doi.org/10.1177/0265659012459526

Hasson, N., & Joffe, V. (2007). The case for dynamic assessment in speech and language therapy. *Child Language Teaching and Therapy, 23*(1), 9-25. https://doi.org/10.1177/0265659007072142

Kapantzoglou, M., Restrepo, M. A., & Thompson, M. S. (2012). Dynamic assessment of word learning skills: Identifying language impairment in bilingual children. *Language, Speech, and Hearing Services in Schools, 43*(1), 81-96. https://doi.org/10.1044/0161-1461(2011/10-0095)

Kohnert, K., Ebert, K., & Pham, G. (2021). *Language disorders in bilingual children and adults* (3rd ed.). Plural Publishing.

Kramer, K., Mallett, P., Schneider, P., & Haywood, D. (2009). Dynamic assessment of narratives with grade 3 students in a First Nations community. *Canadian Journal of Speech and Language Pathology & Audiology. 33*(3), 119-128. http://www.rehabresearch.ualberta.ca/enni/sites/default/files/Kramer%20et%20al%20CJSLPA%20 2009.pdf

Lebeer, J., Birta-Székely, N., Demeter, K., Bohács, K., Candeias, A. A., Sønnesyn, G., Partanen, P., & Dawson, L. (2012). Re-assessing the current assessment practice of children with special education needs in Europe. *School Psychology International, 33*(1), 69-92. https://doi.org/10.1177/0143034311409975

Mirzaei, A., Shakibei, L., & Jafarpour, A. A. (2017). ZPD-Based dynamic assessment and collaborative L2 vocabulary learning. *The Journal of Asia TEFL, 14*(1), 114–129. https://doi.org/10.18823/asiatefl.2017.14.1.8.114

Murphy, R., & Maree, D. (2006) Meta-analysis of dynamic assessment research in South Africa. *Journal of Cognitive Education and Psychology, 6*(1), 32-60.

Patterson, J., Rodriguez, B., & Dale, P. (2013). Response to dynamic language tasks among typically developing Latino preschool students with bilingual experience. *American Journal of Speech-Language Pathology, 22*(1), 103-112. https://doi.org/10.1044/1058-0360

Peña, E., Gillam, R., & Bedore, L. (2014). Dynamic assessment of narrative ability in English accurately identifies language impairment in English language learners. *Journal of Speech, Hearing, and Language Research, 57*(6), 2208-2220. https://doi.org/10.1044/2014_JSLHR-L-13-0151

Peña, E., Gillam, R., Malek, M., Ruiz-Felter, R., Resendiz, M., Fiestas, C., & Sabel, T. (2006). Dynamic assessment of school-age students' narrative ability: An experimental investigation of classification accuracy. *Journal of Speech, Language, and Hearing Research. 49*(5), 1037-1057. http://dx.doi.org/10.1044/1092-4388(2006/074)

Peña, E., Iglesias, A., & Lidz, C. (2001). Reducing test bias through dynamic assessment of students' word learning ability. *American Journal of Speech-Language Pathology, 10*(2), 138-154. http://dx.doi.org/10.1044/1058-0360(2001/014)

Peña, E., Reséndiz, M., & Gillam, R. (2007). The role of clinical judgments of modifiability in the diagnosis of language impairment. *Advances in Speech Language Pathology, 9*(4), 332-345. http://dx.doi.org/10.1080/14417040701413738

Petersen, D. B., Chanthongthip, H., Ukrainetz, T. A., Spencer, T. D., & Steeve, R. W. (2017). Dynamic assessment of narratives: Efficient, accurate identification of language impairment in bilingual students. *Journal of Speech, Language, and Hearing Research, 60*(4), 983-998. https://doi.org/10.1044/2016_JSLHR-L-15-0426

Prasad, A. H. (2015). How do you know when it's a language delay versus a disorder? *Leader Live.* https://leader.pubs.asha.org/do/10.1044/language-delay-versus-a-disorder/full/

Rombouts, E., Maes, B., & Zink, I. (2020). An investigation into the relationship between quality of pantomime gestures and visuospatial skills. *Augmentative and Alternative Communication, 36*(3), 179-189. https://doi.org/10.1080/07434618.2020.1811760

Rudolph, J. M., & Leonard, L. B. (2016). Early language milestones and specific language impairment. *Journal of Early Intervention, 38*(1), 41–58. https://doi.org/10.1177/1053815116633861

Skuy, M., Gewer, A., Osrin, Y., Khunou, D., Fridjon, P., & Rushton, J. P. (2002). Effects of mediated learning experience on Raven's Matrices scores of African and non-African university students in South Africa. *Intelligence, 30*, 221-232.

St. Clair, M. C., Forrest, C. L., Yew, S. G. K., & Gibson, J. L. (2019). Early risk factors and emotional difficulties in children at risk of developmental language disorder: A population cohort study. *Journal of Speech, Language, and Hearing Research, 62*(8), 2750–2771. https://doi.org/10.1044/2018_JSLHR-L-18-0061

Ukrainetz, T. A., Harpell, S., Walsh, C., & Coyle, C. (2000). A preliminary investigation of dynamic assessment with Native American kindergartners. *Language, Speech & Hearing Services in Schools, 31*(2), 142-154. http://dx.doi.org/10.1044/0161-1461.3102.142

Vygotsky, L. S. (1978). *Mind in society: The development of higher psychological processes.* Harvard University Press.

Chapter 5

Ethnographic Assessment of Communication Disorders in Children

Elise Davis-McFarland, PhD, CCC-SLP, ASHA Honors

Ethnography is the scientific description of the customs of individual peoples and cultures (Hammersley & Atkinson, 2019). Ethnographic assessment is a comprehensive approach to evaluation of communication and determination of communication disorders. A thoughtful selection of nonbiased materials allows the evaluator to gather information about the child's cultural influences, family dynamics, communication system, and ability to use language to learn new information. This approach to assessment provides valuable information that can yield a more robust picture of a child's communication system, use of communication in various contexts, and potential for further communication development.

Culture influences a child's language and communication style. Ethnographic assessment is an excellent assessment strategy for any child, but it is especially important for reliable assessment of children with cultural and language differences. It can be a supplement to standardized tests and a method for gathering information about the child's communication development and use. It is a way to learn about family dynamics and provides an opportunity for parents to share their desires for their child's future, as well as their desire and ability to support their child's development.

Speech and language assessments serve three purposes: (1) to determine whether a communication disorder exists; (2) to accurately describe the disorder; and (3) to develop an intervention plan. To accomplish these goals, the assessment must be more comprehensive than the administration of one or two standardized tests. This is especially the case with the culturally and linguistically different child whose first language is not English or who is having trouble with academic progression. The intervention plan's success rests on the accuracy of the assessment and the faithful description of the

Bortz, M. (Ed.). *A Guide to Global Language Assessment: A Lifespan Approach* (pp. 91-109).
DOI: 10.4324/9781003524472-7

child's communication system. Standardized assessments indicate what the child cannot or would not do, while ethnographic assessment can provide a more robust picture of the child's capabilities, learning style, response to instruction, and potential for using language to learn (Davis-McFarland & Dowell, 2000).

Standardized Tests

Several researchers have pointed out the significant issues related to the content and linguistic bias of standardized tests, as well as the fact that low representation of culturally and linguistically different children in standardized tests' normative samples results in culturally and linguistically different children performing below the test mean, which may not be a true indication of their language ability (Dollaghan & Campbell, 1998; Laing & Kamhi, 2003; Plante et al., 2014).

Standardized tests must be given as prescribed, and although notes about a child's demeanor, approach to the assessment situation, and the conditions under which the test was administered can be included in the assessment report, that information will not change the assessment outcomes. Statements about the child's hesitance to respond to a question, strategies they may have used to respond to the test questions, or questions they may have asked during the assessment do not influence their test score or percentile ranking. Issues of content bias, linguistic bias of standardized tests, as well as standardization populations that do not include culturally and linguistically different children have been addressed by several authors and researchers (Horton-Ikard & Weismer, 2007; Laing & Kamhi, 2003; Pearson et al., 2014). Standardized tests are based on multiple assumptions that may not consider the child's unfamiliarity with the test requirements. The tests assume that children are comfortable with the examiner (whom they may never have met), that the child is willing to guess at answers (which may be an unfamiliar concept for the child), that the child understands the tasks and will perform to the best of their ability, that the child is familiar with the information they are asked to provide, and that they are comfortable with the testing experience and the verbal display of knowledge (Roseberry-McKibbin, 2013).

Standardized tests do not provide information about the child's learning style or potential for learning the information the tests purports to assess. The test results reveal only what responses the child provides for the question or the stimulus. Unanswered or incorrectly answered questions may be interpreted as what the child does not know. The clinician may try to surmise from the test results what the child knows, but the test does not indicate what the child is capable of learning. This, and many other issues surrounding administration of standardized tests as well as lack of understanding of the cultural dynamics attendant to children's academic performance, has resulted in an overrepresentation of culturally and linguistically different children in special education and resource classrooms (Dragoo, 2017). These and other issues that come with using standardized tests with children in general and especially culturally and linguistically different children indicate the need for nonbiased evaluation and assessment measures.

Nonbiased Assessments

The use of nonbiased evaluation and assessment measures provides a comprehensive and reliable measure of a child's language development and use. If only standardized tests are used in the assessment, the results may not be comprehensive enough to faithfully reflect the child's current level of development and function, nor the child's capacity for future development. Information including parents' reports about the child's birth, development, and communication as well as the clinician's observations of the child in various contexts (e.g., during play and interaction with family members; a teacher's impressions of the child's academic achievement, behavior, and communication; and any other information that allows a determination of the child's communication system and relevant intervention strategies) can be gathered as part of an ethnographic assessment.

Using ethnographic assessment measures is especially important when a clinician is assessing a child whose nationality, race, or ethnicity is different from the clinician's. Socioeconomic status, home language, and parental attitudes and knowledge influence children's language development and use. Getting the most complete notion of the child's language function may require supplementing standardized test results. In some instances, there may not be standardized tests that are appropriate for the child. Even when there are tests that can be given with confidence, other measures may be necessary to provide a more robust picture of the child's communication development and use. This chapter includes information on language sampling and ethnographic interviewing as measures to be used for nonbiased assessment of children's communication.

This chapter introduces two measures that can be used to evaluate a child's language and language development without fear of bias since the measures are sensitive to the child's culture and language influences. Language sampling allows for assessment of a child's communication using the child's own words. An analysis of what the child says can render a valid assessment of the child's stage of language development. The sample can be used to determine if there are language deficits. Intervention goals for language therapy can also be developed from the sample.

Ethnographic interviewing serves the dual purpose of including the parent or informant in the child's language assessment, while getting additional information about the child's life, interests, language use with family, as well as other information that can be used to develop the most accurate and comprehensive view of the child's language use and ability.

The information in Chapter 4 on dynamic assessment will illustrate how that can be used as part of an ethnographic assessment. Readers will see that completing a dynamic assessment can strengthen the language evaluation results.

Language Sampling

Language sampling analysis has proven to be an ecologically sound method for assessing a child's expressive language ability (Bedore et al., 2010; Davis-McFarland & Dowell, 2000; Ebert & Pham, 2017). According to some researchers, language sampling analysis "may be the only assessment measure that captures a speaker's typical and functional language use" (Miller et al., 2016, p.1). Language samples allow evaluation of a child's language and phonological abilities and conversational skills. Specific language areas including syntax, semantics, morphology, and pragmatics can be assessed as well as the child's phonological repertoire. Information from the sample can also be used to supplement information derived from a standardized test to substantiate or provide additional information about the child's expressive language (American Speech-Language-Hearing Association, 2004). A speech-language therapist can use a language sample to probe specific areas of performance on a standardized test to get a better sense of a child's language proficiency or deficits in specific areas of linguistic production. Another advantage of a language sample is that the speech-language therapist can choose the topic of the engagement used to elicit the child's speech. Language sampling allows the child to use their most natural language in connected discourse as opposed to providing one- or two-word responses to standardized test questions or using short descriptions that do not allow for full assessment of connected discourse. Language samples are also less subject to bias when used with culturally and linguistically different children, especially in place of or to supplement assessment outcomes from standardized tests that do not include a substantial number of culturally linguistically different children in their standardization populations (Bedore et al., 2010; Horton-Ikard, 2010; Stockman, 1996).

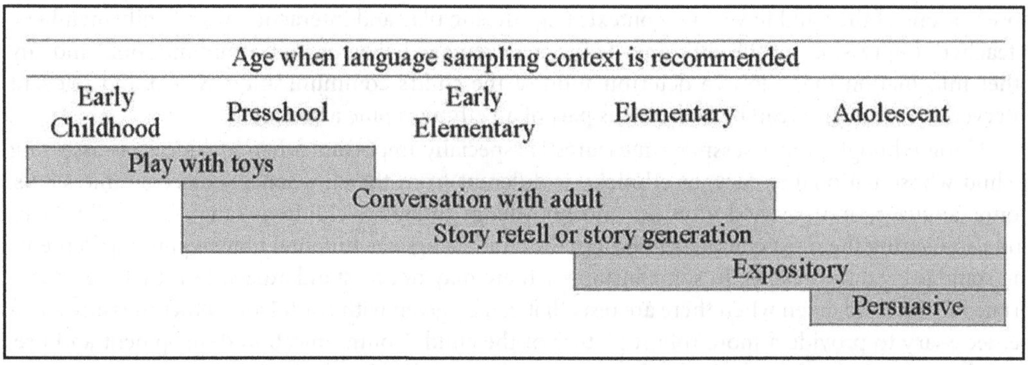

Figure 5-1. Recommended language sample contexts by age. (Reproduced with permission from Pezold, M., Imgrund, C., & Storkel, H. [2020]. Using computer programs for language sample analysis. *Language, Speech, and Hearing Services in Schools, 51*, 103-114. https://doi.org/10.1044/2019_LSHSS-18-0148. License: CC BY-NC-SA 3.0 IGO.)

Assessing Language Structure and Use

Language sampling should be part of any comprehensive language assessment. The process is useful for measuring a wide range of expressive language skills (e.g., mean length of utterance, verbal fluency, overall intelligibility) and difficulties (e.g., repetitions, revisions, grammatical omissions), as well as measures of quality and quantity (see Chapter 6). It is also an excellent way to track the growth of lexical diversity over time (Owens & Leonard, 2002). Even when language sampling is not conducted as part of an original speech-language evaluation, the speech-language therapist can get a sample during initial treatment to establish baseline oral language measures, including number of different words (NDW) as a measure of lexical diversity. The richness of a child's language may depend on the circumstance, environment, or setting in which the sample is elicited. Pezold et al. (2020) recommend that the child's age and developmental stage should determine the context in which the sample is elicited and recorded (Figure 5-1).

Children's language samples allow evaluation of other aspects of oral language including language complexity, narrative skills, perspective-taking, comprehension, imitation, and the ability to follow directions (Prath, 2018). A sample of 50 to 75 utterances is recommended with a recording of the child speaking with at least one other person, in an environment that is comfortable for the child, provides the best sample. Examples of locations for eliciting language samples are at the child's home, school, on the playground with other children, or wherever the child is most likely to feel free to speak and express themself. A recording of the child interacting with family members, teachers, other children, friends, or the speech-language therapist can also provide a good sample of a child's language. Different language activities such as retelling a story, relating a recent experience, describing an object and its uses, giving instructions on how to play a favorite game, or role playing and responding to open-ended questions are activities that can be used to elicit language samples (Davis-McFarland & Dowell, 2000; Prath, 2018; Southwood & Russell, 2004). When necessary for a more comprehensive assessment of a child's language, recordings of the child speaking about different topics with a variety of people provides an opportunity to evaluate how the child's language changes in relation to conversations with various people and in different contexts. The speech-language therapist can select the activities based on knowledge of the child and the assessment's purpose and goals (Davis-McFarland & Dowell, 2000). Language samples can be elicited from children who are toddlers through adolescence so they can be used as a measure of language growth (Rojas & Iglesias, 2010).

Language Sample Analysis

Once the language sample is recorded it must be analyzed to determine the characteristics of the child's language and the stage of the child's language development. The assessment purpose will determine the type of analysis used to assess the child's language. If the purpose of the assessment is to determine whether the child's language is age-appropriate, calculation of the following indicators may be sufficient: mean length of utterance (MLU), total number of words spoken (TNW), clauses per sentence (CPS), and words per sentence (WPS). Using a 50-utterance sample from 385 children of various races and ethnicities between the ages of 3 and 7, researchers were able to demonstrate significant age-related differences in MLU, TNW, CPS, and WPS (Pavelko & Owens, 2019). If a more comprehensive analysis is required, the speech-language therapist can use the language sample to assess various aspects of language including semantics, morphology, syntax, pragmatics, and phonology (Kohnert, 2013). Language sampling can also be used periodically to assess a child's language growth and determine a child's progress during therapy (Rojas & Iglesias, 2010). Developmental Sentence Scoring can be used to further analyze the syntactic structure of the child's language (Lee, 1974). The Narrative Assessment Protocol-2 (Bowles et al., 2020) allows assessment of the language sample's macrostructure and microstructure. Computer-based language analysis systems are also available and require less time for sample analysis. The Child Language Analyses (CLAN; MacWhinney, 2000) and Systematic Analysis of Language Transcripts (SALT; Miller et al., 2016) are computerized analysis systems, and Sampling Utterances and Grammatical Analysis Revised (SUGAR) provides a process for using word processing software for language sample analysis (Pavelko & Owens, 2019). The book *Assessing Grammar: The Language of LSRP* brings together the Language Assessment Remediation Screening Procedure in several different languages and can be useful for English-speaking speech-language therapists who want to elicit and analyze language samples from foreign language speakers (Ball et al., 2012). Additional analysis measures are listed in Chapter 6.

Language sample data is a powerful measure for determining language disorders (Heilmann et al., 2010). Once the language sample is analyzed and the child's developmental language level is determined, language sample analysis is an efficient and effective method for selecting intervention targets. The sample will reveal areas in which the child needs to continue to develop their language skills. Whether the need is for growth in semantics, morphology, syntax, pragmatics, or phonology the sample results, when compared with the language skills of typically developing children (of the test child's age), will provide direction for development of the intervention program.

Language Sampling With Culturally and Linguistically Different Children

Dr. Ida Stockman (1996), in her article on language sample analysis for linguistic minority children, noted:

> LSA (Language Sample Analysis) is valued as an assessment procedure for a linguistically diverse population because it legitimizes the ordinary talk of every community as a clinical resource, whether observed by the speech-language pathologist or a community informant. "Ordinary" refers to language that is routine or familiar to the habits of daily living and interacting. Naturally developed language behavior brings (a) cultural sensitivity, (b) validity, (c) accessibility, and (d) flexibility to the assessment task. (p. 356)

LSA has been shown to be effective in distinguishing language differences from disorders in multilingual children (Boerman et al., 2016). It has been called the gold standard in language assessment with multilingual children (Heilmann et al., 2016). For bilingual children, assessment of only one language is not sufficient unless the assessment results indicate the child does not have a language disorder. Such results indicate that no further testing is required (Gutiérrez-Clellen, 1998). However, if there appears to be a deficit in one language then the other language should be assessed to determine if the child's development of that language is age appropriate (Bedore & Péna, 2008). Failure to assess in both languages violates the U.S. Department of Education (2009) requirement. English monolingual speech-language therapists who are not able to conduct a valid assessment of the child's first language must arrange for an assessment by a speech-language therapist who is conversant in the child's first language. If the child is found to be deficient in that language, the assessment report should include a description of the child's language deficits in both languages. Language samples in both languages will allow for a comparison of the child's strengths and weaknesses in both languages and will provide guidance for development of the intervention program.

Language sampling has been used successfully to assess expressive language development in school-aged Spanish-English bilingual children (Bedore et al., 2010; Ebert & Phamb, 2017). Researchers have also found a positive correlation between standardized tests and language samples with school-aged English-Spanish bilingual children who had identified language disorders (Ebert & Phamb, 2017).

Leadholm and Miller (1992) recommended a remedy to address the issue of culturally and linguistically different children whose scores fall below the norm on standardized tests. They suggested that a "local reference database" be established from language sampling of various culturally and linguistically different children done by speech-language therapists. They recommend that partnerships between school districts and university graduate programs could yield database content to be used in assessment of culturally and linguistically different children. Another study found that the SALT language sample database was effective in differentiating children with language impairment from typically developing children (Heilmann et al., 2010).

Language samples were used to assess African American children's use of cohesive devices during narrative discourse (Horton-Ikard, 2009). The researcher found that typically developing children who spoke African American English used the same category types of cohesive devices as their typically developing peers who spoke Standard American English. Hamilton (2020) recommends that when speech-language therapists use standardized tests with African American children who speak African American English they should elicit a language sample during the assessment process. This allows the clinician to get a meaningful perspective on the child's language in a natural communication context. The sample can be used to write a grammar for the child that indicates the rules the child uses in both African American and Standard American English. This allows the clinician to determine whether the child has a language difference or a deficit and the extent to which the child's language will support purposeful communication, literacy development, and social interactions.

The use of language sample analysis to develop a potent and realistic analysis of a child's speech is presented by Hamilton (2020). When analyzing the language of a culturally and linguistically different child, instead of indicating what mainstream language features the child does not use, the emphasis should be on how the child exhibits the rules of their language or dialect. She uses the example of the analysis of an African American dialect speaking child's language sample.

Instead of this report:

> ...the child exhibits the following linguistic and articulation patterns: dropping of the *-s* in regular plurals, omitting the *-ed* in the past tense, dropping the *-s* in possessives, substitution of /f/ for /θ/ at the ends of words, and substitution of the /d/ for /ð/ at the beginning of words.

Do this report:

> The child exhibits plurals marked by a numerical, past tense marked by intonation and context, possessive marked by owner + thing, the written symbol /th/ pronounced as /f/ at the end of words, and the written symbol for /th/ pronounced as /d/ at the beginning of words. (p. 1)

The child's language sample indicates lack of knowledge of some aspects of mainstream language and phonology; however, the sample also demonstrates the child's mastery of the morphosyntactic and phonological rules of African American dialect. These reveal the child's language competence, which will negate the need for therapy.

Language sampling is a valuable tool in the speech-language therapist's assessment arsenal. Samples can be used to determine the child's developmental language level, to distinguish language differences from disorders, to determine if there is a language disorder, and as a supplement to other tests. Samples taken in different situations or environments and with the child speaking to different people and in different contexts can reveal how the child's language use changes in various situations. All information gathered from a language sample can be used to develop intervention plans, which is a goal of the assessment process. For more information on analysis of multilingual samples see Chapter 6.

Language Sampling in International Settings

The use of language sampling is universal. Clinicians have used language sampling as a language-specific assessment to determine children's language proficiency and to distinguish the language knowledge and use of typically developing children from that of their peers who have language impairments. Researchers have also used language sampling to develop normative data for use in assessments and tests of children's language development and proficiency.

Professor J. van der Linde and Dr. Febe de Wet in a talk at the Speech Base Conference (SA) Programme entitled "How Should I Transcribe a Language Sample" (2021) outlined a process for analysis to children's language samples for children who speak Indigenous South African languages.

Klee et al. (2004) assessed Cantonese children's conversational language to determine the relationship between the children's age and their language development. The researchers' first study included typically developing children ages 28 to 68 months. Twenty-minute language samples were elicited by a Cantonese-speaking research assistant who sat with the children while they played with a doll. The researchers computed each child's MLU and the lexical diversity (D) of the child's language sample. The CLAN computer program (MacWhinney, 2000) was used to calculate MLU and D. The study results indicated children's MLU, and D increased as children matured. Age was a predictor of MLU and D progression.

In a second study, Cantonese children with specific language impairment (SLI) as assessed by standardized language tests had their conversational language abilities assessed for MLU and D with the same play activity as the typically developing children. The children with SLI had significantly lower MLU and D scores than their typically developing peers. The children with SLI had MLU and D scores like younger typically developing children. The researchers concluded that language sampling could be used as one of the measures of SLI in young children.

Thordardottir (2005) developed a method for analyzing language in Quebec French by collecting language samples from 39 French- and English-speaking children ages 21 to 47 months. Sample analysis revealed developmentally sensitive language milestones through the computation of MLU in words and morphemes. Analysis of MLU in morphemes and words revealed they were sensitive measures of lexical and syntactic development. The same elicitation strategies were used for both

English and French; however, the French-speaking children exhibited a higher MLU but smaller vocabulary sizes, and much lower error rates occurred in samples of the French-speaking children. Thordardottir determined that language sample analysis had positive implications for assessment of bilingual children.

Voniati et al. (2021) used language sampling to develop normative data on NDW or word diversity for Greek-Cypriot children. Thirty typically developing children aged 36 to 48 months were enrolled in the study. Each child was seen every 4 months. At each session, the children were engaged in free play activities with their mothers and an age-appropriate set of toys. During each play session the children were recorded, and 50 utterances of their spontaneous speech were analyzed. The recordings yielded typical NDW values for toddlers from 36 to 48 months.

Valian and Eisenberg (1996) recorded 20 Portuguese-speaking 24-month-olds in conversation with their mothers to study competence and performance via an analysis of mean length of utterance in words (MLUW). The children were divided into groups based on their MLUW. The children's use of subjects ranged from 28% in the lowest MLUW group to 57% in the highest group. The children in the highest MLUW group perfectly matched the adult speakers on the MLUW measure. In comparing Portuguese- and English-speaking children, the authors concluded "adult competence about the status of subjects is present at the onset of combinatorial speech, as shown by differential production of subjects" (p. 127).

A study to determine the most effective language sampling method for assessing language development of Afrikaans-speaking boys was undertaken by researchers at Stellenbosch University in South Africa (Southwood & Russell, 2004). Boys between the ages of 5:0 and 5:11 years who were from monolingual Afrikaans-speaking homes were recruited for a study in which number of utterances, variety of syntactic structures, MLU, number of syntactic errors, and the participants' proportion of complex syntactic utterances were used to assess the boys' language maturity and ability. The researchers recorded the boys' spontaneous conversations, speech during free play, and their storytelling during interaction with a researcher. The researchers found that story generation resulted in longer utterances than the other sources of verbalization. The researchers recommended that story generation be used in clinical practice with 5-year-olds to elicit maximum language behaviors.

The successful use of language sampling in international research indicates its utility and reliability with children of various cultural and language backgrounds. In the international studies cited here, language sampling was used to establish language milestones in typically developing children, to reveal differences in the language development of children living in the same province but speaking different languages, to establish normative data for the development of an assessment, as well as to assess children's use of specific parts of speech. Language sampling's broad utility and reliability makes the process an excellent tool for clinical intervention and research.

The following case study illustrates a process for eliciting and using a language sample to assess the language proficiency and intervention needs of a child whose first language is not English.

Case Study: Aalem Abdul

Margaret is a speech-language therapist at Madison Elementary School in Detroit, Michigan. She received a referral for an evaluation for 7-year-old Aalem Abdul. Aalem and his family immigrated from Afghanistan the previous year. Aalem speaks Farsi. His teacher's referral indicated Aalem's limited English proficiency was jeopardizing his progress in learning to read. She said the children in the class complained they did not understand Aalem when he spoke, and she thought his hesitancy to interact with his classmates was because of his limited English skills.

Margaret visited Aalem's class and observed him for 1 hour during reading circle, lunch time, and outdoor play. Aalem was slow to say several words from the word list the teacher was using to teach sight words, but when reading short sentences he was able to read most of the words. At lunch he did not engage in conversation with the other children. If a classmate asked him a question, he answered with one or two words but no more. On the playground he played kickball and seemed to enjoy the game, but he did not converse with anyone.

Margaret researched Farsi and Afghanistan culture. She learned Farsi is an Indo-European language that has 28 Adjad characters rather than an alphabet. There are six Farsi vowels (three long and three short). Most of the Farsi consonant sounds appear in English. Stress is usually on the final syllables of words. There are no definite articles and adjectives that come after the noun as in Spanish. The Afghan culture is conservative. Public embarrassment brings shame, men are responsible for the family's income and welfare, males and females may eat meals separately, and prolonged eye contact between men and women who are not family members is taboo.

Margaret arranged to interview Aalem's parents at their home. Aalem's parents, Tabaan and Bahar Abdul, both spoke some English, but asked their neighbor Aisha who spoke Farsi and English to be there to interpret as needed. When Margaret entered the apartment, she took off her shoes when she saw Bahar was barefoot and her and her husband's shoes were at the wall next to the door. Margaret noticed there was a beautiful tablecloth on the table with embroidery inlay. She told Bahar it was beautiful and asked her to tell her about it. Bahar told her (with some interpretation by Aisha) the tablecloth was made and embroidered by her great-grandmother and passed down to her through the women of her family.

Margaret told Bahar and Tabaan that she came to speak with them about Aalem and Aalem's teacher's request for an assessment. She assured them she wanted them to be partners in Aalem's assessment. Bahar and Tabaan told her about Aalem's birth and his developmental milestones, which all seemed to occur on time: he sat up at 6 months, said his first words at 10 months, and walked at 11 months. He was in good health and has had no ear infections. She said Aalem ate whatever his mother cooked, but he did not like cucumbers or apples. Aalem had two brothers, ages 8 and 10 years. The family spoke Farsi at home. Both parents said they did not feel their English was good enough to be a good model for Aalem, so they did not speak to him in English. Margaret asked if Aalem's speech and language development was like his older brother's at his age. Both parents agreed that it was. When Margaret asked Bahar if she had concerns about Aalem's communication or his progress in school, Bahar said she had no concerns but that Aalem had told her he was afraid to speak English at school because he did not know English as well as his classmates. Tabaan said they came to America hoping for a good life and opportunities for their family. Bahar said she was anxious for Aalem to learn English and do well in school. Margaret explained what an assessment was and what she would be doing with Aalem during his assessment, and that she might ask Bahar and Tabaan to come to the school so she could share the assessment results with them.

The next day Margaret interviewed Aalem. Initially he seemed hesitant to speak, but when Margaret told him she had spoken to his parents and now she wanted to get to know him better he became more conversant. He told her he liked going to school at Madison and he liked his teacher. He said he liked learning English, but that he felt more comfortable speaking Farsi at home with his parents. His classmates sometimes laughed at him when he spoke English, but he said he felt his mastery of English was improving. Margaret explained that for the next couple of days she and another speech-language therapist would be working with him in both Farsi and English to help him learn more English. While they were together, Margaret did a hearing screening, which Aalem passed, and she also completed an oral-peripheral examination, which was negative.

Margaret sent a referral to a speech-language therapist who was fluent in Farsi to conduct a speech and language assessment with Aalem. The school district required standardized test scores for children who were evaluated, so she used the Clinical Evaluation of Language Fundamentals, Fifth Edition (CELF-5) and the Arizona Articulation and Phonology Scale. Aalem's language evaluation indicated his receptive language scores were stronger than his expressive language scores, but both scores were below the mean for his age. He had difficulty forming and understanding compound and complex sentences and generating sentences from picture stimuli. On his articulation test and in connected speech, Aalem demonstrate a t/d substitution, omission of final /l/, and a /t/ substitution for the dental fricatives. Margaret invited Aalem's 10-year-old brother to come and join her and Aalem for a conversation about the family's travel from Afghanistan to Detroit. Margaret recorded their conversation, which included an 80-word language sample for Aalem. She was able to write a grammar that indicated Aalem had mastered many of the English grammar rules except for possessive nouns and irregular verb tenses. He also put adjectives after nouns and stress on the final syllables of words. Both are common in Farsi. The speech-language therapist who evaluated Aalem in Farsi said his language development and articulation and phonological development were age appropriate.

Since Aalem was a fluent Farsi speaker, Margaret was confident in his ability to master English. To add to her confidence, she developed a dynamic assessment that consisted of 10 pictures of items from Aalem's home and classroom. She explained that she wanted him to make sentences about the pictures. She said "I am going to show you a picture. I want you to tell me something about the picture. That is a sentence. I want you to make a sentence. This is a book. The book is on the table. The book is red. The book is large. You decide what you want to tell me about the book. I want a sentence about each picture." After three trials with each of the pictures, Aalem was able to give a sentence about each picture.

Margaret reported that Aalem did not have a language disorder but should receive therapy for his misarticulations and to learn proper syllable stress. She recommended that he receive English as a Second Language (ESL) resource rather than enrollment in ESL courses, and that the teacher select a "buddy" for Aalem to be his conversation partner during lunch and on the playground.

A Discussion of Aalem's Assessment Process

Margaret's observation of Aalem at school allowed her to develop her own impression of his communication skills and interactions with his teacher and classmates. Having the parent interview at Aalem's home allowed a conversation with Aalem's parents in a place that was comfortable for them. It also signaled a genuine interest in Aalem and his family. Following the family's tradition of removing shoes in the house was an indication of her acceptance of their customs. Her notice of the tablecloth and her question about it gave Bahar the opportunity to share information about herself and her family's traditions. All of this gave credence to Margaret's assurance that she and Bahar and Tabaan were partners in Aalem's assessment and empowered them to freely share information in response to the descriptive and structural questions Margaret asked during the interview. The parents' desires to have Aalem exposed to strong English-speaking models and to progress in school helped solidify their partnership with Margaret. Margaret's interview with Aalem allowed him to share his thoughts and feelings about his school experience, his classmates, and his optimism about learning English. Once Aalem shared his information, Margaret had the opportunity to explain the assessment process so he understood its purpose and what would happen.

Margaret knew the CELF-5 evaluation did not give her all the information she needed about Aalem's communication skills, but it revealed areas for growth, ideas for the dynamic assessment, and the need for a language sample. The CELF-5 results were an indication of what aspects of English Aalem had not mastered, but the language sample showed his current mastery of English skills. Having his brother as his conversation partner for the language sample allowed Aalem to speak with someone he was comfortable with while talking about a shared experience. The language sample indicated Aalem was making substantial progress in his mastery of English. The sample results and

Aalem's ability to create English sentences from picture stimuli, in addition to the Farsi evaluation that indicted Aalem had age-appropriate mastery of Farsi, was an assurance that he would continue to master English and make substantial progress in learning to read.

The use of a well-planned ethnographic interview, Margaret's attention to family customs and assuring Aalem's family of their partnership with her, the interview that gave Aalem the opportunity to share his thoughts and ideas, the results of Aalem's Farsi assessment, and Margaret's use of standardized measures to point her to the appropriate unbiased assessments allowed Margaret to identify where Aalem needed intervention and support and gave her confidence that Aalem would become a fluent English speaker.

Two months postassessment Aalem had corrected his t/d substitution and was working on articulation of the interdental fricatives. When Margaret checked with his ESL resource and classroom teachers, they reported Aalem was making progress with his English communication skills and reading mastery. Aalem and Susan, his speech buddy, had bonded and his teacher said she had overheard Aalem teaching some of his classmates Farsi words for objects in the classroom.

The Ethnographic Interview

Parents are a child's first communication partner, so they have a wealth of information about their child's speech and language development and use. One seldom finds a parent who does not remember their child's first word, where they were, and their reaction to that milestone moment. Children have clearly defined roles as family members and their communication ability, characteristics, and style help define their place within the family. A comprehensive assessment of a child's language development and determination of a disorder requires information about the child that goes beyond the tests and observations that are part of the assessment. Information about the child's birth and beginnings, their progress in reaching developmental milestones, their current stage of communication development, as well as the parents' concerns and desires for the child's current and future development are especially important for the assessment's validity. In addition to seeking knowledge about the child's development, the speech-language therapist must begin developing a rapport with the parents to facilitate a solid, supportive relationship between the family and the speech-language therapist if intervention is required.

An Unbiased Approach to Information Gathering

Ethnographic interviewing is an ecologically sound approach to information gathering for a communication assessment and development of an intervention plan in a clinical setting (Jenkins & Rojas, 2020; Westby et al., 2003). The interview is a culturally responsive, family-centered practice that sets the tone for the interviewer's interaction with the parents. It allows for gathering information that will provide a context for the speech-language therapist's evaluation of the child as a family member. By using an ethnographic interview process, the informants are alerted that their input and ideas are valuable information for their child's assessment. It is an approach that honors the family's culture and elicits information about family values and parents' aspirations not only for their child, but also for themselves as parents. The benefits of ethnographic interviewing are threefold: (1) it provides an opportunity to establish a relationship with the family; (2) it provides insight into the child's and family's strengths, desires, and needs; and (3) provides an opportunity to eradicate any preconceived notions the interviewer may have that may prevent a successful assessment of the child and development of a successful intervention plan (Jenkins & Rojas, 2020).

The purpose of a language assessment is to determine if there is a language disorder, and the nature and severity of the disorder. In addition to getting information about the child's medical history and developmental milestones, the speech-language therapist should also get information about the child's place and function within the family, the parents' relationship with the child, their thoughts about the child's communication system and disorder as well as its impact on their child, and their desired outcomes for the assessment and intervention.

The speech-language therapist should go into the interview with the goal of learning as much about the child and family as possible. The speech-language therapist should suspend any preconceived notions and open their mind to what the parent has to say and the information they provide. There should be value in the interview for the parent and the speech-language therapist.

An ethnographic interview is designed to allow a conversation between the parent and speech-language therapist. To achieve the desired outcomes, the interview must be structured to allow a continuous flow of conversation between the parent and the speech-language therapist. During the interview, the speech-language therapist should avoid questions that yield "yes" or "no" answers, but rather pose open-ended questions that allow the parent to provide a narrative. These should be questions that allow the parent to talk more than the speech-language therapist.

Steps for Conducting the Interview

Several things can enhance the speech-language therapist's opportunities to get the best information during the interview:

1. If possible, the interview should be conducted in the parent's home or some other familiar environment. The parent is more likely to feel comfortable conversing with the speech-language therapist if they are interviewed in a familiar place.
2. If the parent agrees, record the interview. This allows the speech-language therapist to devote full attention to what the parent is saying while not being distracted by trying to listen and write. It also allows eye contact with the parent to support development of rapport.
3. The speech-language therapist should begin by explaining the purpose of the interview. "I want to speak with you as part of my language assessment with Aalem, so you can tell me about him and your family. You know Aalem best, so I am interested in speaking with you so we can be partners in his assessment."
4. The interview should begin with a statement or question that helps to build rapport and engage the parent. An example might be "I understand you and the family had a vacation last week. Tell me about it." or "Your garden is lovely. Tell me how you got it started."
5. The speech-language therapist should ask open-ended questions that allow the parent to provide as much information as they are comfortable disclosing. Questions that can be answered with "yes" or "no" yield little information and require the speech-language therapist to ask more questions to get the information necessary to have full understanding of the child and family dynamics. For example, asking "Tell me about mealtime with Aalem" rather than "Is Aalem very talkative during meals?" allows the parent to relate information not only about whether Aalem talks during meals, but they can also provide information about his behavior and demeanor, what he likes and does not like to eat, how long it takes him to eat, whether he is talkative during meals, and what he says.
6. Avoid asking "why" questions that may indicate the parent should have an answer when they may not (Westby et al., 2003). Instead of asking "Why do you think Aalem is quiet during mealtime?" a better choice might be "You mentioned that Aalem is quiet during mealtime and does not participate in the family's conversations. Tell me more about that." This gives the parent an opportunity to say why they think Aalem is quiet during meals as well as provide other information that might be valuable for the assessment and intervention planning.

7. Use *active listening* to ensure hearing and understanding what the parent is saying. The speech-language therapist can indicate to the parent they are paying attention and value the information that is being shared by repeating what the parent says, by nodding affirmatively, by saying "Tell me more" or "Could you say more about that?" etc. Also, if the parent says something that indicates an emotional reaction, the speech-language therapist can acknowledge that by saying "I can hear your frustration" or "Tell me how that made you feel."
8. When appropriate, the speech-language therapist should repeat to the parent what has been said. Reflection can be used when the parent says something that requires further exploration or clarification. An example is this verbatim reflection, "I understand you said Aalem cries sometimes when someone does not understand what he says" as opposed to this paraphrase, "You're saying Aalem is frustrated with a person who doesn't understand him." The verbatim reflection indicates the speech-language therapist has heard what the parent said. This may encourage them to say more without being concerned that you might not understand their point.

The interview provides an opportunity to explore different facets of the child's life and family such as what vocabulary words the child is not likely to know because those words are not used at home, how the child communicates with his playmates versus his family members, whether the child exhibits concern about their communication, if adults seem to notice the child's speech, and whether the parents have concerns about the child's communication. The questions asked during the interview allow the parent to respond in their own style and include whatever information they feel is necessary or important. The interview begins with the speech-language therapist asking open-ended *descriptive* questions, which are designed to elicit information and descriptions of the child's behavior, routines, and experiences as well as information about the family. Descriptive questions are followed by *structural* questions that elicit more specific information about what the parent may have already provided in response to descriptive questions. Table 5-1 provides the types of descriptive and structural questions that can be asked during an ethnographic interview, as well as examples of each.

Interviewing Children

Ethnographic interview questions can also be used with children as part of their assessment process. If the child is mature enough to understand descriptive and structural questions, the interview provides an excellent resource for allowing the child to share their thoughts and feelings. Descriptive questions such as "What is a day at school like for you?" may allow the child to speak about whether and how their peers react to their speech and language. The following question examples allow the child to share their thoughts and feelings about their communication: "Tell me what it's like for you when your teacher calls on you to speak in class" or "Tell me what you think about when someone does not understand what you say" or "Tell me the three things you like most about your speech." The information is a resource for the development of the child's intervention program.

The ethnographic interview provides an excellent opportunity for information gathering and decision making. The interviews can be especially useful when interviewing people whose culture and language may be different from the interviewer's. The descriptive and structural questions are asked in such a way as to encourage parents to talk about their family, culture, and relationships, thus giving the interviewer insight into the important aspects of their and their child's life. The interview also presents the speech-language therapist as a person who is interested in their ideas and wants to develop the best plan to support their child's progress.

This case study illustrates how a culturally responsive ethnographic interview can be used to elicit information for understanding a child's development, parents' desires for their child's future, and the development of the child's communication profile for decision making about intervention.

Table 5-1
Ethnographic Interview Questions

QUESTION CATEGORY	DESCRIPTION	EXAMPLE
	Descriptive	
Grand Tour	To elicit general information about experiences	Describe what a typical day is like for Aalem. or (at the end of the interview) Is there anything else you want to tell me about your family? or Is there anything else you think I should know about Aalem?
Mini Tour	To elicit information about specific events, people, or incidents	Describe what meal time is like for Aalem.
Example	To get an example of something the parent mentioned previously	Give me an example of what Aalem says that makes you think he does not like school.
	Structural	
Experience	To elicit information about an occurrence or experience	Tell me what Aalem does when someone does not understand what he says.
Strict Inclusion	To elicit more information about something that was introduced previously	What has Aalem's teacher told you about his relationships with his classmates?
Cause-Effect	Describes the relationship of two things	What is Aalem's reaction when someone does not understand what he says?
Rationale	Providing reasons for actions	Why do you want Aalem to have speech therapy at home rather than at his school?
Means-End	The relationship of one thing to another	How does Aalem let you know when he does not want to go to school?
Sequence	An order of events	What are the steps for getting Aalem off to school?
Native Language	Seeks to understand terms/phrases used by the informant	What word would you use to describe Aalem's speech?

Data sources: Jenkins & Rojas (2020); Westby et al. (2003).

An Ethnographic Interview in a New Place

Ellen's friend Sandy, a former Peace Corps volunteer, convinced her to travel to Ghana with her for a 1-month vacation. Ellen, who was a speech-language therapist at the local school, decided she was ready for a new experience and agreed to go. Ellen and Sandy flew to the capital city of Accra and spent 4 days recovering from jet lag, spending time in the vast markets across Accra, learning some local customs, and sampling Ghanian food.

During her Peace Corps service, Sandy helped women in a village near Tamale in the Northern region of Ghana start a co-op where the women made handmade kente tablecloths that were sold to tourists in Tamale. She wanted to visit the women she had worked with, so Ellen went with her for the visit. They took a bus from Accra to the Eastern Cape where they were able to get a boat that took them up the Volta River to the Northern Cape and from there to Tamale. While waiting for their bus for the 2-hour ride to the village, Sandy took Ellen to the central mosque, which she said was one of the oldest mosques in Ghana. Sandy told Ellen many people in the region were Muslim and that she had learned a lot about the religion while living in the village.

The first day they were at the village to visit Sandy's friends, Ellen noticed a group of children playing kickball in a field adjacent to the village. After watching for a while one child caught her attention. She was a child with Down syndrome. She appeared to be enjoying the game and she was fully integrated into the group, but she was mainly silent while the children shouted at each other and laughed, and periodically she would sit on the ground as if to rest. Ellen had never expected to meet a child with Down syndrome in Ghana, but she was curious about the child's life and her experiences as a child who was in some ways different from her playmates. Sandy said the girl had been born after she left her work there with the Peace Corps, but that she knew the girl's mother and some of her older children. She agreed to ask the child's mother if Ellen could meet her and her daughter.

Ellen noticed many of the women in the village wore some form of hijab, so as a sign of respect for the family's religion she wrapped her scarf around her head and neck when she went to the family's compound. It was in a large area in the center of the village. The compound was five large huts: one for each of the husband's three wives, a hut for cooking, and one for storage. Sandy went with Ellen to translate during her conversation with the girl named Afua and her mother, Kisi. When Ellen and Sandy entered the hut, Kisi offered them a cup of asana, a drink that was traditionally given to guests. Kisi poured a small amount of her drink on the ground as an offering to the ancestors. Sandy signaled to Ellen that they should do the same so Ellen complied. Kisi signaled for them to sit on the stools that were arranged in a semi-circle in the middle of the hut. Afua sat on a smaller stool next to her mother.

Ellen knew that by conducting an ethnographic interview she could get information about all aspects of Afua's life, her relationships, her health and development, and her speech and language.

Ellen: "Thank you for inviting us into your home. I want to get to know about Afua. There are children like Afua where I live. I work with some of them in my school, and I'd like to know about Afua and how she is doing."

A Discussion of Ellen's Ethnographic Assessment

By conducting an ethnographic interview, Ellen not only gathered information about Afua but she was also able to learn about Kisi's parenting and her relationship with Afua. Afua was accepted as a loved member of her immediate and extended family. Her family understood her needs, and they were aware of the importance of keeping her safe and engaged in village life. Her facial features, stature, poor muscle tone, sleep difference, late milestones, and poor speech and language development were consistent with a diagnosis of Down syndrome.

After their time with Kisi and Afua, Sandy told Ellen the reason Afua was often misunderstood was because Afua had not mastered the tones required to change word meanings. During the interview Ellen made a phonetic transcription of the words Kisi said Afua knew. When Ellen asked Sandy about the Dagbani words Afua knew, she realized the words Afua had mastered were the labials and some of the fricatives of the language but not the alveolar, palatal, velar, or labiovelar sounds.

She was pleased to know Afua was periodically seen by a pediatrician who had determined (by Kisi's description of Afua's checkups and what the doctor told her) that Afua did not have the heart condition that can accompany Down syndrome. Afua was obviously a loved child who was accepted by her family and community. She had forever friends, and her family's plans for her future ensured she would continue to have a good life.

Kisi: "Afua is 10 years old. She was 2 years old before I realized she was different from her four older brothers and sisters."

Ellen: "How did you begin to realize Afua was not like her brothers and sisters?"

Kisi: "Afua's face looked different. Her eyes were different, and she did not seem to understand things like her brothers and sisters had at her age. She began to crawl when she was 13 months old and did not walk until she was 3. I knew she was different, but her father and the village chief told me she was developing in her own way and not to worry. She was not potty trained until she was 4 years old. She has difficulty sleeping through the night and sometimes gets up and wanders outside our hut. The next morning, we might find her in one of my sister wives' huts. She lies down to sleep wherever she wants, but she is always welcome wherever she is."

Ellen noticed while Afua was sitting on the stool next to her mother her back was flexed, her head tipped back, her knees were apart, and her heels lifted—signs for poor muscle tone.

Ellen: "What are most of Afua's days like?"

Kisi: "I usually keep Afua close to me. I need to protect her because she does not communicate very well, and she doesn't always pay attention to things that could hurt her. She also needs more rest than the other children, and she will fall asleep wherever she is. That can be dangerous if she is some place and I don't know where she is.

Ellen: "Give me an example of something that might be dangerous for Afua."

Kisi: "There have been times when Afua plays with other children, she becomes distracted by something she sees in the distance and runs away from the other children to see what it is. She has run out of the village boundaries. Two times Afua got lost in the brush that surrounds the village, and my husband and I feared she would be injured or attacked by animals. I have her stay with me or close to our compound when playing with her sisters. They take care of her. Although she is 10 years old, she is small for her age and her playmates are her 12- and 13-year-old sisters. Afua has not developed her thinking as the other children of her age. Afua goes to the village school and the teacher lets her sit with the children her age, but her work is the same as the teacher gives the younger children.

Ellen: "I saw Afua playing with the other children and she seemed to be having fun. Tell me about her play with the other children."

Kisi: "Everyone here loves Afua. She is always happy, and she makes others happy by paying them compliments. She will point to someone's dress or hijab or something they have and let them know she likes it or thinks it's pretty. Whatever she has she offers to share with others."

Ellen: "Tell me about Afua's speech."

Kisi: "We are Dagbani-speaking people. Afua knows only a few words. I have tried to teach her our language, but her learning is slow. She knows the words for good morning, good night, water, sleep, hungry, and a few others. She does not know how to make the tones that change words, so she is sometimes misunderstood."

Ellen: "Tell me how Afua lets you know what she wants, what she is feeling."

Kisi: "Afua uses gestures and sounds that are similar to the words she wants to use. Our family and others in the village have become accustomed to Afua's words, sounds, and gestures. We pay attention and try to respond to her."

Ellen: "What does Afua do when someone does not understand her?"

Kisi: "Afua is a very patient child who will continue with speaking, using sounds and gestures until we understand her. Sometimes she will fetch me or her sister to help her communicate when speaking to another person."

Ellen: "Tell me about Afua's health."

Kisi: "She is fine. She is healthy. When Afua was 3 years old, the nurse at the clinic in Tamale told me to bring her back to the clinic when a special baby doctor would be there to examine Afua. When I took her, the doctor said he would examine her to see if she was ok. He listened to her heart and asked me some questions about her eating and sleep and play. He told me the name for her condition, but I don't remember it. He said that condition is why her face does not look like her sisters' and why her neck is short and her eyes are different. He said she might not grow to be as tall as her sisters and that she would not learn like the children her age, but she has learned some things slowly over time. Each time that doctor comes I take Afua to him so he can check her."

Ellen: "What do you think Afua's life will be like?"

Kisi: "She will remain here with our family. She is learning to cook and she will know how to dye cloth to sell in the market with me. If she does not marry, she will stay with her father and me and then as her brothers and sisters get older and marry their compounds will be nearby and she will go live with them. She will always be among family and those who know her and will care for her."

References

American Speech-Language-Hearing Association. (2004). *Assessment and evaluation of speech-language disorders in schools.* https://www.asha.org/practice/language samples/components

Ball, M., Crystal, D., & Fletcher, P. (Eds.). (2012). *Assessing grammar: The languages of LARSP.* Multilingual Matters.

Bedore, L., & Peña, E. (2008). Assessment of bilingual children for identification of language impairment: Current findings and implications for practice. *International Journal of Bilingual Education and Bilingualis, 11*(1), 1-29. https://doi.org/10.2167/beb392.0

Bedore, L., Peña, E., Gillam, R., & Ho, T. (2010). Language sample measures and language ability in Spanish English bilingual kindergarteners. *Journal of Communication Disorders, 43*(6), 498-510.

Boerman, T., Leseman, P., Timmermeister, M., Wijnen, F., & Blom, E. (2016). Narrative abilities of monolingual and bilingual children with and without language impairment: Implications for clinical practice. *International Journal of Language & Communication Disorders, 51*(6), 626-638. https://doi.org/10.1111/1460-6984.12234

Bowles, R., Justice, L., Skibble, L., Piasta, S., Kahn, K., & Foster, T. (2020). Development of the narrative assessment protocol 2: A tool for examining young children's narrative skill. *Language, Speech, and Hearing Services in Schools, 51*(2). https://doi.org/10.1044/2019_LSHSS-19-00038

Davis-McFarland, E., & Dowell, B. (2000). Sociocultural issues in assessment and intervention. In L. Watson, E. Crais, & T. Layton (Eds.), *Handbook of early language impairment in children: Assessment and treatment* (pp. 73-110). Delmar.

Dollaghan, C., & Campbell, T. (1998). Nonword repetition and child language impairment. *Journal of Speech and Hearing Research, 41*(5), 1136-1146. https://doi.org/10.1044/jslhr.4105.1136

Dragoo, T. D. (2017). *The Individuals with Disabilities Education Act (IDEA), Part B: Key Statutory and Regulatory Provisions Analyst in Education Policy.* Congressional Research Service.

Ebert, K., & Pham, G. (2017). Synthesizing information from language samples and standardized tests in school-age bilingual assessments. *Language, Speech, and Hearing Services in Schools, 49*(1), 42-55. https://doi.org/10.1044/2016_LSHSS-16-0007

Gutiérrez-Clellen, V. (1998). Syntactic skills of Spanish-speaking children with low school achievement. *Language, Speech, and Hearing Services in Schools, 29*(4). https://doi.org/10.1044/0161-1461.2904.207

Hamilton, M.-B. (2020). An informed lens on African American English. *ASHA Leader, 25*(1). https://doi.org/10.1044/leader.FTR1.25012020.46

Hammersley, M., & Atkinson, P. (2019). *Ethnography: Principles in practice.* Rutledge Group.

Heilmann, J., Miller, J., & Nockerts, A. (2010). Language sampling: Does the length of the transcript matter? *Language, Speech, and Hearing Services in Schools, 41*(4), 393-404. https://doi.org/10.1044/0161-1461(2009/09-0023)

Heilmann, J. J., Rojas, R., Iglesias, A., & Miller, J. F. (2016). Clinical impact of wordless picture storybooks on bilingual narrative language production: A comparison of the "Frog" stories. *International Journal of Language & Communication Disorders, 51*(3), 339-345. https://doi.org/10.1111/1460-6984.12201

Horton-Ikard, R. (2009). Cohesive adequacy in the narrative samples of children who use African American English. *Speech Language and Hearing Services in the Schools, 40*(4), 494-402. https://doi.org/10.1044/0161-1461(2009/07-0070)

Horton-Ikard, R. (2010). Language sample analysis with children who speak non-mainstream dialects of English. *Perspectives on Language Learning and Education.* https://doi.org/10.1044/lle17.1.16

Horton-Ikard, R., & Weismer, S. (2007). A preliminary examination of vocabulary and word learning in African American toddlers from middle and low socioeconomic status homes. *American Journal of Speech-Language Pathology, 16*, 381-392. https://doi.org/10.1044/1058-0360(2007/041)

Jenkins, K., & Rojas, R. (2020). Developing cultural competence from a funds of knowledge framework: Ethnographic interviewing revisited. *SIG 14 Perspectives on Cultural and Linguistic Diversity, 5*(6), 1683-1686. https://doi.org/10.1044/2020_PERSP-20-00081

Karem, R., & Washington, K. (2021). The cultural and diagnostic appropriateness of standardized assessments for dual language learners: A focus on Jamaican preschoolers. *Language, Speech, and Hearing Services in Schools*, 1-20.

Klee, T., Stokes, S. F., Wong, A., Fletcher, P., & Gavin, W. J. (2004). Utterance length and lexical diversity in Cantonese-speaking children with and without specific language impairment. *Journal of Speech, Language, and Hearing Research, 47*(6), 1396-1410. https://doi.org/10.1044/1092-4388(2004/104)

Kohnert, K. (2013). *Language disorders in bilingual children and adults* (2nd ed.). Plural Publishing.

Laing, S. P., & Kamhi, A. (2003). Alternative assessment of language and literacy in culturally and linguistically diverse populations. *Language, Speech, and Hearing Services in the Schools, 34*(1), 44-55. https://doi.org/10.1044/0161-1461(2003/005)

Leadholm, B., & Miller, J. F. (1992). *Language sample analysis: The Wisconsin guide.* Department of Public Instruction.

Lee, L. L. (1974). *Developmental sentence analysis: A grammatical assessment procedure for speech and language clinicians.* Northwestern University Press.

MacWhinney, B. (2000). *The CHILDES project: Tools for analyzing talk* (3rd ed.). Erlbaum.

Miller, J., Andriacchi, K., & Nockerts, A. (2016). Using language sample analysis to assess spoken language production in adolescents. *Speech Language and Hearing Services in the Schools, 47*(2), 99-112. https://doi.org/10.1044/2015_LSHSS-15-0051

Owens, A., & Leonard, L. (2002). Lexical diversity in the spontaneous speech of children with specific language impairment. *Speech, Language, and Hearing Research, 45*(5), 99-112. https://doi.org/10.1044/1092-4388(2002/075)

Pavelko, S., & Owens, R. (2019). Diagnostic accuracy of the Sampling Utterances and Grammatical Analysis Revised (SUGAR) measures for identifying children with language impairment. *Language Speech and Hearing Services in Schools, 50*(2), 211-223. https://doi.org/10.1044/2018_LSHSS-18-0050

Pearson, B. Z., Jackson, J. E., & Wu, H. (2014). Seeking a valid gold standard for an innovative, dialect-neutral language test. *Journal of Speech, Language and Hearing Research, 57*(2), 99-125. https://doi.org/10.1044/2013_JSLHR-L-12-0126

Pezold, M., Imgrund, C., & Storkel, H. (2020). Using computer programs for language sample analysis. *Language, Speech, and Hearing Services in Schools, 51*, 103-114. https://doi.org/10.1044/2019_LSHSS-18-0148

Prath, S. (2018). The how and why of collecting a language sample. *Leader Live.* https://leader.pubs.asha.org/do/10.1044/the-how-and-why-of-collecting-a-langugage-sample/full/

Rojas, R., & Iglesias, A. (2010). Using language sampling to measure language growth. *Perspectives on Language Learning and Education, 17*(1), 24-31. https://doi.org/10.1044/lle17.1.24

Roseberry-McKibbin, C. (2013). *The impact of poverty and homelessness on children's oral and literate language: Practical implications for service delivery.* Presentation at the ASHA Schools Conference.

Southwood, F., & Russell, A. F. (2004). Comparison of conversation, free play, and story generation as methods of language sample elicitation. *Journal of Speech and Hearing Disorders, 47*(2), 366-376. https://doi.org/10.1044/1092-4388(2004/030)

Stockman, I. (1996). The promises and pitfalls of language sample analysis as an assessment tool for linguistic minority children. *Language, Speech, and Hearing Services in Schools, 27*(4), 355-366. https://doi.org/10.1044/0161-1461.2704.355

Thordardottir, E. (2005). Early lexical and syntactic development in Quebec French and English: Implications for cross-linguistic and bilingual assessment. *International Journal of Language & Communication Disorders, 40*(3), 243-278.

Valian, V., & Eisenberg, Z. (1996). The development of syntactic subjects in Portuguese-speaking children. *Journal of Child Language, 23*(1), 103-128. https://doi.org/10.1017/S0305000900010114

van der Linde, J., & de Wet, F. (2021). *How should I transcribe a language sample.* Speech Base Conference (SA) Programme: Contextually relevant speech-language therapy for young children living in Africa: Rethinking early detection, language sample analysis and augmentative and alternative communication.

Voniati, L., Tafiadis, D., Armostis, S., Kosma, E. I., & Chronopoulos, S. K. (2021). Lexical diversity in Cypriot-Greek-speaking toddlers: A preliminary longitudinal study. *Folia Phoniatrica et Logopaedica, 73*(4), 277-288.

Westby, C. Burda, A., & Metha, Z. (2003). Asking the right questions in the right way: Strategies for ethnographic interviewing. *The ASHA Leader, 8*(8), 4-17. https://doi.org/10.1044/leader.FTR3.08082003.4

Chapter 6

New Directions in Language Sample Analysis for Multilingual Contexts

Hanna Ehlert, PhD; Jeannie van der Linde, PhD; Ulrike Lüdtke, PhD; and Juan Bornman, PhD

Introduction

For many speech-language pathologists across the globe, the following case scenario might sound familiar, as it encapsulates the caseload characteristics they are presented with daily:

Katlego is the youngest of Mrs. Madiba's five children. He is 7 years old and in first grade at the same school that his older sisters attend. Mrs. Madiba is confused as the teacher called her to school and said that she is very worried about Katlego's speech and language development, as she often cannot understand him. Although he tries to participate in class and to answer questions, his speech is quite unintelligible. He sometimes struggles to find the right words to express himself and makes mistakes when inflecting verbs. The teacher says that she thinks Katlego understands her and what she is teaching in class, but his speech and language use makes it difficult for her to assess how much he really understands.

Mrs. Madiba explains that at home she noticed that he started speaking later than her other children, but she thought that it might be because he is a boy, as her friends say that boys speak at a later age than girls. She also says that Katlego knows the words, yet when he tries to say them he cannot. For example, when she says to him "Say cat," he cannot repeat the words, although he definitely knows what a cat is. Mrs. Madiba furthermore mentions that Katlego struggles to produce sentences in the correct word order in Sepedi, which is his first language, and he finds it hard to follow instructions in Sepedi. She wonders whether the fact that they speak Sepedi at home while Katlego attends

Bortz, M. (Ed.). *A Guide to Global Language Assessment: A Lifespan Approach* (pp. 111-130).
DOI: 10.4324/9781003524472-8

an English-speaking school perhaps contributes to his unclear speech. The teacher has suggested that Mrs. Madiba take Katlego to the speech-language pathologist at the hospital, as his limited language abilities are currently causing him to fail first grade.

In speech-language therapy, the first step to be taken in the scenario presented here would be to conduct a thorough evaluation of Katlego in both his home language and the language of learning and teaching. This can be challenging, due to several reasons that will be discussed in the next section.

In majority-world countries, access to speech-language therapy services is restricted, as there are not enough speech-language pathologists available to respond to the needs experienced in these countries. In 2017 in South Africa, a majority-world country with a significant disparity in resources, it was estimated that there was a supply–need gap of approximately 2800 speech-language pathologists/audiologists in South Africa (Pillay et al., 2020). This results in extremely large caseloads, which in turn create time limitations, and hence many speech-language pathologists may opt for time-efficient methods of assessment. Moreover, despite the fact that South Africa is a multilingual country with 11 official languages, local speech-language pathologists mostly use either standardized English instruments that are typically developed in the United States, United Kingdom, or Australia (Pascoe et al., 2020) or a standardized Afrikaans translation to assess their clients. Decisions about a child's abilities and needs are made based on comparisons with these norms, even though the tests have not been standardized for the South African population and the child may not be a first-language speaker of English or Afrikaans (Pascoe et al., 2020). Standardized tests usually require children to perform tasks such as looking at visual pictures or listening to verbal prompts and then producing a specific response. The language used and demanded in these standardized tests is not only highly decontextualized but also based on the experiences of children who acted as the normative group (typically monolingual English-speaking children from the United States, United Kingdom, or Australia). As such, it can be argued that these standardized tests do not evaluate South African children's actual use of language in naturally occurring everyday conversational contexts with regular communication partners. For more details regarding the use of standardized and nonstandardized tests, see Chapter 5.

Language sample analysis (LSA), which is widely regarded as the gold standard in speech and language assessment in multilingual contexts (Heilman et al., 2016), is deemed a reliable and valid alternative. For an overview of selected studies in different international settings, see Chapter 5. Since LSA is based on children's language and familiar communicative contexts, it aims to elicit accurate, appropriate, ecologically valid, and unbiased language samples. Yet, the process of LSA—the collection and elicitation of language samples, their transcription, as well as coding and analysis—is quite time consuming. Furthermore, there is often great variability in LSA regarding data collection (i.e., how samples are elicited and collected), transcription, and coding and analysis, all of which complicate its reliable use (Finestack et al., 2014). Figure 6-1 summarizes the three main components of the LSA process.

Before data collection, transcription, coding, and analysis of the language samples, speech-language pathologists must first decide on the specific aim of the assessment, as this will influence all components of the LSA. Assessment can have several goals, for instance, describing the child's language abilities, determining whether the child's language skills are typically developing, whether there is a developmental language disorder present (diagnosis), planning intervention, or evaluating progress with intervention.

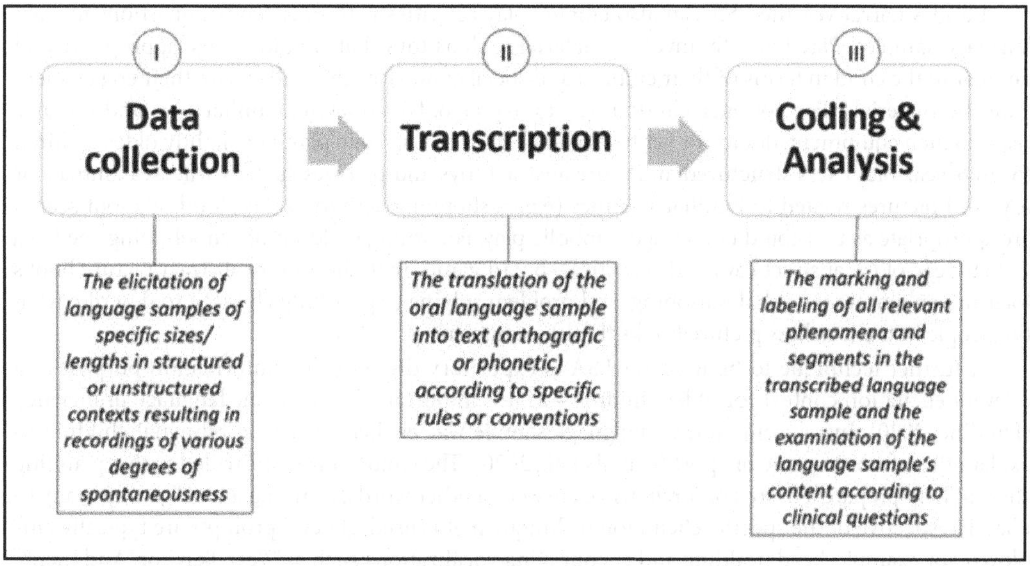

Figure 6-1. The three main components of language sample analysis.

Collection of Samples

The data collected from children form the basis of an LSA. Suitable elicitation contexts provide these children the opportunity to present their language abilities. It is imperative to utilize contexts that are realistic and that accurately represent settings in which functional language is used. One of the first techniques that is used is creating a naturalistic spontaneous conversation in which the child is encouraged to talk, for example, by following the child's interests and asking open-ended follow-up questions (Paradis et al., 2022).

Besides using conversations to elicit language samples, another strategy that is often used is the narrative (personal or fictional). Narratives recount a series of related events around a specific theme (Peets & Bialystok, 2015) and as such constitute a large proportion of children's home and school discourse. Both personal and fictional narratives are also found across cultures (Gress & Hill, 2018). Young children are often taught to provide personal narratives, for example, in "circle time" or "news time," making this a familiar activity to many. Fictional narratives on the other hand have a more direct link to literacy-based language (e.g., wordless storybooks). Peets and Bialystock (2015) reported that both mono- and multilingual speakers reflect similar language proficiency in narratives, while standardized tests often underrepresent the language proficiency of bilingual children.

A third type of narrative that can be included is story retelling. Research has demonstrated that story retelling based on pictorial support, such as pictures or using a silent movie, makes lower cognitive demands on children than telling a story from memory. The pictures help the child to structure a story, and while it minimizes the cognitive (i.e., memory) load, it impacts positively on language proficiency (Kapantzoglou et al., 2017). Pictures are effective because they serve as a common reference for both the adult and the child. They also control the complexity of the story, such as the number of characters and the number and sequence of events in the story. Nevertheless, some researchers warn that although story retelling may provide syntactically more complex samples than conversational discourse (Westerveld & Vidler, 2016), it may not result in an accurate reflection of the child's typical language skills.

Besides narratives, the LSA can also employ play activities with open-ended questions to elicit language samples. Play typically involves material such as toys that should be age appropriate and familiar to the child in terms of their cultural and social context, as this will ensure their engagement with the materials. For younger children (3- to 4-year-olds), concrete, familiar toys and pictures (e.g., kitchen equipment, doctor or vet toys) can be used in symbolic play. For slightly older children (5- to 6-year-olds), less structured and more abstract toys and pictures such as wild/sea animals or toys and pictures related to familiar routines (e.g., a shopping activity or fast-food take-out scene) are appropriate as this could encourage symbolic play. For young children of school-going age (e.g., 7- to 9-year-olds), abstract toys and activities—board games with dice; more abstract picture books focusing on emotions, verbal reasoning, and problem solving (e.g., asking children to describe what the people in the wordless picture books think)—can be used.

A further technique to be used for LSA is expository discourse for information purposes—a relevant elicitation context for older children—as it is important for academic language proficiency (Lundine, 2020). In a recent study, a language sample was elicited by asking bilingual children to explain their favorite game or sport (Cahill et al., 2020). The children were provided with a planning sheet to help prepare a more comprehensive answer, in other words, thinking about "getting ready to play." Irrespective of the specific elicitation technique that is used, general prompts are typically employed, for example, head nodding and encouraging vocalizations such as "Yes/Okay" or "And then?" In summary, conversation tasks are generally considered to be less demanding than narrative tasks, while expository discourse tasks are possibly the most demanding (Paradis et al., 2022).

Software can also be used for data collection, for instance, conversational language samples can be recorded from children in everyday contexts by a device called the Language Environment Analysis (LENA) digital language processor (DLP; Wood et al., 2016). It is a small device that young children can easily wear during everyday activities to capture a day-long language sample. Using speaker recognition software, the LENA DLP device can segment speech by allowing all nonspeech sounds (e.g., TV, radio, silence) to be filtered out, eliminating overlapping speech (multiple speakers at a given moment), and ignoring child nonspeech sounds (e.g., crying, laughing). The utility of this device is further enhanced by the fact that it can typically record up to 16 hours of speech.

When conducting an LSA with multilingual children like Katlego, cross-linguistic comparison may be a desirable goal. If the child's abilities in different languages are to be compared using not-language-specific LSA measures, such as mean length of utterances (MLU), the samples must be elicited in the same contexts—if possible, using the same or comparable material (e.g., story books or set of toys). Additionally, if lexical diversity is to be measured, the samples are required to have the same length because the measures taken are more or less dependent on this feature.

Regarding our case scenario, it is recommended that contextually relevant tasks should be used. In Katlego's case it would be invaluable to use narratives and wordless books that are familiar to Katlego. Narratives may be a viable way of building rapport with Katlego in an effort to obtain a robust language sample, first in his strongest language—most likely Sepedi. It is, however, important to also obtain a sample in his language of learning and teaching (LoLT; McLeod et al., 2017), namely English.

The length of language samples for analysis has been extensively researched and varying findings have been reported in literature (Pezold et al., 2020; Tommerdahl & Kilpatrick, 2014). The proposed sample length in terms of number of words differs greatly and ranges from as little as 50 utterances up to 175 utterance samples (Gavin & Giles, 1996; Pavelko et al., 2016; Pavelko & Owens, 2017; Shipley & McAfee, 2016). Other researchers recommend measuring sample length in terms of minutes, varying from 1 to 2 minutes to 11 minutes (Heilmann et al., 2010; Pavelko et al., 2016; Southwood & Russell, 2004; Tilstra & McMaster, 2007). Nevertheless, the amount of time it takes to collect, transcribe, code, and analyze spontaneous child language samples remains one of the main reasons why speech-language pathologists do not frequently use LSA in practice (Pavelko et al.,

2016). It is therefore important to find ways of streamlining the process by identifying the shortest sample length that still contains the targeted information and renders a representative view on the child's language abilities.

Transcription

Transcription is a uniform checkpoint at which an oral sample is translated into text and/or phonetic symbols. This checkpoint is essential for every language sample before the coding and analysis can follow. As alluded to earlier, orthographic and/or phonetic transcription is imperative to translate the oral language sample into text. Usually, the speech-language pathologist will start by doing an orthographic transcription of at least a section of the speech sample before commencing with the phonetic transcription. Depending on the need, the speech-language pathologist may decide to do either an orthographic transcription or a phonetic transcription. For instance, if the focus is on speech sound production, then a phonetic transcription may be more relevant, whereas a detailed orthographic transcription would suffice when the language use of a child is explored. It is therefore not compulsory to do both in a clinical setting. In research settings, however, conducting both orthographic and phonetic transcriptions is recommended.

Orthographic and phonetic transcriptions can be created in many different ways and saved in many different formats, depending on how they have been created (TextGrid, eaf, etc.). Resources such as Sampling Utterances and Grammatical Analysis Revised (SUGAR; Pavelko & Owens, 2017), Systematic Analysis of Language Transcripts (SALT; Miller & Iglesias, 2012), Computerized Language Analysis (CLAN; MacWhinney, 2000), EUDICO Linguistic Annotator (ELAN; 2022), and PRAAT (Boersma & Weenink, 2022) are available to aid the speech-language pathologist with the LSA (Table 6-1). More specifically, SALT, PRAAT, CLAN, and ELAN can be used for both orthographic and phonetic transcriptions, with ELAN currently being one of the most popular options.

Speech-language pathologists may sometimes opt to classify segments of a word (vowels or consonants) with symbols from the International Phonetic Alphabet (IPA), and at other times choose to evaluate only the overall accuracy of a word or the measure of whole-word matching (Stemberger & Bernhardt, 2020). Deciding what level of detail is required will influence the way the speech-language pathologist transcribes the sample. If the context requires only a "broad" transcription of speech sounds produced, without adding diacritics or refinements (Stemberger & Bernhardt, 2020), a partial transcription of the sample may be opted for. However, if a narrow transcription that includes the coding of details such as sound length, aspiration, glottalization, nasalization, rounding, and degree of fronting is needed (Stemberger & Bernhardt, 2020), the speech-language pathologist may conduct a full sample transcription and also request assistance from other speech-language pathologists to establish a level of interrater agreement between all the transcriptions of the same sample. Narrow transcriptions are frequently used in research settings, whilst broader transcriptions are more common for clinical purposes. Yet, if the speech-language pathologist requires an accurate reflection of a child's phonetic repertoire as well as the speech sound errors, or when they aim to evaluate changes during or after treatment, a narrow transcription will provide more precise information about speech sound production (Wren et al., 2020). The type of transcript will thus inform the selection of more specific treatment strategies as well as subtle changes or improvements due to intervention (Wren et al., 2020).

A position paper by Cruz-Ferreira (2012), entitled *Multilingual Children With Speech Sound Disorders*, is a helpful guideline that describes the principles and practices needed when working with multilingual children with speech difficulties. This document specifically mentions phonetic transcription, which is regarded as playing a key role in the assessment and management of multilingual children with speech difficulties:

Table 6-1

Resources Supporting Language Sample Analysis

RESOURCE	DESCRIPTION	USED FOR
SUGAR (Sampling Utterances and Grammatical Analysis Revised)	Protocol that utilizes regular word processing software for the linguistic analysis of language samples with an associated set of measures	Manual coding and automated analysis (language: focus grammar)
SALT (Systematic Analysis of Language Transcripts)	Software for distributional and linguistic analysis of language samples with an associated transcription and coding format (English and Spanish only)	Data collection, manual transcription, manual/automated coding, and automated analysis (language)
CLAN (Computerized Language Analysis)	Open-source software for distributional and linguistic analysis of language samples with an associated transcription and coding format CHAT (Codes for the Human Analysis of Transcripts)	Manual transcription, manual/automated coding, and automated analysis (language)
PRAAT (Dutch for "speech")	Open-source software for editing, annotation, and phonetic analysis (e.g., intensity, pitch height, duration, or formants) of speech samples	Manual coding and automated analysis (speech)
ELAN (EUDICO Linguistic Annotator)	Open-source software for creating and modifying transcriptions and annotations for audio and video data in a particular format	Manual transcription and manual coding

> Speech and language therapists receive sufficient training in the International Phonetic Alphabet (IPA, 1999), the Extensions to the IPA ... and prosody to ensure they are competent in transcribing speech, both typical and disordered, in their own languages and the languages of the children within their communities. Specific training should also address multilingual speech acquisition compared with monolingual speech acquisition in cross-linguistic contexts ... and apply this knowledge to the identification of children with speech sound disorders. (Cruz-Ferreira, 2012, p. 3)

In multilingual contexts like South Africa, speech-language pathologists often fail to master phonetic transcription due to challenges such as time constraints or limited knowledge of the 11 official languages, and this results in them using binary correct/incorrect classification systems (Munson & Brinkman, 2004) when analyzing speech samples. Understanding the level of skill and proficiency needed to transcribe speech from other languages helps determine the degree to which a speech-language pathologist can successfully manage multilingual children (Wren et al., 2020). The clinician must be sufficiently trained to use diacritics from their own language, but also needs to be familiar with the full IPA (Wren et al., 2020) as children's language and speech may be influenced by all the other languages that they are exposed to.

The transcription of language samples is integral to speech-language pathology practice (Pascoe et al., 2020; Stemberger & Bernhardt, 2020). Apart from allowing speech-language pathologists to determine whether changes in speech and language samples have occurred over time or in response to intervention, transcription also enables the speech-language pathologist to break down language-specific constraints by focusing on speech using a common, internationally intelligible alphabet (Stemberger & Bernhardt, 2020). Transcribing multilingual samples allows speech-language pathologists to explore the commonalities and diversity in speech and language production—both within and across languages (Stemberger & Bernhardt, 2020).

Considering the previous challenges, certain strategies can be recommended to aid speech-language pathologists in the transcription of speech and language samples:

- Use a video stimulus as it offers both visual and auditory cues to reflect how speech perception typically takes place. Transcribing with auditory information only and with multiple talkers is also advocated to assist transcribers in developing their phonetic transcription skills (Stemberger & Bernhardt, 2020).
- Record any visually salient information during the elicitation of the language sample (e.g., tongue protrusion or lateralization, labiodental contact, lip rounding, lip spreading, jaw movement), as such detail will enhance later transcription (Stemberger & Bernhardt, 2020).
- Undergo practical training in phonetics using the entire IPA as it will enable transcribers to analyze multiple languages. However, even if transcribers expand their repertoire of speech sound categories through phonetic training, their ability to transcribe in a "foreign" language will not have the same accuracy level as that of a native speaker of that language. Thus, biases may lead to differences in the transcription of units that are close to the boundaries, even though other robust units may be transcribed in the same way (Stemberger & Bernhardt, 2020).
- Use "seeing speech resources" such as sketches of the phonology and phonetics of different languages, for example, those published as illustrations of the IPA, as articles in the *Journal of the International Phonetic Association*, or as chapters in the *Handbook of the International Phonetic Association* (IPA, 1999). Although IPA charts can also be used, a drawback of these is that only a few environments are illustrated (i.e., a consonant produced in word-initial position and between /a/; Stemberger & Bernhardt, 2020). Transcribers therefore cannot hear the sound paired with other vowels or in consonant sequences in different locations in words (Stemberger & Bernhardt, 2020). Furthermore, the fact that all sounds are produced by a single speaker using hyper-articulated speech is not an accurate representation of sound production in spontaneous speech samples. The "seeing speech resource" also provides the transcriber with sagittal views of either a schematic drawing, MRI image, or raw ultrasound images (Stemberger & Bernhardt, 2020). The schematic representation is often most informative as it provides clear details that transcribers find less distracting than real images (Stemberger & Bernhardt, 2020).
- Find human resources in the multilingual context, for instance, interpreters and first-language speakers who can assist in the transcription process by providing more information on the context, language(s), etc.

In the case of Katlego it will be helpful to start with orthographic transcriptions of both language samples. Should the speech-language pathologist not be proficient in the child's L1, the strategies as outlined previously can be utilized to aid the clinician. Phonetic transcriptions will supplement information and assist with diagnosis. Should the speech-language pathologist find this too time consuming, partial phonetic transcriptions of utterances in both languages can be considered.

Coding and Analysis of Multilingual Samples

The core of the LSA process is analysis of the linguistic content of the sample. Very different aspects of communication and language can be evaluated using language samples, including focusing on the child only or on a communicative dyad. The latter includes samples of caregiver–child interaction, the child's ability to engage in conversational or expository discourse, the child's narrative abilities, and the child's language development focusing on form, content, and use (Nippold, 2021; Ramírez-Esparza et al., 2014). Standard LSA includes grammatical measures, lexical measures, and measures of verbal fluency (Miller et al., 2019). A variety of LSA measures that give the speech-language pathologist a good overview of a child's language development at different ages can be computed from coded transcripts. These measures include general outcome measures that yield a single quantitative score of overall proficiency (e.g., mean length of utterance [MLU]; Brown, 1973), specific measures that make a more detailed assessment of components within a specific skill set (e.g., phrase elements; Owens et al., 2018), and a combination of overall and specific measures by means of language sampling programs (e.g., Developmental Sentence Scoring [DSS]; Lee, 1974; and the Index of Productive Syntax/IPSyn; Scarborough, 1990).

Best assessment practice for multilingual children involves evaluating performance in each language the child uses (Bedore & Peña, 2008; Kohnert, 2010). This reasonable and desirable goal poses challenges for multilingual language sample analysis. Challenges relate to the knowledge that is needed to code and analyze relevant aspects of a sample for assessment and intervention planning in each of the child's languages, the handling of multilingual phenomena such as code switching, as well as the validity of LSA measures for multilingual children. Therefore, speech-language pathologists should gain a basic understanding of language typology (e.g., different phonological systems, word orders, or morphological structures) and a comprehensive understanding of how multilingual children develop skills in each language. Adequate language-specific knowledge is needed on the differences between the speech and language structures of multilingual children with typical development and those of multilingual children with developmental language disorders (DLDs). If evidence on specific speech and language structures is limited, typological language-specific information should be gathered to hypothesize about possible cross-linguistic transfer. Knowledge of the different languages' phonetic inventories is needed in terms of their grammar and rough placement on the analytic (not-inflected) and synthetic (inflected) continuum. If sufficient evidence is available, areas of expected difficulty for multilingual children with various language abilities can be anticipated, bearing in mind that these areas might differ for each language. For example, in heavily inflected languages such as Spanish, Polish, or German, noun-verb agreement is critical to understand meaning. In contrast, languages more toward the analytic pole, such as English, Chinese, or Vietnamese, rely stronger on word order rules to derive meaning (Gutiérrez-Clellen et al., 2000). This information could guide the selection of measures for analysis of the sample to explore aspects of clinical relevance—which might be morphological marking in one language and word order in another. Therefore, when planning an LSA for an individual child, the exploration of prior learning experiences is required to select areas of interest and select target measures in the different languages.

Prior to collecting samples, information should be gathered on the child's learning environment, quantity and quality of exposure to each language, contexts of use, relative proficiency in each language across situations/domains, and language dominance, as all these aspects might influence multilingual language acquisition besides age (Unsworth, 2016). Primary caregivers (i.e., parents) or teachers could be valuable sources of information in this regard. In addition to planning the analysis of the sample, this complementary information may guide the interpretation of LSA measures with bilingual children. For example, if children are assessed in their nondominant language, they may not perform within age expectations, even when compared to their multilingual peers (Ebert, 2020).

Specific measures have been developed for all the purposes that LSA can be utilized for, and many of them are tailored for use with multilingual children. Measures can be divided along a continuum of less language-dependent ones (macrostructural measures), more language-dependent ones, and even dialect-dependent ones (microstructural measures). Macrostructural measures include the evaluation of genre-specific features, such as elements of story grammar or features of explanations, as well as aspects of pragmatic abilities (Govindarajan & Paradis, 2019; Peets & Bialystock, 2015). Microstructural measures target various linguistic levels such as phonology, morphology, or lexicon. Table 6-2 shows examples of language-dependent measures focused on assessing the quantity and quality of utterances by multilingual children.

The first step is the coding of relevant aspects in a sample that can subsequently be analyzed. In general, coding schemes are language specific, as languages vary greatly in their structural features. Detail in coding depends on the aspects of interest in analysis. In addition, measures can be calculated using different units of communication and these units may even be defined differently in some cases. Commonly coded units of LSA measures are utterances, words, morphemes, syllables, or phonemes. A basic annotation in the speech analysis of multilingual children can include the marking of utterances that involve code switching.

If only broad measures are to be calculated, then coding might focus on marking utterances as grammatical or ungrammatical, or linking verb forms to their word roots to ensure that measures of word use are not inflated by the presence of multiple forms of a single word. However, a broad coding of utterances as grammatical or ungrammatical already requires the prior definition of "ungrammaticality" in each language, for example, in the form of a list of errors (Bedore et al., 2010). If the sample analysis aims to gain more detailed insights (e.g., grammatical abilities), various structures must be coded, such as verb tense markers or noun plural, along with various error types. These may differ for each of the child's languages, according to their specific grammatical structure and previous knowledge on the feature's respective relevance in the assessment of DLD.

SALT (Miller & Iglesias, 2012) and CLAN (MacWhinney, 2000) offer coding schemes for several languages and have distinct conventions to segment utterances and label features of typologically diverse languages. For example, word roots and pronominal clitics, relevant for inflected languages such as Spanish, can be identified in SALT conventions. For English and Spanish, these options are even automated in SALT (Rojas & Iglesias, 2006). Furthermore, both software applications offer the assignment of individual codes by users. Thus, coding is influenced by the sample's language, but if the analysis aims for a cross-linguistic perspective, it may need to be aligned to allow comparison across languages (Ebert, 2020).

A unique feature of LSA with multilingual children is that the samples might include code switching. Code switching can be coded, for example in CHAT, but for the sake of convenience these parts may often be excluded from the analysis. This reduces the number of utterances available for analysis, but usually only by a small portion, as researchers in their studies on LSA in assessment contexts (Bedore et al., 2010; Gutiérrez-Clellen et al., 2009) report about 5% to 15% utterances that involve code switching. If sentences with code switching are kept in the sample for analysis, these utterances should not be scored as demonstrating errors, for example, in morphological analysis (Gutiérrez-Clellen, 2000). Further, frequency and type of code switches should not be used as an indicator of DLD, as they occur similarly among multilingual children with various language abilities (Kapantzoglou et al., 2021).

As illustrated in Table 6-2, LSA measures of different depth can be utilized. Linguistic analysis software such as SALT or CLAN, designed to support LSA, offers a variety of different measures for these two objectives, for instance, MLU in words or morphemes, number of different words (NDW), and Type/Token Ratio (TTR; including variants), provided that the samples have been transcribed and coded according to the software's respective conventions.

Table 6-2
Examples of LSA Measures of Utterance Quantity and Quality in Multilingual Children

MEASURES OF QUANTITY	Productivity • Mean Length of Utterance (MLU; Ooi & Wong, 2012; Rojas & Iglesias, 2013; Simon-Cereijido & Gutierrez-Clellen, 2007; Spoelman & Bol, 2012) • Length of the Longest Utterance produced in Words (LU-W; Guiberson, 2020) • Average length of the three longest utternances/C-units (Altman et al., 2016; Guiberson, 2020) • Total Number of Words (TNW; Altman et al., 2016; Guiberson, 2020; Wood et al., 2016) • Total number of Utterances (UTT; Bedore et al., 2010) • Tense and Agreement Productivity (TAP) score (Potapova et al., 2018)
	Fluency • Words Produced per Minute (WPM; Rojas & Iglesias, 2013)
MEASURES OF QUALITY	Complexity • Lexical diversity: ◦ Number of Different Words (NDW; Altman et al., 2016; Bedore et al., 2010; Rojas & Iglesias, 2013; Tsimpli et al., 2016; Washington et al., 2019) ◦ Type/Token Ratio (TTR; Otwinowska et al., 2020) and variants: Moving-Average Type/Token Ratio (MATTR; Hiebert & Rojas, 2021); Average Type/Token Ratio (D/VocD; Ooi & Wong, 2012) • Syntactic diversity: ◦ Clausal density (ratio measure; Cahill et al., 2020; Paradis et al., 2022) ◦ Ratio of subordinate clauses to total number of C-units (Tsimpli et al., 2016) ◦ Complex sentence types (Paradis et al., 2022) ◦ Subordination index/types of subordination (Dam et al., 2020; Kapantzoglou et al., 2017) • Morphological diversity: ◦ Tense Marker Total (TMT; Potapova et al., 2018)
	Accuracy • Percentage of utterances in the sample that are grammatically correct/grammatically incorrect (Bedore et al., 2010; Kapantzoglou et al., 2017; Simon-Cereijido & Gutiérrez-Clellen, 2007) • Error type: ◦ Grammar: ▪ Omission/commission errors (Castilla-Earls et al., 2022) ▪ Composite tense/agreement accuracy measure (Potapova et al., 2018) ▪ Counts of specific errors (e.g., gender, number, classifier, verb tense marking; Dam et al., 2020; Spoelman & Bol, 2012) ◦ Lexicon: ▪ Use of general-purpose verbs (Altman et al., 2016) ◦ Articulation: ▪ Phonological error patterns (Jasso & Potratz, 2020)

While productivity measures of quantity are often included in a LSA, measures of utterance quality such as complexity or accuracy allow more detailed insights into a child's language development and use. Moreover, one language may be the primary focus or, alternatively, comparing all the child's languages may be aimed at. The aspects of interest in each language can either be the same (e.g., productivity/complexity) or language dependent (e.g., the mastery of specific morphosyntactic features or phonemes). For treatment planning, language-specific measures regarding target structures, as well as more detailed measures of complexity are more useful than broader measures of productivity (Cahill et al., 2020).

Besides language, speech may also be a focus of the sample analysis. This can provide the opportunity to compare the child's phonetic inventory and phonological error patterns to those identified in single-word assessment tasks. In addition, the consistency of possible errors can be evaluated across multiple contexts, while other segmental or suprasegmental problems may be revealed and the child's intelligibility can be rated in connected speech (Jasso & Potratz, 2020). Extending the LSA to this area with multilingual children may potentially improve diagnostic accuracy when the two languages of bilingual children are combined, as has been shown for single-word assessment (Fabiano-Smith et al., 2021). Restricting the focus to this area in LSA is the challenge of phonetic transcription (which for multilingual children must be extended to different languages, as has been outlined in the previous section).

Although Table 6-2 outlines a variety of measures for assessing the quantity and quality of utterances by multilingual children, many of these lack supporting evidence and research involving diverse groups of multilingual children should be explored in the future. The applicability of specific LSA measures with multilingual children also needs to be considered carefully. The popular productivity measure MLU, for example, cannot be used for multilingual children where typological differences in inflectional complexity may cause differences in scores. These differences occur as the number of words may be higher in less inflected languages, and therefore MLU is deemed too broad to gain clear insights on complexity (Gutiérrez-Clellen et al., 2000; Otwinowska & Opaki, 2020). Calculating MLU for multilingual children in words instead of morphemes—as is usually done for monolingual English-speaking children—is a way to address this problem of typological differences, as it is less language-dependent and simplifies cross-linguistic comparison (Castilla-Earls, 2022; Ebert, 2020; Otwinowska & Opaki, 2020; Potapova et al., 2018). Another example of multilingual specifications involves measures of morphosyntactic accuracy in the form of language-specific error calculations. These must be based on language typology and research into the adaptation of language-specific markers of DLD for multilingual children (Rothweiler et al., 2012). Regarding vocabulary measures as used with monolingual children, LSA in this area focuses mainly on lexical diversity with NDW being the most popular measure of complexity in studies with multilingual children (Altman et al., 2016; Bedore et al., 2010; Rojas & Iglesias, 2013; Tsimpli et al., 2016; Washington et al., 2019). Code switching could play a more important role in the evaluation of lexical diversity than in other LSA measures used with multilingual children. In a longitudinal study of Spanish/English-speaking children from preschool to early school age, Hiebert and Rojas (2021) found that the inclusion or exclusion of parts of this phenomenon had an impact on Moving-Average Type/Token Ratio (MATTR) and therefore on the assessment of these children's expressive language abilities.

If the cross-linguistic comparison of language-specific measures is a goal of assessment, the typological distance between the two languages should be kept in mind and comparison of distant languages should be made with caution (Otwinowska & Opaki, 2020). Furthermore, it requires the measures to use the same unit of analysis in both languages. For MLU in particular, the mean length should be calculated in words, because this unit avoids language-specific rule sets for calculation. It also allows the analysis of codeswitched passages in the sample and yields more reliable results for different dialects in inflected languages such as Spanish (Gutiérrez-Clellen, 2000). Due to the existence of specific language structures, such as various constructions of sentences, cross-linguistic differences must be expected if language-specific measures are utilized.

Returning to our case sample, it has been evident that Katlego shows signs of a DLD, as his speech and language are affected in both his home language and LoLT. Understanding how to differentiate between children with typical language development and those with DLD (e.g., Katlego) is one of the main goals of assessment. Since standardized testing is often not an available or suitable option for multilingual children, the LSA should be the preferred assessment method.

When diagnosing DLD, norms for monolingual children cannot be applied to multilingual children, even when the same language is assessed. Furthermore, it is inappropriate to apply measures or developmental norms developed for one language to another language, as the characteristics of the other language are not taken into consideration. This principle applies to assessment in general and not just to LSA. Some studies, however, indicate that LSA measures (such as narratives) are less language-dependent at a macrostructure level (Ebert, 2020). To effectively identify children with DLD, assessment measures must be accurate (i.e., highly sensitive and specific, valid, and reliable; Dollaghan & Horner, 2011).

Many LSA measures have been applied in research to draw a comparison between typically developing multilingual children and those with DLD. Yet, the application remains limited due to barriers such as the variability in study characteristics (including age of the participants and the sampling context), few accuracy studies conducted, and contradictory findings on macrostructural and microstructural measures (Altman et al., 2016; Fichman et al., 2016; Govindarajan & Paradis, 2019; Kapantzoglou et al., 2017; Lazewnik et al., 2019; Paradis et al., 2022; Tsimpli et al., 2016). Confounding factors such as language exposure, language proficiency, as well as age of the children have been reported (Ebert, 2020; Paradis et al., 2022).

To simplify differential diagnosis, the developmental stage in the target language and DLD characteristics at certain developmental stages should be considered. Several studies discuss the differences between LSA measures for earlier and later stages of development or language proficiency (Castilla-Earls et al., 2022; Govindarajan & Paradis, 2019; Lazewnik et al., 2019; Ooi & Wong, 2012). In earlier stages of development where abilities in a given language are just emerging, productivity measures (e.g., MLU or TAP), certain error types (e.g., omission errors) and macrostructural measures (e.g., story grammar elements) may be more appropriate to identify language disorders (Castilla-Earls et al., 2022; Govindarajan & Paradis, 2019; Lazewnik et al., 2019; Ooi & Wong, 2012). This is due to the characteristics of language abilities in emerging stages. As stated earlier, MLU is not seen as a measure of complexity, but as a measure of productivity. However, for earlier stages of development it may serve as a measure of grammatical complexity because utterances are formed before grammatical knowledge is refined and therefore MLU could potentially differentiate between multilingual children with and without DLD (Bedore et al., 2010; Ooi & Wong, 2012). Practical measures that can even be transcribed in real time include length of the longest utterance or the average of the three longest utterances produced in words. These measures have been proven to reflect the MLU in mono- and multilingual children (Guiberson, 2020) and may be valuable for speech-language pathologists due to their convenience of coding—provided that additional research provides more evidence on their validity and diagnostic accuracy (Altman et al., 2016).

The type of errors made by multilingual children is linked to their utterance length. With emerging language abilities, children make more omission errors in contrast to commission errors (e.g., substitutions and additions) when they increase their utterance length (Castilla-Earls et al., 2022). Lack of competence in creating narrative macrostructures may also suggest DLD in the early stages (more so in the second language), as story grammar skills can potentially be shared between languages and therefore develop at a faster rate than more language-dependent microstructural aspects (Govindarajan & Paradis, 2019). In contrast, composite accuracy measures that are associated with mastery of specific language structures may be better suited for capturing later stages of development, for example in morphosyntax (Rispoli & Hadley, 2018). When language abilities are emerging, they might be biased by repetitions or formulaic constructions that could lead to an overestimation of abilities (Potapova et al., 2018). Conversely, the diagnostic power of measures of productivity, such as MLU, is discussed controversially in the literature for later stages of development when overall language productivity of children with and without DLD may sometimes show greater overlap (Eisenberg et al., 2001; Eisenberg & Guo, 2013).

Speech and language characteristics for the different age groups can also assist with differential diagnosis. Multilingual children with DLD often exhibit morphosyntactic deficits from the age of 3.5 and older (Simon-Cereijido & Gutiérrez-Clellen, 2007; Kapantzoglou et al., 2017; Paradis et al., 2022; Rothweiler et al., 2012; Spoelman & Bol, 2012) when compared to their monolingual peers. The types of error vary across languages, but often include aspects of morphological verb features or complex syntactic constructions (Cahill et al., 2020; Paradis et al., 2022). Therefore, measures targeting grammar may assist more with the differential diagnosis of DLD than do measures of productivity such as MLU in LSA (Castilla-Earls et al., 2022; Kapantzoglou et al., 2017; Paradis et al., 2022, Verhoeven et al., 2011). More specifically, measures of syntactic complexity, such as clausal density or subordination index, have shown the power to differentiate between groups of typically developing multilingual children and children with DLD (Kapantzoglou et al., 2017; Paradis et al., 2022). In other words, the use of complex syntax measures is less likely to over-identify a language difference as a language disorder (Cahill et al., 2020; Paradis et al., 2017, 2022).

Measures of morphosyntactic accuracy, such as the percentage of grammatical/ungrammatical utterances or specific grammatical errors, are also appropriate to aid with the differential diagnosis of DLD (Altman et al., 2016; Simon-Cereijido & Gutiérrez-Clellen, 2007; Verhoeven et al., 2011). However, specific grammatical errors may vary across languages and may be linked to language experience (Verhoeven et al., 2011). When comparing the accuracy measures, the percentage of correctness may be deemed more universal and easier to code reliably, while specific error measures are more powerful but need evidence-based linguistic adaptation (Ebert, 2020).

Finally, language-specific developmental norms are needed for multilingual children. If database comparison (besides comparing language norms) is desired, the elicitation context of the sample and the developmental history of the children must match, as these may influence the calculation and outcome of measures (Wood et al., 2016). Some of the software programs provide database samples, for instance, SALT provides samples of English/Spanish-speaking children (Pezold et al., 2020). In the case of Katlego, very little is known about multilingual child language development with emphasis on language norms for Sepedi as his home language and English as the LoLT.

Before Katlego's assessment, the speech-language pathologist must decide which LSA measures will be relevant to achieve the objective of assessment. Katlego's level of proficiency in English, the LoLT, should also be considered as this would influence the applicability of some of the measures. As mentioned earlier, some measures are more suitable in the early and later stages of developing a language respectively. Since Katlego speaks English at school, the selection of macrostructural measures of narrative ability could potentially be useful as they are less language-dependent and informative—especially in earlier stages of language development. Complementing these with language-specific microstructural measures of grammatical accuracy or syntactical complexity in both English and Sepedi could add valuable information for diagnosing DLD and for deciding on how to support Katlego in his multilanguage development. For an example how to report multilingual language use, see Chapter 5.

In conclusion, to address all three main components of LSA, the following guidelines should be considered:

- All the multilingual child's languages should be targeted in LSA. Interpreters or native speakers can be of assistance in all three components of the process.
- In collecting data for LSA with multilingual children, age-dependent, contextually relevant, as well as familiar tasks should be favored.

- If multilingual children are to be compared across and within languages using LSA, age, language typology, language learning experience, sampling contexts and utterance length, as well as measure units must be considered carefully.
- Orthographic transcriptions should be compiled of samples in all the child's languages. Phonetic transcriptions will supplement this information and assist with diagnosis.
- Coding must be language specific and follow the requirements of the subsequent analysis.
- Analysis should not be based on singular measures but on a carefully selected bouquet of measures.
- Measures should be selected to fit the focus of assessment, language typology, and the individual child's characteristics, such as early or later stages of development.
- All diagnostic observations should be cross-validated. Integrating information from the LSA, standardized assessment and caregiver/teacher reports can enhance diagnostic accuracy and thus guide clinical decision making.

Potential Benefits and Challenges of Automation for Language Sample Analysis With Multilingual Children

Even though the advantages of LSA in general (and especially in assessing multilingual children) are evident, the time it takes to record, transcribe, annotate, and analyze a sample of child speech and/or language is a significant drawback constantly indicated in the previous sections. Therefore, (partial) automation as one aspect of future development of the method could be key to facilitating routine implementation. With automatic speech recognition becoming more popular in tools such as Siri (Apple) or Alexa (Google), these technological advances extend the possibilities of digital assistance for the evaluation of human language (Kothalkar et al., 2018). An automated support—especially for the most time-intensive component of transcription—could save resources and improve the method's clinical practicability profoundly. Besides increasing process efficiency, automation would also allow the inclusion of audio and text parameters into analysis and strengthen the method's ecological validity by enabling the collection of spontaneous samples in natural communication settings (e.g., at home or in school). These possibilities apply to monolingual as well as multilingual children. For the latter, automation and the resulting possibility of more unrestricted LSA hold additional benefits:

- Ecologically valid information can be obtained about the child's use of all their languages in various everyday settings (i.e., relative proficiency).
- The artificial separation of the child's languages in different elicitation sessions for assessment purposes is no longer required.
- The multilingual learning environment can be evaluated.
- Support is provided for the transcription (and possibly annotation and analysis) of languages that the clinician does not speak.
- Cross-linguistic comparisons are facilitated when large (several-hour-long) samples can be collected, because the burden of manual transcription is lifted.

The potential of introducing automatic speech recognition software into the process of LSA for assessing multilingual children's speech and language is evident. However, although technology has made huge advances over the past decades, the application of LSA to child language and clinical contexts is still in its early stages. To capture the challenges of automatic speech recognition and processing when applied to children, one has to understand how these programs work and how they are developed. Automatic speech recognition is the technology able to convert speech (verbal audio data) to text by analyzing the shape of the speech wave. Automatic speech recognition and subsequent natural language processing are based on machine learning applications, which rely heavily on the input data. These algorithms match the input (e.g., speech) with a set of alternatives (e.g., phones, letters, words) based on input characteristics by employing a set of human-made rules. Lastly, they apply so-called "deep learning" to detect underlying patterns of data solely by using labeled examples of the respective tasks (e.g., manually transcribed audio recording; Alharbi et al., 2021). Both depend on appropriate data to train the models, deep learning models in particular. This is the main cause of delays in the development of automatic speech recognition and processing software for children. Child speech training data is not as available as adult data, and because of children's higher intra- and interspeaker variability (Potamianos & Narayanan, 2003) machine learning models need more data to perform automatic speech recognition and processing accurately.

The lack of suitable data becomes even more evident when considering multilingual children, as in this chapter where Katlego's story was shared. To process more than one language in a recording and possibly even in a singular utterance (as in the case of code switching), the model as a whole or its components need to be trained with multilingual data. An early approach for dealing with multilingual input involved the construction of universal phone sets by pooling all phoneme units of different languages (Schultz & Waibel, 2001). However, this was a very demanding task and has led to an enormous number of acoustic units challenging automatic speech recognition of specific language pairs. Later approaches are implementing feature sharing between models in a more well-conceived way, so that each language can maintain its own phone set (Burget et al., 2010).

Combining language-independent and language-dependent measures remains a popular approach (Huang et al., 2013), and special attention has been given to the differences in available language resources to train models for automatic speech recognition. For Western languages such as English, Spanish, or German, many resources are available—at least for adult speech. Many other languages (e.g., on the African continent) are highly underresourced, but the careful addition of training data from well- or better-resourced languages to a limited training set in the underresourced language should benefit the performance of automatic speech recognition. Deciding which languages to include in the development of models for underresourced languages needs further investigation. Although phonetic overlap may play a role (Tachbelie et al., 2020), other language or recording characteristics should also be considered (van der Westhuizen et al., 2021). To conclude, the potential benefit of automated support for the time-consuming LSA component of transcription is clear. Research therefore focuses on solutions to bypass the exponentiating sparseness of child data (and specifically multilingual child data) by exploring variations in software design.

One example of efforts being taken to provide automated support for language sample analysis is the TALC-project (Tools for Analyzing Language and Communication) of the Leibniz Lab for Relational Communication Research, led by Ulrike Lüdtke, Bodo Rosenhahn, and Jörn Ostermann. In an interdisciplinary, international collaboration, researchers from Germany (Hanna Ehlert, Edith Beaulac, Lars Rumberg, and Christopher Gebauer, Leibniz University Hannover) and South Africa (Juan Bornman, Jeannie van der Linde, University of Pretoria; Febe de Wet, North-West University) are combining expertise from speech-language pathology, computational linguistics, and information technology to develop a system that will support language sample analysis with the use of machine learning models. In the TALC-project, automatic speech recognition software is designed to perform (semi)automatic transcription, annotation, and analysis of child language samples recorded in natural contexts. The software will be trained with data from monolingual children in the beginning, starting with German and Afrikaans, as those are the project languages with the most existing language resources. However, the project's ultimate aim is to enable automated support for language sample analysis with multilingual children as well. To achieve this, spontaneous child data are being collected and specifically processed by the project's researchers to fit the needs of automatic speech recognition development for child speech.

Conclusion

Although LSA is deemed the gold standard for speech and language assessment in multilingual children, the development and identification of measures specifically tailored for such children remains a challenge. In our case scenario, Katlego needs to be assessed by taking samples from both his first language (Sepedi) and his LoLT (English). Since the LSA process may be time consuming, we outlined important guidelines to be considered by speech-language pathologists when they plan and analyze the language samples of multilingual children. Differential diagnoses of DLD and differences in second language acquisition using LSA were also outlined. Most studies involving multilingual children assess the language development of children with English as a second language and Spanish as their first. Unfortunately, developmental language norms for Katlego do not (yet) exist, which is not a unique occurrence in minority-world countries. Future research should be conducted on automated LSA to support speech-language pathologists globally in their quest to routinely implement this potentially informative method in their clinical practice.

References

Alharbi, S., Lrazgan, M., Alrashed, A., Alnomasi, T., Almojel, R., Alharbi, R., Alharbi, S., Alturki, S., Alshehri, F., & Almojil, M. (2021). Automatic speech recognition: Systematic literature review. *IEEE Access, 9*, 131858-131876.

Altman, C., Armon-Lotem, S., Fichman, S., & Walters, J. (2016). Macrostructure, microstructure, and mental state terms in the narratives of English–Hebrew bilingual preschool children with and without specific language impairment. *Applied Psycholinguistics, 37*, 165-193.

Bedore, L. M. & Peña, E. D. (2008). Assessment of bilingual children for identification of language impairment: Current findings and implications for practice. *International Journal of Bilingual Education and Bilingualism, 11*(1), 1-29. https://doi.org/10.2167/beb392.0

Bedore, L. M., Peña, E. D., Gillam, R. B., & Hoa, T.-H. (2010). Language sample measures and language ability in Spanish English bilingual kindergarteners. *Journal of Communication Disorders, 43*(6), 498-510. https://doi/org/10.1016/j.jcomdis.2010.05.002

Boersma, P., & Weenink, D. (2022). *PRAAT: Doing phonetics by computer* (Version 6.2.12) [Computer software]. http://www.praat.org/

Brown, R. A. (1973). *First language: The early stages.* Harvard University Press.

Burget, L., Schwarz, P., Agarwal, M., Akyazi, P., Feng, K., Ghoshal, A., Glembek, O., Goel, N., Karafiát, M., Povey, D., Rastrow, A., Rose, R., & Thomas, S. (2010). Multilingual acoustic modeling for speech recognition based on subspace Gaussian mixture models. *2010 International Conference on Acoustics, Speech and Signal Processing*, Dallas, Texas, USA, 2010, pp. 4334-4337. https://doi.org/10.1109/ICASSP.2010.5495646

Cahill, P., Cleave, P., Asp, E., Squires, B., & Kay-Raining Bird, E. (2020). Measuring the complex syntax of school-aged children in language sample analysis: A known-groups validation study. *International Journal of Language & Communication Disorders, 55*(5), 765-776.

Castilla-Earls, A., Francis, D. J., & Iglesias, A. (2022). The complex role of utterance length on grammaticality: Multivariate multilevel analysis of English and Spanish utterances of first-grade English learners. *Journal of Speech, Language, and Hearing Research, 65*, 238-252.

Cruz-Ferreira, M. (2012). *Multilingual children with speech sound disorders.* Position paper. www.csu.edu.au/research/multilingual-speech/position-paper

Dam, Q., Pham, G., Potapova, I., & Pruitt-Lorda, S. (2020). Grammatical characteristics of Vietnamese and English in developing bilingual children. *American Journal of Speech-Language Pathology, 29,* 1212-1225.

Dollaghan, C. A., & Horner, E. A. (2011). Bilingual language assessment: A meta-analysis of diagnostic accuracy. *Journal of Speech, Language, and Hearing Research, 54,* 1077-1088.

Ebert, K. J. (2020). Language sample analysis with bilingual children: Translating research into practice. *Topics in Language Disorders, 40*(2), 182-201.

Eisenberg, S., & Guo, L.-Y. (2013). Differentiating children with and without language impairment based on grammaticality. *Language, Speech, and Hearing Services in Schools, 44*(1), 20-31. https://doi.org/10.1044/0161-1461(2012/11-0089)

Eisenberg, S., McGovern Fersko, T., & Lundgren C. (2001). The use of MLU for identifying language impairment in preschool children: A review. *American Journal of Speech-Language Pathology, 10,* 323-334. https://doi.org/10.1044/1058-0360(2001/028)

ELAN (Version 6.3) [Computer software]. (2022). *Nijmegen: Max Planck Institute for Psycholinguistics, The Language Archive.* https://archive.mpi.nl/tla/elan

Fabiano-Smith, L., Privette, C., & An, L. (2021). Phonological measures for bilingual Spanish/English-speaking preschoolers: The language combination effect. *Journal of Speech, Language, and Hearing Research, 64,* 3942-3968.

Fichman, S., Altman, C., Voloskovich, A., Armon-Lotem, S., & Walters, J. (2016). Story grammar elements and causal relations in the narratives of Russian-Hebrew bilingual children with SLI and typical language development. *Journal of Communication Disorders, 69,* 72-93.

Finestack, L. H., Payesteh, B., Rentmeester Disher, J., & Julien, H. M. (2014). Reporting child language sampling procedures. *Journal of Speech, Language, and Hearing Research, 57*(6), 2274-2279. https://doi.org/10.1044/2014_JSLHR-L-14-0093

Gavin, W. J., & Giles, L. (1996). Sample size effects on temporal reliability of language sample measures of preschool children. *Journal of Speech, Language, and Hearing Research, 39*(6), 1258-1262. https://doi.org/10.1044/jshr.3906.1258

Govindarajan, K., & Paradis, J. (2019). Narrative abilities of bilingual children with and without developmental language disorder (SLI): Differentiation and the role of age and input factors. *Journal of Communication Disorders, 77,* 1-16.

Gress, K. C., & Hill, E. A. (2018). Language difference or disorder: How do you know? *MinneTESOL Journal, 34*(1), 1-11.

Guiberson, M. (2020). Alternatives to traditional language sample measures with emergent bilingual preschoolers. *Topics in Language Disorders, 40*(2), e1-e6.

Gutiérrez-Clellen, V. F., Restrepo, M., Bedore, L., Peña, E., & Anderson, R. (2000). Language sample analysis in Spanish-speaking children: Methodological considerations. *Language, Speech, and Hearing Services in Schools, 31,* 88-98.

Gutiérrez-Clellen, V. F., Simon-Cereijido, G., & Erickson Leone, A. (2009). Code-switching in bilingual children with specific language impairment. *International Journal of Bilingualism, 13*(1), 91-109.

Heilmann, J., Nockerts, A., & Miller, J. F. (2010). Language sampling: Does the length of the transcript matter? *Language, Speech, and Hearing Services in Schools, 41*(4), 393-404. https://doi.org/10.1044/0161-1461(2009/09-0023)

Heilmann, J., Rojas, R., Iglesias, A., & Miller, J. F. (2016). Clinical impact of wordless picture storybooks on bilingual narrative language production: A comparison of the 'Frog' stories. *International Journal of Language and Communication Disorders, 51*(3), 339-345. https://doi.org/10.1111/1460-6984.12201

Hiebert, L., & Rojas, R. (2021). A longitudinal study of Spanish language growth and loss in young Spanish-English bilingual children. *Journal of Communication Disorders, 92,* 106110.

Huang, J.-T., Li, J., Yu, D., Deng, L., & Gong, Y. (2013). Cross-language knowledge transfer using multilingual deep neural network with shared hidden layers. ICASSP, IEEE, pp. 7304-7308.

International Phonetic Association. (1999). *Handbook of the International Phonetic Association: A guide to the use of the international phonetic alphabet.* Cambridge University Press.

Jasso, J., & Potratz, J. R. (2020). Assessing speech sound disorders in school-age children from diverse language backgrounds: A tutorial with three case studies. *ASHA Perspectives, 5,* 714-725.

Kapantzoglou, M., Esparza Brown, J., Cycyk, L. M., & Fergadiotis, G. (2021). Code-switching and language proficiency in bilingual children with and without developmental language disorder. *Journal of Speech, Language, and Hearing Research, 64*(5), 1605-1620.

Kapantzoglou, M., Fergadiotis, G., & Restrepo, M. A. (2017). Language sample analysis and elicitation technique effects in bilingual children with and without language impairment. *Journal of Speech, Language, and Hearing Research, 60,* 2852-2864.

Kohnert, K. (2010). Bilingual children with primary language impairment: Issues, evidence and implications for clinical actions. *Journal of Communication Disorders, 43*(6), 456-473. https://doi.org/10.1016/j.jcomdis.2010.02

Kothalkar, P. V., Rudolph, J., Dollaghan, C., McGlothlin, J., Campbell, T. F., & Hansen, J. H. (2018). Automatic screening to detect "at risk" child speech samples using a clinical group verification framework. *40th Annual International Conference of the IEEE Engineering in Medicine and Biology Society (EMBC),* pp. 4909-4913.

Lazewnik, C., Creaghead, N. A., Breit Smith, A., Prendeville, J.-A., Raisor-Becker, L., & Silbert, N. (2019). Identifiers of language impairment for Spanish–English dual language learners. *Language, Speech, and Hearing Services in Schools, 50,* 126-137.

Lee, L.L. (1974). *Developmental sentence scoring.* Northwestern University Press.

Lundine, J. P. (2020). Assessing expository discourse abilities across elementary, middle, and high school. *Topics in Language Disorders, 40*(2), 149-165.

MacWhinney, B. (2000). *The CHILDES project: Tools for analyzing talk* (3rd ed.). Erlbaum.

McLeod, S., Verdon, S., Baker, E., Ball, M. J., Ballard, E., David, A. B., Bernhardt, M., Bérubé, D., Blumenthal, M., Bowen, C., Brosseau-Lapré, F., Bunta, F., Crowe, K., Cruz-Ferreira, M., Davis, B., Fox-Boyer, A., Gildersleeve-Neumann, C., Grech, H., ... Zharkova, N. (2017). Tutorial: Speech assessment for multilingual children who do not speak the same language(s) as the speech-language pathologist. *American Journal of Speech-Language Pathology, 26*(3), 691-708.

Miller, J. F., Andriacchi, K., & Nockerts, A. (2019). *Assessing language production using SALT software. A clinician's guide to language sample analysis.* SALT Software LLC.

Miller, J., & Iglesias, A. (2012). *Systematic Analysis of Language Transcripts (SALT)* [Computer software]. SALT Software LLC. https://www.saltsoftware.com/

Munson, B., & Brinkman, K. N. (2004). The effect of multiple presentations on judgments of children's speech production accuracy. *American Journal of Speech-Language Pathology, 13,* 341-354.

Nippold, M. A. (2021). *Language sampling with children and adolescents.* Plural Publishing.

Ooi, C. C.-W., & Wong, A. M.-Y. (2012). Assessing bilingual Chinese-English young children in Malaysia using language sample measures. *International Journal of Speech-Language Pathology, 14*(6), 499-508. https://doi.org/10.3109/17549507.2012.712159

Otwinowska, A., Mieszkowska, K., Białecka-Pikul, M., Opacki, M., & Haman, E. (2020). Retelling a model story improves the narratives of Polish-English bilingual children. *International Journal of Bilingual Education and Bilingualism, 23*(9), 1083-1107. https://doi/org/10.1080/13670050.2018.1434124

Otwinowska, A., & Opaki, M. (2020). Polish–English bilingual children overuse referential markers: MLU inflation in Polish-language narratives. *First Language,* 1-25. https://doi.org/10.1177/0142723720933769

Owens, R. E., Pavelko, S. L., & Bambinelli, D. (2018). Moving beyond mean length of utterance: Analyzing language samples to identify intervention targets. *ASHA Wire.* https://doi.org/10.1044/persp3.SIG1.5

Paradis, J., Rusk, B., Duncan, T. S., & Govindarajan, K. (2017). Children's second language acquisition of English complex syntax: The role of age, input, and cognitive factors. *Annual Review of Applied Linguistics, 37,* 148-167. https://doi/org/10.1017/S0267190517000022

Paradis, J., Sorensen Duncan, T., Thomlinson, S., & Rusk, B. (2022). Does the use of complex sentences differentiate between bilinguals with and without DLD? Evidence from conversational and narrative tasks. *Frontiers in Education, 6,* 804088. https://doi/org/10.3389/feduc.2021.804088

Pascoe, M., Mahura, O., & Rossouw, K. (2020). Transcribing and transforming: Towards inclusive, multilingual child speech training for South African speech-language therapy students. *Folia Phoniatrica et Logopaedica, 72*(2), 108-119. https://doi/org/10.1159/00049942

Pavelko, S. L., & Owens, R. E. (2017). Sampling Utterances and Grammatical Analysis Revised (SUGAR): New normative values for language sample analysis measures. *Language, Speech, and Hearing Services in Schools, 48*(3), 197-215. https://doi.org/10.1044/2017_LSHSS-17-0022

Pavelko, S. L., Owens, R. E., Ireland, M., & Hans-Vaughn, D. L. (2016). Use of language sample analysis by school-based SLPs: Results of a nationwide survey. *Language, Speech, and Hearing Services in Schools, 47,* 246-258. https://doi.org/10.1044/2016_LSHSS-15-0044

Peets, K. F., & Bialystock, E. (2015). Academic discourse: Dissociating standardized and conversational measures of language proficiency in bilingual kindergarteners. *Applied Psycholinguistics, 36,* 437-461. https://doi:10.1017/S0142716413000301

Pezold, M. J., Imgrund, C. M., & Storkel, H. L. (2020). Using computer programs for language sample analysis. *Language, Speech, and Hearing Services in Schools, 51,* 103-114. https://doi.org/10.1044/2019_LSHSS-18-0148

Pillay, M., Tiwari, R., Kathard, H., & Chikte, U. (2020). Sustainable workforce: South African audiologists and speech therapists. *Human Resources for Health, 18*(47), 1-13. https://doi.org/10.1186/s12960-020-00488-6

Potamianos, A., & Narayanan, S. (2003). Robust recognition of children's speech. *IEEE Transactions on Speech and Audio Processing, 11*(6), 603-616.

Potapova, I., Kelly, S., Combiths, P. N., & Pruitt-Lorda, S. L. (2018). Evaluating English morpheme accuracy, diversity, and productivity measures in language samples of developing bilinguals. *Language, Speech, and Hearing Services in Schools, 49,* 260-276. https://doi.org/10.1044/2017_LSHSS-17-0026

Ramírez-Esparza, N., García-Sierra, A., & Kuhl, P. K. (2014). Look who's talking: Speech style and social context in language input to infants are linked to concurrent and future speech development. *Developmental Science, 17*(6), 880-891. https://doi.org/10.1111/desc.12172

Rispoli, M., & Hadley, P. A. (2018). Let's be explicit about the psycholinguistic bases of developmental measures: A response to Leonard, Haebig, Deevy, and Brown (2017). *Journal of Speech, Language, and Hearing Research, 61,* 1455-1459. https://doi.org/10.1044/2018_JSLHR-L-17-0488

Rojas, R., & Iglesias, A. (2006). Bilingual (Spanish-English) narrative language analyses: Why and how? *Communication Disorders and Sciences in Culturally and Linguistically Diverse Populations, 13*(1), 3-8. https://doi.org/10.1044/cds13.1.3

Rojas, R., & Iglesias, A. (2013). The language growth of Spanish-speaking English language learners. *Child Development, 84*(2), 630-646. https://doi.org/10.1111/j.1467-8624.2012.01871.x

Rothweiler, M., Chilla, S., & Clahsen, H. (2012). Subject–verb agreement in specific language impairment: A study of monolingual and bilingual German-speaking children. *Bilingualism: Language and Cognition, 15*(1), 39-57. https://doi:10.1017/S136672891100037X

Scarborough, H. S. (1990). Index of productive syntax. *Applied Psycholinguistics, 11,* 1-22.

Schultz, T., & Waibel, A. (2001). Language-independent and language adaptive acoustic modeling for speech recognition. *Speech Communication, 35*(1), 31-51. https://doi.org/10.1016/S0167-6393(00)00094-7

Shipley, K. G., & McAfee, J. G. (2016). *Assessment in speech-language pathology* (5th ed.). Cengage Learning.

Simon-Cereijido, G., & Gutiérrez-Clellen, V. F. (2007). Spontaneous language markers of Spanish language impairment. *Applied Psycholinguistics, 28*(2), 317-339. https://doi:10.1017/S0142716407070166

Southwood, F., & Russell, A. F. (2004). Comparison of conversation, free play, and story generation as methods of language sample elicitation. *Journal of Speech, Language, and Hearing Research, 47*(2), 366-376. https://doi.org/10.1044/1092-4388(2004/030)

Spoelman, M., & Bol, G. W. (2012). The use of subject–verb agreement and verb argument structure in monolingual and bilingual children with specific language impairment. *Clinical Linguistics and Phonetics, 26*(4), 357-379. https://doi.org/10.3109/02699206.2011.637658

Stemberger, J. P., & Bernhardt, B. M. (2020). Phonetic transcription for speech-language pathology in the 21st century. *Folia Phoniatrica et Logopaedica, 72*(suppl 2), 75-83. https://doi/org/10.1159/000500701

Tachbelie, M. Y., Abate, S. T., & Schultz, T. (2020). Development of multilingual ASR using GlobalPhone for Less-Resourced Languages: The case of Ethiopian languages. *Proceedings of the INTERSPEECH*, 1032-1036.

Tilstra, J., & McMaster, K. (2007). Productivity, fluency, and grammaticality measures from narratives: Potential indicators of language proficiency? *Communication Disorder Quarterly, 29*(1), 43-53. https://doi.org/10.1177/1525740108314866

Tommerdahl, J., & Kilpatrick, C. D. (2014). The reliability of morphological analyses in language samples. *Language Testing, 31*(1), 3-18. https://doi.org/10.1177/0265532213485570

Tsimpli, I. M., Peristeri, E., & Andreou, M. (2016). Narrative production in monolingual and bilingual children with specific language impairment. *Applied Psycholinguistics, 37,* 195-216. https://doi:10.1017/S0142716415000478

Unsworth, S. (2016). Early child L2 acquisition: Age or input effects? Neither, or both? *Journal of Child Language, 43,* 608-634. https://doi/org/10.1017/S030500091500080X

van der Westhuizen, E., Padhi, T., & Niessler, T. (2021). Multilingual training set selection for ASR in under-resourced Malian languages. In A. Karpov & R. Potapova (Eds.), *SPECOM 2021, LNAI 12997* (pp. 749-760).

Verhoeven, L., Steenge, J., & von Balkom, H. (2011). Verb morphology as clinical marker of specific language impairment: Evidence from first and second language learners. *Research in Developmental Disabilities, 32*(3), 1186-1193.

Washington, K. N., Fritz, K., Crowe, K., Kelly, B., & Wright Karema, R. (2019). Bilingual preschoolers' spontaneous productions: Considering Jamaican Creole and English. *Language, Speech, and Hearing Services in Schools, 50,* 179-195.

Westerveld, M. F., & Vidler, K. (2016). Spoken language samples of Australian children in conversation, narration and exposition. *International Journal of Speech-Language Pathology, 18*(3), 288-298. https://doi/org/10.3109/17549507.2016.1159332

Wood, C., Diehm, E. A., & Callender, M. F. (2016). An investigation of language environment analysis measures for Spanish–English bilingual preschoolers from migrant low socioeconomic status backgrounds. *Language, Speech, and Hearing Services in Schools, 47,* 123-134.

Wren, Y., McLeod, S., & Verdon, S. (2020). Transcription of children's speech. *Folia Phoniatrica et Logopaedica, 72*(2), 73-74.

Chapter 7

Assessment of Narratives

A Global Perspective

Marleen F. Westerveld, PhD, FSPA, CPSP
and Carol Westby, PhD, CCC-SLP

Introduction

Narrative discourse is foundational to all social and academic interactions across the lifespan, from sharing a past personal experience with a friend, to writing a fictional story at school, to reminiscing about a holiday 20 years ago. Narrative discourse is a complex task, which requires integration of linguistic, cognitive, and social skills and can be defined as "an account of experience or events that are temporally sequenced and convey some meaning" (Engel, 1995). By this definition, different narrative genres exist, including personal narratives and fictional narratives (McCabe et al., 2008). Personal narratives, defined as accounts of personally experienced events, are one of the most spontaneous and earliest developing forms of discourse (Preece, 1987). Fictional story generation or retelling is less spontaneous and may be considered more difficult for children to produce (Hughes et al., 1997). The importance of differentiating between personal narratives and fictional narratives when discussing narrative assessment also comes from research involving children with language disorders (McCabe et al., 2008), in which children with language disorders demonstrate significant differences in performance across the two genres on measures of length and cohesion, with the quality of a child's performance in one genre only mild-moderately correlated with the child's performance on the other genre.

Bortz, M. (Ed.). *A Guide to Global Language Assessment: A Lifespan Approach* (pp. 131-153).
DOI: 10.4324/9781003524472-9

Assessment of narrative skills should be the cornerstone of the speech-language pathologist's assessment battery for diagnosing language disorders (Hughes et al., 1997) in children, adolescents, and adults (Steel et al., 2021). However, assessment methods need to take numerous factors into consideration, including the client's age and language ability, and also whether the client is from a culturally and/or linguistically diverse background (Paradis, 2016; Rollins et al., 2000). Importantly, narratives are a universal genre, a primary mode of thought. Persons in *all* cultures tell personal and fictional stories, and regardless of a child's cultural and/or linguistic background, the ability to tell a coherent story is critical for participating in everyday activities at home, school, or in the community.

In this chapter, our main focus is on narrative assessment in children, from preschool to adolescence. However, evidence supports extrapolating the findings from the developmental literature to adults, particularly when focusing on the structural organization of narratives (Whitworth et al., 2015). We will start this chapter by considering how children typically develop personal and fictional narratives, followed by an overview of different assessment methods. We then turn our attention to narrative assessment of individuals from culturally and linguistically diverse backgrounds.

Personal Narratives

As outlined by Labov and Waletzky (1967), personal narratives serve two functions: (1) to tell the listener about an event that has happened to the narrator, and (2) to convey to the listener how meaningful the event was to the narrator. As defined by Reese et al. (2011), "a coherent personal narrative is one that *makes sense* to a naïve listener—not just in terms of understanding when, where, and what event took place but also with respect to understanding the meaning of that event to the narrator" (p. 425). Personal narratives make up more than half of children's conversations (Peterson & McCabe, 1983), with competence in personal narrative skills crucial for supporting social interactions underpinning social and psychological well-being (Westby & Culatta, 2016).

Children generally develop the ability to produce past personal event narratives during the preschool period, often scaffolded by their parents. When describing the typical sequence in which children develop their ability to produce a personal narrative, one needs to not only consider what elements the child includes (when, where, what happened, past tense actions, resolution) but also whether the personal narrative is coherent. Results from research into the development of personal narrative proficiency show a general developmental trend (Peterson & McCabe, 1983; Reese et al., 2011). Peterson and McCabe described the development of personal narratives in children ages 4 to 9, using high-point analysis. They found that 3.5-year-olds produced two-event narratives; 4-year-olds produced more than two past events, even though the events were often out of sequence; by age 5, children produced past tense events in a logical order and included a "high point" (i.e., a climax), but no resolution; by age 6, many children were able to produce a classic narrative, containing at least two past events, a climax, and a resolution. Reese et al. (2011) appraised personal narratives on three dimensions: context, chronology, and theme. Their results indicated that preschoolers showed little evidence of coherence; and although their narratives were on topic, few children included contextual information and chronology was poor. School-aged children (ages 6 and 8) provided some context information and better performance on chronology. By adolescence, students began to develop causal coherence in their stories, making links between their actions and their personality or sense of identity (Habermas & Silveira, 2008). This is an important aspect of personal narratives in adults.

Fictional Narratives

Research investigating oral narrative ability in preschool and school-aged children has clearly demonstrated the importance of fictional narrative proficiency for academic and social success, both concurrently and longitudinally (Bishop & Edmundson, 1987; Boudreau, 2008; Feagans & Appelbaum, 1986; Griffin et al., 2004). To illustrate, children who demonstrate better oral narrative skills during the preschool years show better oral language and reading comprehension skills during the early school years; conversely, children who struggle producing well-structured oral narratives are at increased risk of academic underachievement. Considering narrative skills are strongly associated with reading comprehension throughout the school years (Babayiğit et al., 2021), assessment of fictional narratives is a critical component of language assessment in school-aged children.

The ability to produce fictional narratives gradually develops during the preschool years. To produce oral narratives, children need adequate skills across several language domains, at word-, sentence-, and text-level. At word- and sentence-level (also referred to as microstructure level), children need adequate skills in semantics (vocabulary) and syntax. Although vocabulary and syntactic structures, as measured on standardized language tests, are foundational for narrative skills, they are insufficient for explaining narrative structure and use. At macrostructure level, children need to demonstrate the ability to produce a coherent, well-sequenced narrative containing important story grammar elements including setting, initiating event (or problem), internal response (or goal), attempts, and resolution (Stein & Glenn, 1979). At macrostructure level, problem-oriented narratives can be defined as a sequence of goal-directed actions by the protagonist to solve a problem (Trabasso et al., 1992). At age 3, children may produce descriptive statements unrelated to the overall problem of the narrative; by age 4, children start including goal-directed attempts, but may sequence them temporally as opposed to causally. By 5 years of age, children start to organize their narratives around a goal and plan. Beyond the preschool years, children continue to develop their narrative skills, with 9-year-olds producing well-structured, goal-oriented narratives across multiple episodes.

Although much of the research has focused on fictional narrative *production*, the importance of narrative *comprehension* should not be ignored (Boudreau, 2008; Skarakis-Doyle & Dempsey, 2008). From a theoretical perspective, narrative comprehension and production are linked (Kintsch, 2005). According to the construction-integration model, one may hypothesize that oral narrative comprehension relies on the activation of mental models (schemas) of stories in long-term memory. These mental models help guide the listener's understanding of the overall structure of the story, as well as the characters' actions, which in turn facilitate story recall. To fully understand a narrative, the listener requires both factual and inferential comprehension, with inferential comprehension comprising the ability to (1) infer causal relationships between events or actions described in the story; (2) identify the internal states of the character (related to the goal); and (3) draw on background knowledge to fill "gaps" in the story or to make predictions (Kintsch, 2005; Rapp & van den Broek, 2005). From a developmental perspective, 4-year-old children show the ability to answer questions about the protagonist's main problem (Filiatrault-Veilleux et al., 2016) and can draw mental state inferences (Ford & Milosky, 2003). By 6 years of age, children are able to deduce consequences of actions/events as well as the actions needed to solve the problem. They may also be able to predict what will happen next (Adams et al., 2009).

Narrative Assessment Methods

Personal Narratives

It is important to distinguish between personal narratives and scripts. As described by Hughes et al. (1997), scripts are accounts of familiar, routine events and are generally told in the timeless present tense. An example of a script is when the child tells you what generally happens when they go to kindergarten or when they get up in the morning. Personal narratives tap into one particular experience and are told in the past tense, for example, when the child tells you what happened when they went to kindergarten that morning.

Assessment of Personal Narratives

Assessment of personal narratives can be conducted in a variety of ways, although the impact of specific elicitation methods on children's personal narrative production skills has not been well researched. Peterson and McCabe (1983) suggested using a conversational map technique in which the examiner provides the child with a short prompting narrative (e.g., "I went to the doctor because I had a sore throat"), followed by the question, "Did anything like that ever happen to you?", to encourage the child to share one of their own personal experiences. Prompts included experiences such as illness, bee stings, car accidents, holidays, and pet adventures. In an adaptation of this task, Westerveld and colleagues successfully used a series of photos with short prompting narratives to encourage children to share their own experiences (Westerveld et al., 2004; Westerveld & Vidler, 2016). The overall idea is to prompt the child to share an experience that is meaningful to them (Peterson & McCabe, 1983), regardless of the elicitation method.

Prompt Topics. Peterson and McCabe (1983) used the conversational map technique with children ages 3.5 to 9.5, and evaluated which prompts were more successful than others. Successful prompts tapped "stand-out" experiences as opposed to those that children engage in regularly (which are more likely to elicit scripts). The most successful prompts for eliciting lengthy narratives included trips, car wrecks, hospitalizations, and pets. Fivush et al. (2003) asked 5- to 12-year-old children raised in violent communities to narrate both positive and negative experiences. Interestingly, children produced more coherent narratives, containing more information about their thoughts and feelings, when referring to negative experiences. In contrast more descriptive detail was included when narrating positive experiences.

Tasks. With 3- and 4-year-old children, researchers successfully engaged children in a pretend zoo activity and prompted the children approximately 2 weeks later to "tell me everything that happened when you went to the pretend zoo" (Reese & Newcombe, 2007). Other tasks that have been used successfully include prompting children to recount special events selected by their mothers (4- to 6-year-olds), listing and describing positive and negative personal experiences related to school (6- to 14-year-olds), and recalling negative and/or positive experiences or something that happened "to change your life and is still really important" (11- to 14-year-olds; Reese et al., 2010, 2011).

When eliciting personal narratives, the aim is to engage the child in the task, to minimize self-consciousness, and to encourage the child to produce a meaningful narrative. Table 7-1 presents a summary of factors that need to be considered when eliciting personal narratives from children, with examples of elicitation stimuli.

Table 7-1
Considerations for Stimuli When Eliciting Personal Narratives

STIMULI	CONSIDERATIONS
Engaging the child/adolescent/adult in conversation. Child may spontaneously produce personal narratives.	This method may be time consuming. Most spontaneous. The child may not produce any personal narratives.
Use of scripted prompts (in general): "Tell me about an exciting experience you have had; a scary experience."	Consider including both positive and negative experiences; for older students, a life-changing experience. Some prompts are likely to elicit scripts (e.g., birthday parties, trips).
Scripted prompts embedded in conversation (no pictures): "I took my cat to the vet last summer and when the vet was about to give him a shot, my cat took off and ran around the office. Do you have any cats or other pets?" (If necessary: "Did anything ever happen to your __ ?") (Peterson & McCabe, 1983, p. 16).	May reduce the child's self-consciousness.
Scripted prompts with generic photos: "This little girl had to go to the doctor, because she had a bad cough. Have you ever been to the doctor?" "These children went to the beach in the summer holidays. They dug a big hole and waited for the sea to fill it up! Have you ever been to the beach? What happened last time you went to the beach?" (Westerveld et al., 2004).	Child may choose to describe the picture rather than a past personal event. May be more time efficient than prompts embedded in conversation. Picture scenes may not be familiar to some children (e.g., snow, beach, mountains).
Social problem-solving prompt: "Tell me a story about a time someone asked you to do something you knew you weren't supposed to do. Tell me what you were thinking and how you solved the problem" (e.g., Noel & Westby, 2014). "Tell me the story of a time when someone wanted your help and you didn't want to give it to them." "Tell me what you were thinking and how you solved the problem."	These prompts are best for older elementary students and adolescents. They require that students have a meta-awareness of their behavior. These could also be useful for adults with traumatic brain injury as a way of assessing their executive functioning.
Written prompts: "Tell me about the most important moment in your life. How did that moment change you?" "Write about a time when you felt successful. What happened that led to your success?" "Think about the best day you have ever had. What happened on that day that made it so great?"	May work well with older children or adults, who may not mind/prefer this more formal approach. Written prompts often ask the person to reflect on or evaluate the experience.

Analyzing Personal Narrative Skills

Analysis of a child's personal narrative performance can be at microstructure and/or macrostructure level. Commonly used microstructure measures include (1) semantics: number of different words; (2) syntax: mean length of utterances (MLU), clausal density, or subordination index; (3) morphology: MLU in morphemes; as well as (4) verbal fluency (mazing behavior); and (5) verbal productivity—total number of words or number of utterances. However, other measures may better capture the quality or coherence of the personal narrative. One example of a tool for evaluating coherence is the Narrative Assessment Profile (NAP; Peterson & McCabe, 1983) that covers the following aspects: topic maintenance, event sequencing, informativeness, referencing, conjunctive cohesion, and fluency. Other approaches for evaluating personal narratives at macrostructure level include high-point analysis (as outlined previously) and story grammar analysis (i.e., inclusion of setting, character/s, problem, plan, actions, resolution, and conclusion). Considering the fact not all personal narratives are goal-directed with clear actions, resolutions, and conclusions, we agree with Hughes et al. (1997) that a story grammar approach, such as the one used in the Narrative Language Measures (NLM; Petersen & Spencer, 2012), is more suitable for analyzing fictional narratives. Table 7-2 provides an overview of some of the tools and methods that are available for analyzing personal narratives at macrostructure level.

Fictional Narratives

It is important to acknowledge the impact of the elicitation context (comprehension, generation vs. retell) as well as the elicitation condition (e.g., picture support, use of a model story, auditory vs. oral presentation) on children's oral narrative performance, as the level and type of support provided may influence an individual's performance at both microstructure and macrostructure level. This is particularly important if the aim of the assessment is to describe a child's strengths and challenges in narrative skills (across microstructure and macrostructure measures).

Assessment of Fictional Narratives

We will first discuss some of the factors that need to be taken into consideration when assessing fictional narratives. We will then summarize the different types of microstructure and macrostructure level supports that can be provided when eliciting fictional narratives.

Generation or retell. The first choice is whether to use a story generation (i.e., asking someone to tell a story without listening to a story first) or retell task (e.g., asking someone to retell a story after listening to story). Although generation tasks may be considered more spontaneous, the advantage to using a retell task is that retold narratives are generally longer, contain longer utterances, and comprise a higher number of different words (Westerveld & Gillon, 2010b). Moreover, story retells contain more story grammar elements and complete episode structures and are easier to score (Merritt & Liles, 1989). In contrast, story retells are influenced by the complexity of the model story (Holloway, 1986) and the story itself may not conform to the child's cultural expectations (Gutiérrez-Clellen & Quinn, 1993), which we will discuss in more detail later.

Table 7-2
Tools for Analyzing Personal Narrative Samples at Macrostructure Level

TOOLS/MEASURES	ELEMENTS	COMMENTS REGARDING AGE GROUPS/CULTURES
Narrative Assessment Profile (NAP; Bliss et al., 1998) Personal narratives are scored on six elements.	• Topic maintenance • Event sequencing • Informativeness • Referencing • Conjunctive cohesion • Fluency	The NAP has been used with child and adult populations (e.g., Bearman et al., 2021; Biddle et al., 1996).
Narrative Coherence Coding Scheme (NCCS; Reese et al., 2011) Each element of coherence is scored (levels 0 to 3).	• Context • Chronology • Theme	The NCCS has been used with individuals aged between 3 and 60 years, across a range of English-speaking countries.
High Point Analysis (Peterson & McCabe, 1983) Personal narratives are scored and categorized according to inclusion of the elements.	• Past tense events • Logical/causal sequence • Narrated sequence mirrors actual sequence • High point (concentration of evaluative comments) • Resolution	There seems to be developmental trend between ages 3.5 and 6 in English-speaking children.
Adapted from Labov and Waletzky (1967) and Peterson and McCabe (1983), as described in Rollins et al. (2000)	• Orientation • Action • Evaluation • Resolution • Coda	Evidence that children from a range of cultures include all elements (except resolution; see Rollins et al., 2000). Authors suggest asking a member of the child's culture to appraise the child's personal narrative for quality/inclusion of the elements and/or observing child and parent co-construct a narrative and observe which elements are highlighted by the parent for inclusion.
Narrative Language Measures (NLM; Petersen & Spencer, 2012) Macrostructure (and microstructure) elements scored on 0- to 3-point scale.	• Character • Setting • Problem • Plan/attempt • Consequence • Ending • Emotion	Pre-K to third-grade students are asked to generate a personal narrative based on a model narrative they listened to. May not be suitable for analyzing personal narratives that are not goal-oriented.

The use of picture stimuli. There are numerous options regarding the use of pictures (or not) prior to and/or during the story retell or generation task. When asking children to generate a story, evidence supports the use of a complex wordless picture book over a single-scene picture (Pearce, 2003), with children producing longer, more informative, and more complex stories in the picture book condition. Another consideration is whether to allow the child to refer to the pictures when retelling a story (see also Mills, 2015). Although allowing the child to refer to the pictures when retelling a story is less dependent on the child's memory of the story, research suggests children produce more complex language and use more specific vocabulary when retelling a story (based on four pictures; 160 words) without the support of pictures (Masterson & Kamhi, 1991). However, contrasting results were found by Westerveld and Heilmann (2012) with children in the picture support condition producing longer stories, containing more different words and a higher narrative structure score than children who did not have access to the pictures. There were no differences in syntactic complexity. The most likely explanation for these differences at microstructure level is the much longer stories used in the Westerveld and Heilmann study (*Frog, Where Are You?* [Mayer, 1969]; 515 words, 29 pictures).

Allowing a child to refer to the pictures when telling a story may mask a child's difficulty comprehending a story (Reuterskiöld Wagner et al., 1999). In a study of 5-year-olds, no correlations were found between children's story grammar scores (i.e., macrostructure level performance) and their ability to answer questions, leading the authors to conclude that the children may have been able to obtain story grammar points without fully understanding the causal links depicted in the story. This may also explain the findings by Westerveld and Heilmann (2012), who found that children obtained higher macrostructure scores when retelling a story in a picture support condition.

The types of stories. Because the main aim of fictional narrative assessment is to evaluate whether the child can produce a well-sequenced, goal-directed story containing all essential story grammar elements, most assessment tasks contain problem-based stories (Hudson & Shapiro, 1991) or goal-oriented story starters (Cain, 2003). One of the most frequently used stories is the wordless picture book *Frog, Where Are You?* (Mayer, 1969), which has been used with children and adults in many countries around the world, including children with developmental language disorder (DLD) and autism spectrum disorder (Berman & Slobin, 1994; Heilmann et al., 2010; Norbury & Bishop, 2003; Strömqvist & Verhoven, 2004; Westerveld & Heilmann, 2012).

Other considerations. Other factors influencing the child's narrative production skills include the number of exposures to the model story and the use of a naïve listener (Liles, 1985; Masterson & Kamhi, 1991), with children producing more complex sentences containing more specific vocabulary in the naïve listener situation (i.e., the examiner is unfamiliar to the story). Finally, the speech pathologist needs to be aware of potential linguistic trade-offs, which Crystal (1987) referred to as the bucket theory. Consistent with a limited capacity working memory model, if cognitive processing is required for one linguistic operation (e.g., to access and retain the story structure model during retelling), less capacity may be available for other linguistic operations, such as grammatical complexity or verbal fluency.

Deciding the level of support. Table 7-3 provides a summary overview of considerations regarding microstructure and macrostructure task supports when eliciting a story retell from children. Microstructure supports involve providing children with models of the types of words, temporal and causal connectives, and syntactic patterns to use when telling the story. Macrostructure supports may be provided either by verbally modelling a story that contains all the narrative macrostructure elements (e.g., character, setting, initiating event/problem, response, plan, consequence, resolution) or by providing a picture story sequence that would include the macrostructure elements. Although all the narrative macrostructure elements may be in the picture story sequence, children must interpret the pictures appropriately if they are to include the elements in the story they tell. Hence, retelling a story which they listened to while looking at a picture sequence provides the most microstructure and macrostructure support. In contrast, generating a story from a story prompt (e.g., "Tell me a story about the dog that learned to fly"), a story starter (e.g., "I dug quickly and then my shovel hit something hard"), or a single picture provides the least microstructure and macrostructure support.

With younger children or children with known DLD, you may decide to use tasks or stimuli that provide more micro- and macrostructure support such as retells with picture support. Use of story retells or stimuli with picture sequences may provide too much support for older or more capable students, resulting in not identifying possible narrative difficulties. For older or more capable students, story generation with limited support (a story starter statement or a single picture) may be more informative of their narrative skills. These tasks and stimuli place a higher cognitive load on students, as they require more working memory. Students must have internalized knowledge of narrative macrostructure, be able to organize the macrostructure, and produce the appropriate microstructure sentences to coherently convey the story content. For students who are being evaluated for DLD, it is beneficial to use a variety of narrative tasks and stimuli to determine how they respond to various levels of support. This information is useful in determining intervention strategies.

Analyzing Fictional Narrative Skills

At microstructure level, the most common measures to appraise performance include (1) semantics: number of different words; (2) syntax: MLU, clausal density, or subordination index; (3) morphology: MLU in morphemes; as well as (4) verbal fluency (mazing behavior); and (5) verbal productivity: total number of words or number of utterances (Ebert & Scott, 2014; Scott & Windsor, 2000; Westerveld & Gillon, 2010a). At macrostructure level, numerous coding schemes have been put forward, including the Narrative Scoring Scheme (Heilmann et al., 2010), Oral Narrative Quality (Westerveld & Gillon, 2010a), the Strong Narrative Assessment Protocol (Strong, 1998), and the Monitoring Indices of Scholarly Language (MISL; Gillam & Gillam, 2015). Other methods include counting the number of story grammar components and the number of episodes (Merritt & Liles, 1989). Finally, Westby (2005) devised a decision tree for determining a child's level of narrative organization. Figure 7-1 shows the hierarchical stages of narrative development from the decision tree that evaluates the child's narrative level: an inability to sequence more than one event (descriptive sequence), a temporally related sequence of a series of events (action sequence), a causally related sequence of events (reactive sequence), a story that implies goal-directed behavior by the protagonist (abbreviated episode), a story with specific references to intentional behavior (complete episode), and an elaborated story (e.g., complex, multiple episode, embedded episode). The micro- and macrostructure narrative measures used with children are also appropriate for adults (Whitworth et al., 2015), including those with aphasia and traumatic brain injury (Marini et al., 2011). Adults with traumatic brain injury may have normal lexical and grammatical skills, but they are likely to produce narratives with increased errors of cohesion and coherence due to the frequent interruption of ongoing utterances, derailments, and extraneous utterances that made their discourse vague and difficult to understand.

Table 7-3
Considerations for Stimuli When Eliciting Fictional Narratives From Children

STIMULI	TASK SUPPORT/ REQUIREMENTS	EXAMPLE OF A TASK
Picture sequence, story retell	Macro- and microstructures provided, complexity of the model story will influence the child's performance, child relies on memory of the story, pictures reduce working memory load	The child is asked to retell a story after listening to a story depicted in a picture sequence, for example, using the Multilingual Assessment Instrument for Narratives (MAIN; see https://main.leibniz-zas.de/).
Picture sequence, story generation after listening to a different story	Macro- and microstructures provided, complexity of the model story will influence the child's performance, child does not rely on memory of the story, pictures reduce working memory load	The child is asked to generate their own story after listening to a different but similar story sequence (e.g., MAIN).
Picture sequence, story generation	Pictures provide macrostructure but child must recognize the story schema, pictures reduce working memory load, child must generate microstructures	The child is asked to generate a story based on a picture sequence, for example, the Edmonton Narrative Norms Instrument (ENNI; Schneider et al., 2005) or the MAIN.
Wordless picture book, story retell with pictures	Macro- and microstructures provided, complexity and length of the model story will influence the child's performance, child relies on memory of the story, pictures reduce working memory load	Child is shown the wordless picture book *Frog, Where Are You?* (Mayer, 1969) and asked to listen to the story while viewing the pictures. The child is then asked to retell the story with the pictures as support.
Wordless picture book, story retell without pictures	Macro- and microstructures provided, complexity and length of the model story will influence the child's performance, two exposures of the story may reduce child's reliance on memory of the story, child needs to draw on internalized story schema when retelling the story	Child is shown a wordless picture book and asked to listen to the story while viewing the pictures. The child is then asked to retell the story without the pictures as support (e.g., Westerveld & Gillon, 2002).
Wordless picture book, story generation	Pictures provide macrostructure but child must recognize the story schema, pictures reduce working memory load, greater working memory load than picture sequence	Child is shown the wordless picture book *Frog, Where Are You?* (Mayer, 1969) and is asked to look through the pictures of the book once, before telling the story in their own words.
Video, story generation	Videos give students more cues for interpreting the story macrostructure than wordless picture books, watching the video twice may reduce memory demands	Pixar shorts are particularly useful for eliciting story generation for students across ages.

(continued)

Table 7-3 (continued)
Considerations for Stimuli When Eliciting Fictional Narratives From Children

STIMULI	TASK SUPPORT/ REQUIREMENTS	EXAMPLE OF A TASK
Single scene picture, story generation	Child must draw on internalized story schema, child must simultaneously generate the macro- and microstructures; high working memory load	The child is shown a single picture (e.g., the alien story from the *Test of Narrative Language* [Gillam & Pearson, 2017], and asked to tell a story.
Retell story from auditory only stimuli (one exposure)	Macro- and microstructures provided, complexity of the model story will influence the child's performance, child relies on memory of the story	Child listens to a verbally presented story (without pictures) and is asked to retell the story (see Schneider & Dubé, 2005).
Story title, story generation	Child must draw on internalized story schema, child must simultaneously generate the macro- and microstructures, high working memory load	The child is asked to generate a story when provided with a story title, for example, "Elephant Is Lonely."

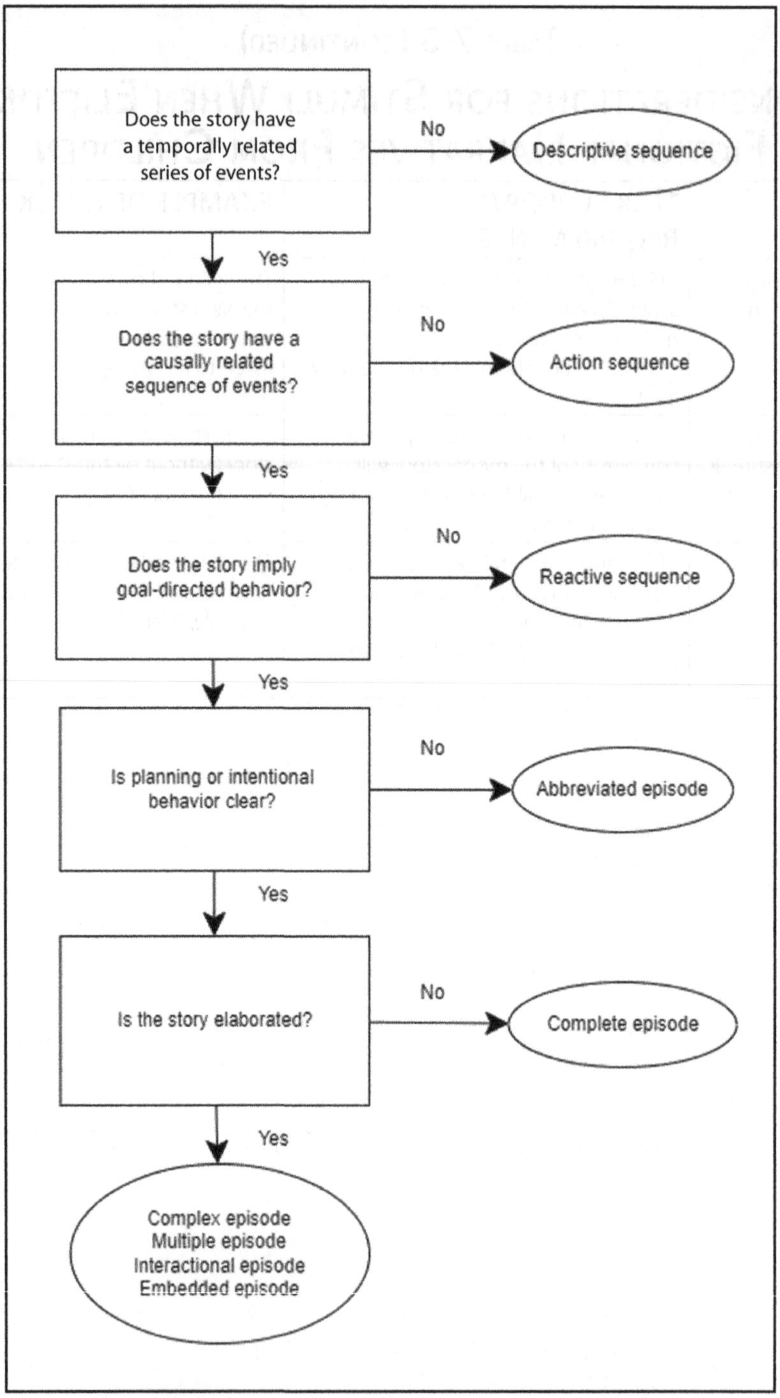

Figure 7-1. Developmental hierarchy of narrative structure from least to most complex (Story Grammar Decision Tree). (Kamhi, A. G., & Catts, H., *Language and reading disabilities* [3rd ed.], © 2012. Reprinted by permission of Pearson Education, Inc.)

Narrative Skills of Children From Culturally and/or Linguistically Diverse Backgrounds

As outlined in Chapter 2 (Westby, 2024), conducting language assessments of multilingual speakers and/or of those from culturally diverse backgrounds may be particularly challenging, with a real risk of under- or overidentifying children as language disordered. The risk of using standardized tests to identify language disorders in children from culturally and linguistically diverse backgrounds has been well researched (Paul et al., 2018; Pearce & Williams, 2013) and the argument for using more ecologically valid discourse-level language tasks, such as narrative tasks, has been well established (McCabe & Bliss, 2003).

Fictional Narratives

At macrostructure level, research generally demonstrates the universal nature of the structural organization (i.e., macrostructure) of a story (Berman & Slobin, 1994), with typically developing children showing the ability to apply their knowledge of the macrostructure of a story obtained in their L1, to their L2 (Hipfner-Boucher et al., 2015; Westerveld, 2014). However, children's performance on these tasks may still appear "disordered" if children from culturally diverse backgrounds are unfamiliar with the overall organization of the narrative, potentially resulting in challenges with macrostructure aspects when telling or retelling a story or when producing personal narratives. Interestingly, a study by Pearce and Flanagan (2020) investigating the narrative retell skills of young school-aged Indigenous Australian children compared to their non-Indigenous peers found no group differences in story complexity (macrostructure elements) using three different protocols: a story retell without pictures (Westerveld & Gillon, 2010a), a story retell with pictures, and a story generation (using pictures) specifically designed to minimize cultural challenges. These results were unexpected, considering traditional Aboriginal Australian story style is nonlinear and nonhierarchical, with significant emphasis on people and place. The authors hypothesized that perhaps the exposure to problem-oriented and goal-directed stories during their (limited) time at school influenced these children's narrative performance. However, another potential explanation is that the children may have responded to the cultural expectations of their listener with respect to the amount of information to include, the stylistic strategies to use, or the sequence in which the narrative should be told (Gutiérrez-Clellen & Quinn, 1993). All children were assessed at school, using traditional narrative tasks as opposed to a more culturally appropriate yarning approach, using an interactional, conversational style as opposed to a more direct "testing" style (Lewis et al., 2017).

Personal Narratives

When asking children to produce personal event narratives, some narrative themes are common across cultures such as themes of villains, lack or loss, trickery, or hero journeys. Yet stories across cultures can vary in a number of ways: who tells stories, how children are socialized to tell stories, and the functions, content, structure, and style of stories. Moreover, "social cognitive theory adopts an agentic perspective to human development" (Bandura, 2002, p. 269). According to this theory there are three modes of agency: personal agency exercised individually, proxy agency in which one attempts to influence others to reach desired outcomes, and collective agency in which people act cooperatively to help shape the future (Bandura, 2002). Of interest is that although people may demonstrate all three agencies when sharing personal stories, the relative contribution of each of these agencies may vary across cultures. For example, personal narratives produced by people from collectivist cultures may demonstrate relatively stronger collective agency than those produced by people from individualistically oriented cultures. In clinical practice one must consider how all of these factors may influence data collection and analyses, while avoiding biased generalizations. We agree that when working with children from cultures other than one's own, collaboration with participants from that culture is essential. Unfortunately, in reality, that is not always possible. Table 7-4 shows examples of these narrative variations across cultures (Chang & McCabe, 2013; Rollins et al., 2000; Westby, 2021).

Narrative Skills of Bilingual Children

Evaluation of bilingual children's narrative skills at microstructure level needs to consider the child's proficiency in their L1 and L2. As summarized by Paradis (2016), if children speak a minority language at home, after 2 years of exposure to English—regardless of their L1 background—approximately 65% of children score as well as their monolingual English-speaking peers on a standardized test of receptive vocabulary. Children's rate of morphological development is even more highly dependent on their L1, with only 45% of children meeting monolingual age-based expectations after more than 2 years of exposure to English. In contrast, after 3 years of exposure to English, 100% of children reached monolingual age expectations on a macrostructure measure of narrative performance (Paradis, 2016). Considering the importance of vocabulary and morphosyntactic skills when producing a narrative, it is not surprising that bilingual children tend to score relatively low on narrative microstructure measures (e.g., sentence length) compared to their monolingual peers, despite adequate performance at macrostructure level (Paradis & Kirova, 2014).

When assessing bilingual children, assessment in both languages is highly recommended, but not always feasible due to the high number of language combinations clinicians may encounter in daily practice (Boerma & Blom, 2017). Results from Boerma and Blom's research suggest that a combination of two unbiased language assessments (nonword repetition task and analysis of a child's narrative skills at macrostructure level), combined with results from a parent report questionnaire (e.g., presence of speech, language, learning or literacy problems in the family), showed excellent diagnostic validity in monolingual children (94% sensitivity, 93% specificity). In a bilingual group, a combination of the parent report measure, a nonword repetition task and narrative comprehension and production (at macrostructure level) showed high diagnostic validity (sensitivity and specificity 97%) in the bilingual group.

Table 7-4

Considerations for Stimuli When Eliciting Fictional Narratives From Children

NARRATIVE VARIATIONS	EXAMPLES
Who tells stories	Any child or adult, only adults, children of a particular age/gender
How children are socialized to telling stories	By watching and listening to adults tell stories, by reminiscing with adults, in scaffolded conversational interactions with adults, in a monologue vs. co-constructed with others, in scaffolded interactions with story books
Functions of stories	To entertain, teach, gossip, explain, warn, share experiences, display knowledge, reflect on self, recount experience
Content/themes of stories	Universal (villainy, lack/loss, trickery, hero journey), culturally/gender-specific themes
Type of character agency portrayed in the personal narrative	Direct personal agency (individual self) • People bring their influence to bear directly on themselves and their environment in managing their lives • Proxy agency (relational self) • People rely on others to act on one's behalf to secure desired outcomes Collective agency (collective self) • People act together to shape their future • Exercised through socially coordinated and interdependent methods
Structure of stories	Linear (explicit temporal-causal sequence), digressive (extraneous material for elaboration), topic-centered vs. topic associative; circular/indirect, goal-directed agency to achieve vs. focus on accepting/adjusting
Style of stories	Very accurate factually, exaggeration for interest, content conveyed only through words vs. content also conveyed through prosody, intonation, repetitions, sound effects (e.g., Gee, 1989; Heath, 1983)

Examples of Global Initiatives

Global TALES

The Global TALES (Talking About Lived Experiences in Stories) project is an initiative of the Child Language Committee (CLC) of the International Association of Communication Sciences and Disorders (IALP). In this project, an international team of researchers (including Australia, New Zealand, United Kingdom, United States, Russia, Israel, Cyprus, and Greece) set out to investigate methods for eliciting and analyzing children's personal event narratives. The aim of this project is to develop global tools and approaches to support interventions for this important skill in children with significant challenges in their learning, including those with language disorders.

During 2018 and 2019, the CLC developed an elicitation protocol (the Global TALES protocol; Westerveld et al., 2020) and conducted a pilot study in which the protocol was used to elicit personal narratives from monolingual 10-year-old children from 10 different countries, across eight different languages (Westerveld et al., 2022). The protocol is freely available from https://osf.io/ztqg6/. When developing the protocol, the following features were taken into account:

1. *Pictures.* It was decided not to use pictures to avoid cultural bias.
2. *Topic prompts.* The prompts covered a range of feelings and emotions, both positive and negative, including excited/happy, worried/confused, annoyed/angry, and feeling proud. It also contained two prompts in which children were asked about a time they had a problem and an event that was important to them.
3. *Generation.* To avoid cultural bias children were not provided with a model personal narrative, they were simply asked to "tell a story."

One important aspect of piloting the project was to obtain feedback from researchers regarding the process of adapting the protocol for use in their own country or language. The main issue was translation. Although no significant difficulties were reported, some researchers opted not to use word-for-word translation, but translated the prompts for meaning instead. Others reported using a process of back-translation. There were some language-specific translation challenges. For example, the word "annoyed" was not easily translated into Portuguese; the word "worried" was not easily understood by Icelandic children. (For research updates, please visit https://osf.io/ztqg6)

Multilingual Assessment Instrument for Narratives

The Multilingual Assessment Instrument for Narratives (MAIN) was specifically developed for assessing fictional narrative skills in children who acquire one or more languages from birth or from an early age. All resources are freely available from the website https://main.leibniz-zas.de/. As described on the website, "It contains four parallel stories, each with a carefully designed six-picture sequence based on a multidimensional model of story organization. The stories are controlled for cognitive and linguistic complexity, parallelism in macrostructure and microstructure, as well as for cultural appropriateness and robustness." Each story comprises three episodes, and the basic structure of each story consists of setting, goal, attempt, and outcome. When eliciting the story, the examiner can: (1) ask the child to generate a story (with the pictures), (2) ask the child to retell a story after listening to the story, and (3) generate their own story after listening to a different, but similar story sequence (i.e., baby birds, baby goats). The assessment task also contains 10 comprehension questions. The way the task is administered ensures that the child thinks the examiner has not seen the pictures before, thus promoting a naïve listener situation.

The assessment underwent more than 200 revisions, was piloted in more than 12 countries, and has been used with more than 500 mono- and bilingual children, ages 3 to 10, across 15 different language combinations. At macrostructure level, the stories are analyzed for story structure components, structural complexity, and internal mental state terms. At microstructure level, analysis focuses on narrative length and lexis, morphosyntactic complexity and discourse cohesion, and syntactic complexity (Gagarina et al., 2016). Finally, story comprehension questions assess goals and internal states as well as background knowledge. The test can be used to assess the child's narrative language proficiency across languages by using parallel stories several days apart.

The results to date clearly indicate this tool is suitable for assessing macrostructural narrative abilities in diverse cultures and regions of the world (Armon-Lotem et al., 2015). However, not all studies that used the MAIN protocol found similar macrostructure scores across children's L1 and L2 (Kapalková et al., 2016), with amount of exposure to L2 a potential factor.

A detailed explanation on how to adapt MAIN to other languages is described in Bohnacker and Gagarina (2019). We will review some of the main considerations.

- *Generation or retell.* The MAIN assessment contains both a generation and a retell task. Kunnari et al. (2016) recommend that the story generation task may provide better insight into a child's ability to independently produce a narrative, which may be particularly useful for children who do not have an equal balance between L1 and L2.
- *Pictures.* There are four MAIN picture story sets, with all stories using six-picture stimuli. Two of the four-story sets involve a human character and all four have animals: a cat, a dog, baby birds, or baby goats. As outlined by the authors, the objects and characters were chosen to suit a variety of cross-cultural environments and piloted in a range of countries. As a result, some changes were made to the pictures such as adjusting the skin color of the boy, adjusting the colors of the animals, or replacing certain items (i.e., chicken legs rather than sausages). The stories/pictures have been successfully used in at least 20 different languages across the world. It is interesting to note that some researchers requested more substantial changes to the pictures to better suit their cultural environment, although no specifics are provided.
- *Other considerations.* The task itself conforms to a Western-style assessment methodology in which a child is asked to generate or retell a story in the presence of an examiner. The picture sequence itself contains a goal-directed story schema that may not conform to different story telling styles such as "yarning" that is explained by Lewis et al. (2017) or a Hawaiian "talk story" (Boggs, 1985).

Adapting Narrative Protocols

Based on the current evidence, we suggest clinicians and researchers take a range of factors into account when adapting/translating fictional and/or personal narrative protocols for use in different countries (cultures and/or languages). These considerations are summarized in Table 7-5.

Table 7-5
Factors to Consider When Adapting Narrative Protocols for Use Across the Globe

	CONSIDERATION	EXAMPLES
Fictional Narratives		
Pictures	Are the pictures culturally appropriate? Consider if the child can identify with the main character/s, the setting, the actions of the characters.	In some Indigenous cultures you cannot tell stories of animals when they are hibernating.
Use of model story/picture sequence	Does the model story adhere to the structure of a story children typically engage in? Goal-directed stories are not commonly used in all cultures.	Traditional Aboriginal Australian story style is nonlinear and nonhierarchical, with significant emphasis on people and place. Place is also an important aspect of the story in Southwest American Indian stories.
Vocabulary	Is there a translation equivalent? When translated, does the word carry the same meaning?	"Annoyed" is not easy to translate in Portuguese.
Syntax	When translating the model story, does it affect the morphosyntactic complexity? Are temporal/causal relationships explicitly stated?	Many languages have a different morphological system (e.g., Hebrew). In some cultures people are expected to infer the causal relationships (e.g., Mandarin Chinese).
Administration	Does the administration conform to cultural expectations?	Consider if the child identifies with the examiner, the examiner's culture. The child produces the story independently or the child produces the story collaboratively (with a peer/examiner).
Personal Narratives		
Pictures	Are the pictures culturally appropriate? Can the child identify with the scene?	Beach (or snow) pictures for children living in Outback Queensland may not be appropriate.
Prompts	Are the prompts culturally appropriate? Is there content that cannot be shared with those not from the culture?	For example, theme parks and school trips may not be appropriate. Korean children reported it was not appropriate to talk about being annoyed with a person.
Use of a model narrative	Does the model adhere to the structure of a personal event narrative children typically produce?	Personal stories in Western cultures focus on the storyteller and their perspective; In Eastern cultures personal stories give more attention to others involved in the event and the storyteller may tell the story from an observer perspective.
Administration	Is it in line with cultural norms to produce a personal event narrative to an unfamiliar adult?	Consider involving someone from the same culture.

Conclusion

In this chapter we highlighted the importance of assessing both fictional *and* personal narratives. Although the importance of fictional narratives to classroom participation and academic achievement has been well established, analysis of personal narratives provides insight into a person's ability to use language to connect with others, a vital communication skill for participating in society, and closely linked with socioemotional well-being.

We emphasize the need for careful consideration of elicitation methods and tasks to obtain accurate, reliable, and representative narrative samples from individuals across the lifespan and from a range of cultural and/or linguistic backgrounds. Furthermore, we argued for a developmental perspective on the use of stimuli, with some individuals requiring more micro (linguistic) or macro (story schema) support than others. Throughout this chapter we encouraged evidence-based reflective practice by focusing on the most important factors to consider when assessing and/or analyzing narrative skills of children, adolescents, and adults.

References

Adams, C., Clarke, E., & Haynes, R. (2009). Inference and sentence comprehension in children with specific or pragmatic language impairments. *International Journal of Language & Communication Disorders, 44*(3), 301-318. https://doi.org/10.1080/13682820802051788

Armon-Lotem, S., de Jong, J., & Meir, N. (2015). *Assessing multilingual children: Disentangling bilingualism from language impairment.* Multilingual Matters.

Babayiğit, S., Roulstone, S., & Wren, Y. (2021). Linguistic comprehension and narrative skills predict reading ability: A 9-year longitudinal study. *British Journal of Educational Psychology, 91*(1), 148-168,

Bandura, A. (2002). Social cognitive theory in cultural context. *Applied Psychology, 51*(2), 269-290.

Bearman, M., Westerveld, M., Brubacher, S. P., & Powell, M. (2021). The ability of adults with limited expressive language to engage in open-ended interviews about personal experiences. *Psychiatry, Psychology, and Law,* 29(2), 241-255. https://doi.org/10.1080/13218719.2021.1904453

Berman, L., & Slobin, D. (1994). *Relating events in narrative: Across linguistic developmental study.* Lawrence Erlbaum Associates. Inc., Publishers.

Biddle, K. R., McCabe, A., & Bliss, L. S. (1996). Narrative skills following traumatic brain injury in children and adults. *Journal of Communication Disorders, 29*(6), 447-469. https://doi.org/10.1016/0021-9924(95)00038-0

Bishop, D. V. M., & Edmundson, A. (1987). Language-impaired 4-year-olds: Distinguishing transient form persistent impairment. *Journal of Speech and Hearing Disorders, 52,* 156-173.

Bliss, L. S., McCabe, A., & Miranda, A. E. (1998). Narrative assessment profile: Discourse analysis for school-age children. *Journal of Communication Disorders, 31,* 347-363.

Boerma, T., & Blom, E. (2017). Assessment of bilingual children: What if testing both languages is not possible? *Journal of Communication Disorders, 66,* 65-76. https://doi.org/https://doi.org/10.1016/j.jcomdis.2017.04.001

Boggs, S. T. (1985). *Speaking, relating, and learning: A study of Hawaiian children at home and at school.* Greenwood Publishing Group.

Bohnacker, U., & Gagarina, N. (2019). Background on MAIN—Revised, how to use it and adapt it to other languages. *ZAS Papers in Linguistics, 63,* iv-xii.

Boudreau, D. (2008). Narrative abilities: Advances in research and implications for clinical practice. *Topics in Language Disorders, 28*(2), 99-114.

Cain, K. (2003). Text comprehension and its relation to coherence and cohesion in children's fictional narratives. *British Journal of Developmental Psychology, 21,* 335-351. https://doi.org/10.1348/026151003322277739

Chang, C.-J., & McCabe, A. (2013). Evaluation in Mandarin Chinese children's personal narratives. *Chinese Language Narration: Culture, Cognition, and Emotion, 19,* 33-56.

Crystal, D. (1987). Towards a "bucket" theory of language disability: Taking account of interaction between linguistic levels. *Clinical Linguistics and Phonetics, 1,* 7-22.

Ebert, K. D., & Scott, C. M. (2014). Relationships between narrative language samples and norm-referenced test scores in language assessments of school-age children. *Language, Speech, and Hearing Services in Schools, 45*(4), 337-350. https://doi.org/10.1044/2014_LSHSS-14-0034

Engel, S. (1995). *The stories children tell: Making sense of narratives in childhood.* W. H. Freeman.

Feagans, L., & Appelbaum, M. I. (1986). Validation of language subtypes in learning disabled children. *Journal of Educational Psychology, 78,* 358-364.

Filiatrault-Veilleux, P., Bouchard, C., Trudeau, N., & Desmarais, C. (2016). Comprehension of inferences in a narrative in 3- to 6-year-old children. *Journal of Speech, Language, and Hearing Research, 59*(5), 1099-1110. https://doi.org/10.1044/2016_JSLHR-L-15-0252

Fivush, R., Hazzard, A., McDermott Sales, J., Sarfati, D., & Brown, T. (2003). Creating coherence out of chaos? Children's narratives of emotionally positive and negative events. *Applied Cognitive Psychology, 17*(1), 1-19. https://doi.org/10.1002/acp.854

Ford, J. A., & Milosky, L. M. (2003). Inferring emotional reactions in social situations: Differences in children with language impairment [Research Support, U.S. Gov't, P.H.S.]. *Journal of Speech, Language, and Hearing Research, 46*(1), 21-30. https://doi.org/10.1044/1092-4388(2003/002)

Gagarina, N., Klop, D., Tsimpli, I. M., & Walters, J. (2016). Narrative abilities in bilingual children. *Applied Psycholinguistics, 37*(1), 11-17. https://doi.org/10.1017/S0142716415000399

Gee, J. P. (1989). Two styles of narrative construction and their linguistic and educational implications. *Discourse Processes, 12*(3), 287-307.

Gillam, S., & Gillam, R. (2015). *Monitoring indices of scholarly language.* https://cdn-links.lww.com/permalink/tld/a/tld_2015_12_07_sandra_1500023_sdc2.pdf

Gillam, R. B., & Pearson, N. A. (2017). *Test of Narrative Language—2.* Pro-Ed.

Griffin, T. M., Hemphill, L., Camp, L., & Palmer Wolf, D. (2004). Oral discourse in the preschool years and later literacy skills. *First Language, 24,* 123-127. https://doi.org/10.1177/0142723704042369

Gutiérrez-Clellen, V. F., & Quinn, R. (1993). Assessing narratives of children from diverse cultural/linguistic groups. *Language, Speech, and Hearing Services in Schools, 24*(1), 2-9.

Habermas, T., & Silveira, C. D. (2008). The development of global coherence in life narratives across adolescence: Temporal, causal, and thematic aspects. *Developmental Psychology, 44*(3), 707-721. https://doi.org/10.1037/0012-1649.44.3.707

Heath, S. B. (1983). *Ways with words: Language, life, and work in communities and classrooms.* Cambridge University Press.

Heilmann, J., Miller, J. F., Nockerts, A., & Dunaway, C. (2010). Properties of the Narrative Scoring Scheme using narrative retells in young school-age children. *American Journal of Speech-Language Pathology, 19*(2), 154-166. https://doi.org/10.1044/1058-0360(2009/08-0024)

Hipfner-Boucher, K., Milburn, T., Weitzman, E., Greenberg, J., Pelletier, J., & Girolametto, L. (2015). Narrative abilities in subgroups of English language learners and monolingual peers. *International Journal of Bilingualism, 19*(6), 677-692. https://doi.org/10.1177/1367006914534330

Holloway, K. F. C. (1986). The effects of basal readers on oral language structures: A description of complexity. *Journal of Psycholinguistic Research, 15,* 141-151.

Hudson, J. A., & Shapiro, L. R. (1991). From knowing to telling: The development of children's scripts, stories, and personal narratives. In A. McCabe & C. Peterson (Eds.), *Developing narrative structure* (pp. 89-136). Lawrence Erlbaum.

Hughes, D., McGillivray, L., & Schmidek, M. (1997). *Guide to narrative language: Procedures for assessment.* Thinking Publications.

Kapalková, S., Polišenská, K., Marková, L., & Fenton, J. (2016). Narrative abilities in early successive bilingual Slovak–English children: A cross-language comparison. *Applied Psycholinguistics, 37*(1), 145-164. https://doi.org/10.1017/S0142716415000454

Kintsch, W. (2005). An overview of top-down and bottom-up effects in comprehension: The CI perspective. *Discourse Processes, 39*(2-3), 125-128. https://doi.org/10.1080/0163853X.2005.9651676

Kunnari, S., Välimaa, T., & Laukkanen-Nevala, P. (2016). Macrostructure in the narratives of monolingual Finnish and bilingual Finnish–Swedish children. *Applied Psycholinguistics, 37*(1), 123-144,

Labov, W., & Waletzky, J. (1967). Narrative analysis: Oral versions of personal experience [in J. Helm (Ed.). Essays on the verbal and visual arts (pp. 12-44). University of Washington Press.]. *Journal of Narrative and Life History, 7*(1997), 3-38.

Lewis, T., Hill, A. E., Bond, C., & Nelson, A. (2017). Yarning: Assessing Proppa ways. *Journal of Clinical Practice in Speech Language Pathology, 19*(1), 14-18.

Liles, B. Z. (1985). Cohesion in the narratives of normal and language-disordered children. *Journal of Speech and Hearing Research, 28*, 123-133.

Marini, A., Galetto, V., Zampieri, E., Vorano, L., Zettin, M., & Carlmagno, S. (2011). Narrative language in traumatic brain injury. *Neuropsychologia, 49*(10), 2904-2910. https://doi.org/10.1016/j.neuropsychologia.2011.06.017

Masterson, J. J., & Kamhi, A. G. (1991). The effects of sampling conditions on sentence production in normal, reading-disabled, and language-disabled children. *Journal of Speech and Hearing Research, 34*, 549-558.

Mayer, M. (1969). *Frog, where are you?* Penguin Putnam.

McCabe, A., & Bliss, L. S. (2003). *Patterns of narrative discourse. A multicultural lifespan approach.* Allyn & Bacon.

McCabe, A., Bliss, L., Barra, G., & Bennett, M. (2008). Comparison of personal versus fictional narratives of children with language impairment. *American Journal of Speech-Language Pathology, 17*(2), 194-206. https://doi.org/10.1044/1058-0360(2008/019)

Merritt, D. D., & Liles, B. Z. (1989). Narrative analysis: Clinical applications of story generation and story retelling. *Journal of Speech and Hearing Disorders, 54*, 429-438.

Mills, M. T. (2015). The effects of visual stimuli on the spoken narrative performance of school-age African American children. *Language, Speech, and Hearing Services in Schools, 46*(4), 337-351. https://doi.org/10.1044/2015_LSHSS-14-0070

Noel, K. K., & Westby, C. (2014). Applying theory of mind concepts when designing interventions targeting social cognition among youth offenders. *Topics in Language Disorders, 34*(4), 344-361.

Norbury, C. F., & Bishop, D. V. M. (2003). Narrative skills of children with communication impairments. *International Journal of Language & Communication Disorders, 38*(3), 287-313. https://doi.org/10.1080/136820310000108133

Paradis, J. (2016). The development of English as a second language with and without specific language impairment: Clinical implications. *Journal of Speech, Language, and Hearing Research, 59*(1), 171-182. https://doi.org/doi:10.1044/2015_JSLHR-L-15-0008

Paradis, J., & Kirova, A. (2014). English second-language learners in preschool: Profile effects in their English abilities and the role of home language environment. *International Journal of Behavioral Development, 38*(4), 342-349. https://doi.org/10.1177/0165025414530630

Paul, R., Norbury, C. F., & Gosse, C. (2018). *Language disorders from infancy through adolescence. Listening, speaking, reading, writing, and communicating* (5th ed.). Mosby Elsevier.

Pearce, W. M. (2003). Does the choice of stimulus affect the complexity of children's oral narratives? *Advances in Speech-Language Pathology, 5*(2), 95-103.

Pearce, W. M., & Flanagan, K. (2020). Story-telling abilities of young indigenous and non-indigenous Australian children across three protocols. *International Journal of Speech-Language Pathology, 22*(2), 206-215. https://doi.org/10.1080/17549507.2019.1648550

Pearce, W. M., & Williams, C. (2013). The cultural appropriateness and diagnostic usefulness of standardized language assessments for indigenous Australian children. *International Journal of Speech-Language Pathology, 15*(4), 429-440. https://doi.org/10.3109/17549507.2012.762043

Petersen, D. B., & Spencer, T. D. (2012). The narrative language measures: Tools for language screening, progress monitoring, and intervention planning. *Perspectives on Language Learning and Education, 19*(4), 119-129.

Peterson, C., & McCabe, A. (1983). *Developmental psycholinguistics: Three ways of looking at a child's narrative.* Plenum.

Preece, A. (1987). The range of narrative forms conversationally produced by young children. *Journal of Child Language, 14*, 353-373.

Rapp, D. N., & van den Broek, P. (2005). Dynamic text comprehension: An integrative view of reading. *Current Directions in Psychological Science, 14*(5), 276-279.

Reese, E., & Newcombe, R. (2007). Training mothers in elaborative reminiscing enhances children's autobiographical memory and narrative. *Child Development, 78*(4), 1153-1170. https://doi.org/10.1111/j.1467-8624.2007.01058.x

Reese, E., Yan, C., Jack, F., & Hayne, H. (2010). Emerging identities: Narrative and self from early childhood to early adolescence. In *Narrative development in adolescence* (pp. 22-43). Springer.

Reese, E., Haden, C. A., Baker-Ward, L., Bauer, P., Fivush, R., & Ornstein, P. A. (2011). Coherence of personal narratives across the lifespan: A multidimensional model and coding method. *Journal of Cognition and Development, 12*(4), 424-462. https://doi.org/10.1080/15248372.2011.587854

Reuterskiöld Wagner, C., Sahlen, B., & Nettelbladt, U. (1999). What's the story? Narration and comprehension in Swedish preschool children with language impairment. *Child Language Teaching & Therapy, 15*(2), 113-137. https://doi.org/doi:10.1177/026565909901500202

Rollins, P. R., McCabe, A., & Bliss, L. (2000). Culturally sensitive assessment of narrative skills in children. *Seminars in Speech & Language, 21*(3), 223-233.

Schneider, P., & Dubé, R. V. (2005). Story presentation effects on children's retell content. *American Journal of Speech-Language Pathology, 14*(1), 52-60.

Schneider, P., Dubé, R. V., & Hayward, D. (2005). *The Edmonton Narrative Norms Instrument.* http://www.rehab-research.ualberta.ca/enni.

Scott, C. M., & Windsor, J. (2000). General language performance measures in spoken and written narrative and expository discourse of school-age children with language learning disabilities. *Journal of Speech, Language, and Hearing Research, 43*(2), 324-339.

Skarakis-Doyle, E., & Dempsey, L. (2008). Assessing story comprehension in preschool children. *Topics in Language Disorders, 28*(2), 131-148.

Steel, J., Elbourn, E., & Togher, L. (2021). Narrative discourse intervention after traumatic brain injury: A systematic review of the literature. *Topics in Language Disorders, 41*(1), 47-72.

Stein, N., & Glenn, C. (1979). An analysis of story comprehension in elementary school children. In R. O. Freedle (Ed.), *New directions in discourse processing* (Vol. 2, pp. 53-120). Ablex.

Strömqvist, S., & Verhoven, L. (2004). Typological and contextual perspectives on narrative development. In *Typological and Contextual Perspectives* (pp. 3-14). Psychology Press.

Strong, C. J. (1998). *The Strong Narrative Assessment Profile.* Thinking Publications.

Trabasso, T., Stein, N. L., Rodkin, P. C., Park Munger, M., & Baughn, C. R. (1992). Knowledge of goals and plans in the on-line narration of events. *Cognitive Development, 7*(2), 133-170. https://doi.org/10.1016/0885-2014(92)90009-g

Westby, C. (2021). The influence of culture on storytelling. In C. Deam (Ed.), *Story frames for teaching literacy: Enhancing student learning through the power of storytelling* (pp. 241-256). Brookes.

Westby, C. (2024). The ICF framework and global assessment. In M. Bortz (Ed.), *A guide to global language assessment: A lifespan approach.* SLACK Incorporated.

Westby, C. E. (2005). Assessing and remediating text comprehension problems. In H. W. Catts & A. G. Kamhi (Eds.), *Language and reading disabilities* (2nd ed., pp. 157-232). Pearson Education.

Westby, C., & Culatta, B. (2016). Telling tales: Personal event narratives and life stories. *Language, Speech, and Hearing Services in Schools, 47,* 260-282. https://doi.org/10.1044/2016_LSHSS-15-0073

Westerveld, M., & Gillon, G. (2002). *Westerveld and Gillon language sampling protocol.* University of Canterbury: Department of Speech and Language Therapy. https://www.marleenwesterveld.com

Westerveld, M., Nelson, N., Fernandes, F. D. M., Ferman, S., Gillon, G., McKean, C., Petinou, K., Tumanova, T., Vognidroukas, I., Westby, C., Theodrorou, E., Moonsamy, S., Einarsdottir, J. T., & Quinanilla Cobian, M. A. (2023, August 21). *Global TALES Project Protocol 2018.* https://doi.org/10.17605/OSF.IO/6TA5G

Westerveld, M. F., Gillon, G. T., & Miller, J. F. (2004). Spoken language samples of New Zealand children in conversation and narration. *Advances in Speech-Language Pathology, 6*(4), 195-208. https://doi.org/10.1080/14417040400010140

Westerveld, M. F., & Gillon, G. T. (2010a). Profiling oral narrative ability in young school-aged children. *International Journal of Speech-Language Pathology, 12*(3), 178-189. https://doi.org/10.3109/17549500903194125

Westerveld, M. F., & Gillon, G. T. (2010b). Oral narrative context effects on poor readers' spoken language performance: Story retelling, story generation, and personal narratives. *International Journal of Speech-Language Pathology, 12*(2), 132-141. https://doi.org/10.3109/17549500903414440

Westerveld, M. F., & Heilmann, J. J. (2012). The effects of geographic location and picture support on children's story retelling performance. *Asia Pacific Journal of Speech, Language and Hearing, 15*(2), 129-143. https://doi.org/10.1179/jslh.2012.15.2.129

Westerveld, M. F. (2014). Emergent literacy performance across two languages: Assessing four-year-old bilingual children. *International Journal of Bilingual Education and Bilingualism, 17*(5), 526-543. https://doi.org/10.1080/13670050.2013.835302

Westerveld, M. F., & Vidler, K. (2016). Spoken language samples of Australian children in conversation, narration and exposition. *International Journal of Speech-Language Pathology, 18*(3), 288-298. https://doi.org/10.3109/17549507.2016.1159332

Westerveld, M. F., Lyons, R., Nelson, N. W., Chen, K. M. Claessen, M., Ferman, S., Fernandes, F. D. M., Gillon, G. T., Kawar, K., Kuvač Kraljević, J., Petinou, K., Theodorou, E., Tumanova, T., Vogandroukas, I., & Westby, C. (2022). Global TALES feasibility study: Personal narratives in 10-year-old children around the world. *PLoS ONE, 17*(8), e0273114. https://doi.org/10.1371/journal.pone.0273114

Whitworth, A., Claessen, M., Leitão, S., & Webster, J. (2015). Beyond narrative: Is there an implicit structure to the way in which adults organise their discourse? *Clinical Linguistics & Phonetics, 29*(6), 455-481. https://doi.org/10.3109/02699206.2015.1020450

Part III

SPECIFIC EXAMPLES OF GLOBAL ASSESSMENTS

Chapter 8

Partnering to Develop a Community-Based Measure of Expressive Language in Guatemala

Lisa Domby, MS, CCC-SLP
and Maria Elizabeth Jaramillo, MS, MPH, CCC-SLP

Introduction

Our experience in communication disorders, bilingualism, cross-cultural service delivery, global health, and collaboration with colleagues in Guatemala led us to develop the *Prueba brillo de lenguaje expresivo y relatos personales* (Brillo Assessment of Spanish Grammar and Personal Narratives; Brillo), with the aim of supporting Spanish-language development outcomes of Guatemalan children. We incorporated methodologies from education, global health, psychology, and anthropology to increase our confidence that our measure is appropriate for the local community.

A language assessment measure should reflect local cultural and linguistic variables. Engaging directly with the community increases the likelihood that stimulus items and instructions will be culturally and linguistically appropriate. By cultivating competencies for effective global engagement, we can collaborate to develop tools that adequately address the needs of the population served, overcoming common barriers in lower-resource settings. Guatemala is culturally and linguistically rich, with 22 Mayan languages, two additional Indigenous languages, and Spanish as the official language. The Instituto Nacional de Estadística Guatemala estimates the 2020 population at approximately 17 million, with 6 million belonging to Indigenous ethnic groups. The name Guatemala is derived from the K'iche Mayan word for "many trees," Cuauhtēmallān. When Spaniards invaded Guatemala in 1524, they imposed Spanish language and cultural standards, along with suppression of Mayan

Bortz, M. (Ed.). *A Guide to Global Language Assessment: A Lifespan Approach* (pp. 157-175).
DOI: 10.4324/9781003524472-11

people and their languages and complex cultural practices (Grandin et al., 2011). The Academia de Lenguas Mayas de Guatemala (ALMG), formally recognized in 1990, promotes preservation of Mayan languages, standardized written language systems for these languages, and support for bilingual education. Most speakers of Mayan languages also speak Spanish, which is spoken by around 93% of the population of Guatemala. In remote areas, Spanish is less likely to be spoken. The primary author has collaborated with interpreters and cultural liaisons when working with Tz'utujil speakers in Sololá and Kaqchikel speakers in Sacatepéquez.

The American Speech-Language-Hearing Association Ad Hoc Committee to Develop Guidance for Members and Students Engaging Globally in Clinical, Scholarly, and Other Professional Activities (Hallowell et al., 2021) recommends a checklist to guide ethical global engagement. This chapter outlines implementation of each principle on the checklist as we developed an assessment measure of Spanish grammar and narrative language in Guatemala. We illustrate our process of cultural and linguistic adaptation of a child language assessment procedure and discuss cultural influences pertaining to narrative language production.

Engaging Host Partners in Program Design and Determination of the Non–United States Participants' Needs and Desires

The Brillo assessment described in this chapter developed from an ongoing professional collaboration with Lcda. Leticia Lopez, a Guatemalan psychologist and speech-language therapist who is the founder of Collegio Brillo de Sol, an inclusive nongovernmental school serving children with special education needs. The school's mission is to transform the lives of children through education and rehabilitation by attending to the humanity of each child in a way that respects their individuality and unique learning needs. As a result of a conversation regarding misdiagnosis of children with speech and language impairment, Lcda. Lopez requested assistance with developing an assessment tool to measure and document language learning for Guatemalan children in the local area.

The assessment process is central to educational and rehabilitative services for children with language disorders in school settings. There are many barriers to providing services for developmental delays to children in lower- and middle-resource countries, among which are the lack of appropriate assessments and trained professionals to administer assessments (Maulik & Darmstadt, 2007; Small et al., 2019). Most research that impacts health and educational outcomes for children with developmental disabilities is conducted in high-resource countries, while the majority of the world's children live in lower- and middle-resource countries (Durkin et al., 2015; Erskine, 2016; Wallace et al., 2012).

Considering Resource Implications and Addressing Related Ethical Concerns

When administering diagnostic measures, it is important to consider whether they were developed and normed for communities that share the same cultural, linguistic, and socioeconomic characteristics. It is equally important to consider the level of education and training of the individuals who will administer, score, and interpret the assessment tool. A key barrier common among limited resource settings is lack of access to advanced training programs for professionals who would administer developmental assessments such as those created for use in the United States context (Hartley & Newton, 2009). Collaborative methods improve awareness of local needs and our ability to serve these populations. Engaging the community that we serve in the development of assessment measures increases our confidence that the measure meets the assessment needs of that community.

Attending to Sustainability and Continuity

To build sustainable services for people with communication disorders in developing countries, speech-language pathologists can function to build capacity of other service providers rather than functioning solely as clinicians working with individual clients (Wickenden, 2013). Through principles of effective global engagement, we can build collaborative partnerships and increase local service capacity. We utilized competencies proposed by Hyter et al. (2017) to guide our attitudes and dispositions, knowledge, and skills as we engaged in the process of developing a culturally and linguistically responsive language assessment measure in Guatemala. (These competencies are explained in Chapter 1, Introduction.) We considered the goals of the assessment tool as well as the barriers to language assessment for the context of our partner community.

The culmination of this project is a language assessment measure that can be administered by Guatemalan speech-language therapists and special education teachers. This project furthered our understanding of the complex process of cultural and linguistic adaptation of a child language assessment. Importantly, we characterized the goals and perceptions of local partners as we collaborated in this process. Additionally, we engaged in a broader dialogue on cultural aspects of narrative production and assessment. This project illustrates how competent engagement can guide our research and service in global contexts. Our methods for this project were intentionally designed to gather input to ensure local goals are met and the tool is appropriately implemented.

Ensuring Reciprocity and Mutuality

Willingness to provide services and engage with others from a posture of reciprocity is more likely to yield effective global engagement (Hyter et al., 2017). Cultural humility and self-awareness facilitate our ability to work in partnership to improve services to marginalized populations. Speech-language pathologists can effectively engage in global exchange of knowledge and skills by collaborating in needs assessment to ensure reciprocity and sustainability.

The need for an authentic measure of Spanish grammar and narrative language development in Guatemala and the inception of the project emerged, and continues to be guided, through a professional collaboration with the Director of Brillo de Sol. Most speech-language therapists *(terapistas de lenguaje)* in Guatemala do not have access to standardized language assessment measures. Importantly, the current level of training in Guatemala does not meet examiner qualifications for these measures, such as coursework in statistics and psychometrics. They may rely on measures intended for pass/fail screening of speech and language development. Thus, speech-language services may target goals that are not optimal for the characteristics of the individual child.

Considering Brillo de Sol's emphasis on healthy emotional and social expression, we discussed the functional relevance of personal narrative skills and their importance in the development of social and academic language (Chapter 7; Westby & Culatta, 2016). We also discussed potential methods of collecting and analyzing expressive language that are appropriate for the level of training of Guatemalan speech-language therapists.

Considering Resource Implications and Addressing Related Ethical Concerns

We hosted an informal "lunch and learn" workshop for Guatemalan teachers, speech-language therapists, and university speech-language students during which we illustrated various procedures for eliciting and analyzing personal narratives. Prior to the workshop, each teacher had been asked to identify one child in their class who they would describe as having well-developed language skills. We obtained brief narratives from each child about their school experiences. The workshop participants read these narratives aloud and discussed their impressions of the children's language development based on the narrative sample. This helped to establish a shared impression of typical expected language expression at each grade level. Workshop participants shared their ideas for incorporating personal narratives in the classroom.

Written handouts explained the impact of personal narrative skills on development of social and academic language. The handouts also included strategies and techniques for developing personal narrative skills. Prior to the workshop, we asked a Guatemalan resource teacher to review the handouts for appropriate local terminology.

Characterizing the goals and perceptions of local educators enabled us to establish a working relationship and provide a space for community input in the planning of this project, as well as to engage in a broader dialogue on cultural influences of narrative production and assessment. Overall, participants agreed that an assessment tool that elicits personal narratives would be beneficial in characterizing and developing children's language abilities.

Designing Formative and Summative Impact Assessments and Associated Steps for Responsiveness

Considering Options

The Brillo de Sol Director indicated the school would benefit from access to an assessment tool that, in addition to eliciting personal narratives, would also elicit specific grammatical elements of Spanish. We considered whether the Spanish Structured Photographic Expressive Language Test (Spanish SPELT-3; Langdon, 2012) might be appropriate for use in Guatemala. Although the Spanish SPELT-3 was created in Spanish, it is intended for use in the United States. Upon examining the stimulus photographs used in this assessment, it was clear that many were not relevant or appropriate for Guatemalan culture and daily life. For example, some photos depict prices in U.S. dollars and the "poolside" photo shows children in a swimming pool, which may not be familiar to rural children in Guatemala. On the other hand, many of the elicitation prompts were appropriate, if adjustments could be made to the photographs and some of the words and phrases. The SPELT-3 also thoroughly probes for Spanish grammatical morphemes. We reached out to the SPELT-3 author (Langdon, 2012), who granted permission for us to adapt the protocol.

Adapting Test Items

We considered which scenarios, associated photographs, and stimulus prompts would need to be entirely substituted and which would simply need to be modified. When we returned to Guatemala, we photographed scenes depicting daily life in the local area, including children interacting with teachers, staff, and one another. Table 8-1 compares an original image stimulus and associated elicitation items from the Spanish SPELT-3 (Langdon, 2012) with the corresponding image stimulus and elicitation items included in the Brillo assessment. The original "arcade" photograph from the Spanish SPELT-3 depicted activities that are uncommon in daily Guatemalan life. We substituted this activity for *saltando a la cuerda* (jumping rope), a common activity experienced by school-aged children.

In addition to eliciting grammatical elements in phrase completion tasks as in the Spanish SPELT-3, we wanted to utilize the same photographs for eliciting personal narratives as well. Narratives are told in all cultures, while types of narratives, reasons they are told, content and structure, and the way children are socialized to produce narratives can vary. Life stories influence problem solving and self-regulation strategies (Westby & Culatta, 2016). In individualist cultures (e.g., the United States), parents and teachers support reminiscing about details and feelings about the past and children typically refer to themselves in their stories. In collectivist cultures (e.g., Guatemala), children may produce shorter narratives with minimal actions and event sequencing, while they may include more details about social aspects of engagement (Hyter & Salas-Provance, 2019; Westby & Culatta, 2016).

Table 8-2 includes a list of all 12 pictured scenarios and their associated prompts for eliciting narrative language. When adapting our methodology for other cultural and language environments, it is important to consider whether these scenarios are representative of children's communication activities in the local setting.

When developing an assessment of expressive language, it is important to include grammatical forms that are representative of the target language. Table 8-3 lists Spanish grammatical structures and the expected age of acquisition (Langdon, 2012). The 12 scenarios include phrase completion prompts that elicit grammatical structures of Spanish shown in Table 8-3.

Table 8-1
Modification of Assessment Prompts

SPANISH SPELT-3 (LANGDON, 2012)	**BRILLO ASSESSMENT OF SPANISH GRAMMAR AND PERSONAL NARRATIVES**
9. Arcade 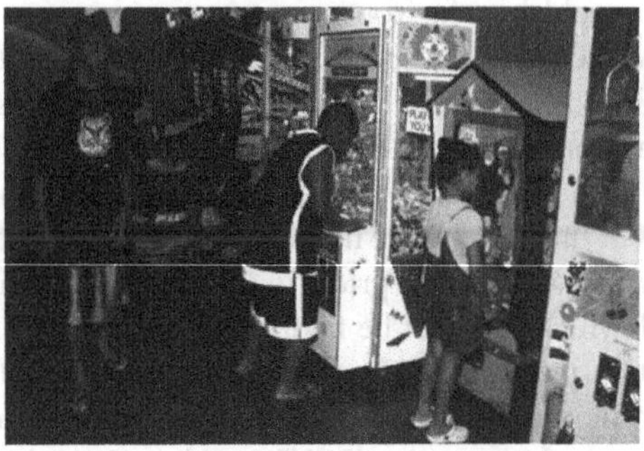	*9. Saltando a la cuerda (jumping rope)* 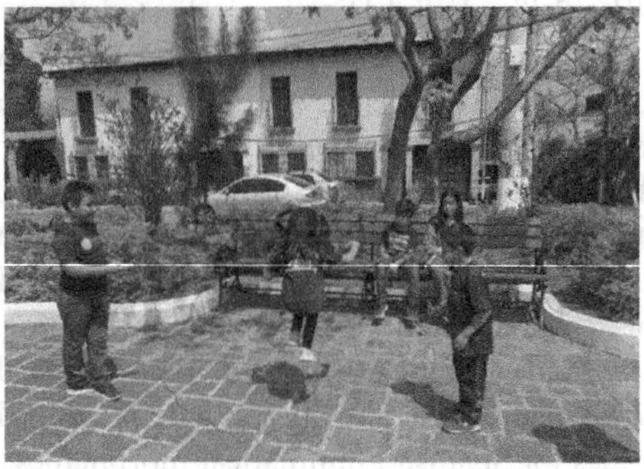
44. *(Señale los tres niños que están jugando)* (Point to the three children who are playing) *¿Qué hacen estos tres niños?* What are these three children doing?	44. *(Señale los tres niños que están saltando a la cuerda)* (Point to the three children who are jumping rope) *¿Que hacen estos tres niños?* What are these three children doing?
45. *(Señale los tres niños al frente)* (Point to the three children in front) *Los pantalones de los niños …* The boys' pants …	45. *(Señale los tres niños al frente)* (Point to the three children in front) *Las camisetas de los niños …* The kids' t-shirts …
46. *(Señale al niño que no está jugando)* (Point to the child who is not playing) *¿Por qué no juega este niño?* Why isn't this boy playing?	46. *(Señale a la niña sentada en el banco)* (Point to the girl sitting on the bench) *¿Por qué no juega esta niña?* Why isn't this girl playing?
47. *Los niños no traen calcetas (calcetines, medias) porque …* The children are not wearing socks because …	47. *Los niños no traen chanclas porque …* The children are not wearing slippers/flipflops because …
48. *(Señale los tres niños parados y luego el niño sentado atrás)* (Point to the children who are standing and then to the child sitting behind them) *Estos niños están parados pero este niño …* These children are standing but this boy is …	48. *(Señale los tres niños parados y luego el niño sentado atrás)* (Point to the children who are standing and then to the child sitting behind them) *Estos niños están parados pero este niño …* These children are standing but this boy is …

The left column depicts an original image stimulus and the associated elicitation prompts from the Spanish Structured Photographic Expressive Language Test (Spanish SPELT-3). Reproduced with permission from Langdon, H. (2012). *Spanish Structured Photographic Expressive Language Test* (3rd ed.). Janelle Publications.
Aligned horizontally on the right are the corresponding image stimulus and elicitation prompts included in the Brillo Assessment of Spanish Grammar and Personal Narratives. When elicitation prompts were relevant to both photograph stimuli, the original Spanish SPELT-3 prompts were also used in the Brillo. Prompts 45, 46, and 47 were adapted for the photographed Guatemalan context.

Table 8-2
Descriptions of Photographed Scenarios and Prompts Used to Elicit Narratives

#	SCENARIO	NARRATIVE ELICITATION PROMPT
1	*Niños en la oficina* Children in the school office	*Cuéntame sobre una vez cuando fuiste a la oficina.* Tell me about a time when you went to the office.
2	*Maestra enseñando* Teacher teaching	*Ella es maestra. En su trabajo ella enseña a los niños. ¿Cuándo tu seas mayor, qué trabajo te gustaría tener? ¿Por qué? ¿Qué harías en ese trabajo?* She's a teacher. It's her job to teach children. Tell me about the kind of work you want to do when you are grown. Why? What will you do at this job?
3	*Niños trabajando en un proyecto* Children working on a project	*Dime sobre un proyecto que hiciste en grupo.* Tell me about a project that you did in a group.
4	*Niños que salen de la escuela* Children leaving school	*Cuéntame lo que te gusta hacer después de la escuela.* Tell me about what you like to do after school.
5	*Comida* Mealtime	*¿De que van a hablar los niños mientras comen?* What will the children talk about while they are eating?
6	*Refacción* Snack time	*Este niño no come nada porque quería tortillas. ¿Qué pasos necesita para hacer tortillas?* This child isn't eating because he wanted tortillas. What are the steps for making tortillas?
7	*En el huerto* In the garden	*¿Por que es importante tener un huerto?* *¿Qué te gusta hacer en el huerto?* Why is it important to have a garden? What do you like to do in the garden?
8	*Gasolinera* Gas station	*Este señor necesita gasolina antes de ir de viaje. ¿A donde te gustaría ir a ti de viaje?¿Qué te gustaría hacer?¿Con quién?* This man needs to get gas before going on a trip. Where would you like to go on a trip? What would you like to do? Who would you go with?
9	*Saltando a la cuerda* Jumping rope	*Describe tu juego favorito. ¿Como se juega?* Tell me about your favorite game and how you play it.
10	*En clase* In the classroom	*Descríbeme a tu mejor amigo (amiga) y que les gusta hacer a ustedes?* Tell me about your best friend and what you like to do together.
11	*Una excursión* Field trip	*Cuéntame sobre una vez cuando fuiste en una salida escolar.* Tell me about a time when you went on a field trip.
12	*Ayudando a una amiga* Helping a friend	*Cuéntame sobre una vez cuando le ayudaste a alguien, o cuando alguien te ayudó? ¿Cómo le ayudaste?* Tell me about a time when you helped someone or when someone helped you. How did you help them?

Table 8-3
Target Grammatical Structures and Expected Age of Acquisition

LAS FRASES NOMINALES (NOUN PHRASES)	AGE OF ACQUISITION (YEARS)
Artículos (Articles)	By 4
Posesivos (Possessives)	By 4
Plurales cortos (Short plurals)	By 4
Plurales largos (Long plurals)	By 4
Preposiciones (Prepositions)	By 4
Géneros de adjetivos (Gender in adjectives)	By 4
Géneros de pronombres (Gender in pronouns)	By 4
Número de verbos (Number agreement)	By 4
LAS FRASES VERBALES (VERB PHRASES)	**AGE OF ACQUISITION (YEARS)**
Infinitivo (Infinitive)	Begins at 2
Indicativo (Indicative)	Begins at 2
Progresivo (Progressive)	Begins at 2
Imperativo (Imperative)	By 3
Imperfecto (Imperfect)	By 3-4
Pretérito regular (Regular preterite)	By 4
Pretérito irregular (Irregular preterite)	By 4-5
Futuro perifrástico (Periphrastic future)	By 3-4
Cópula (Copula)	By 2-3
El presente subjuntivo (Present subjunctive)	By 3
Condicional (Conditional)	By 3-4
Condicional pasado (Past conditional)	By 6-7
TIPOS DE ORACIONES (SENTENCE TYPES)	**AGE OF ACQUISITION (YEARS)**
Activo/declarativo (Active/declarative)	By 3
Negativo (Negative)	By 3
Interrogativo (Interrogative)	By 3

Reproduced with permission from Langdon, H. (2012). *Spanish Structured Photographic Expressive Language Test* (3rd ed.). Janelle Publications.

Table 8-4 lists the functions and pragmatic intent of the stimulus items, as presented in the Spanish SPELT-3 (Langdon, 2012). Examples from the Brillo protocol illustrate how each function/intent is represented.

Table 8-4
Target Functions/Pragmatic Intent

FUNCTION/INTENT	SELECTED PROMPTS AND EXAMPLE RESPONSES
Commenting	*La motociclista tuvo que esperar su turno en fila porque … (había otro carro en frente)* The motorcyclist had to wait his turn in line because … (there was another car in front)
Describing	*Los niños están … (en la oficina)* The children are … (in the office)
Explaining	*Los niños están allí porque …(van a aprender)* The children are here because … (they're going to learn)
Hypothesizing	*Sin el agua, las plantas … (no podrían crecer)* Without water, the plants … (won't grow)
Informing	*Los niños están en la oficina porque … (les van a dar sus premios)* The children are in the office because … (they're going to get their prizes)
Naming	*Estos son … (platos, huevos, frijoles)* These are … (plates, eggs, beans)
Negating	*Tres personas tienen gorras pero los otros niños … (no tienen)* Three children are wearing hats but the other children … (aren't)
Questioning	*¿Cómo les pregunta la niña a los niños si quieren agua? (¿Quieren que les traigan agua?)* How would the girl ask the other children if they want water? (Do you want me to bring you some water?)

Scenario Example

The prompt, "Tell me about a time when you helped someone or someone helped you," is recommended for eliciting a personal narrative from a child (Westby & Culatta, 2016). We included "Helping a friend" (Figure 8-1) as a scenario.

In the "Helping a friend" scenario, the following grammatical forms are elicited. The expected grammatical form and example responses are provided.

- *Las niñas le ayudan a que ella* … The girls help her …
  - Verb + number agreement (e.g., *camine* or walk)
- *¿Como está el clima? El día está asoleado. El sol está* … How is the weather? It's a sunny day. The sun is …
  - Adjective or adverb (e.g., *asoleado, caliente* or shining, hot)
- *¿Que están haciendo ellas?* … What are they doing?
  - Gerund (e.g., *caminando, ayudando* or helping, going)
- (Point to backpack) *¿Que lleva en su espalda?* … What is she wearing on her back?
  - Article (e.g., *una mochila, su mochila, la mochila* or a backpack, her backpack, the backpack)
- *El carro es de su abuelo. La mochila es* … The car belongs to her grandfather. The backpack is …
  - Possessive (e.g., *de ella, de la niña, suya* or hers/the girl's)

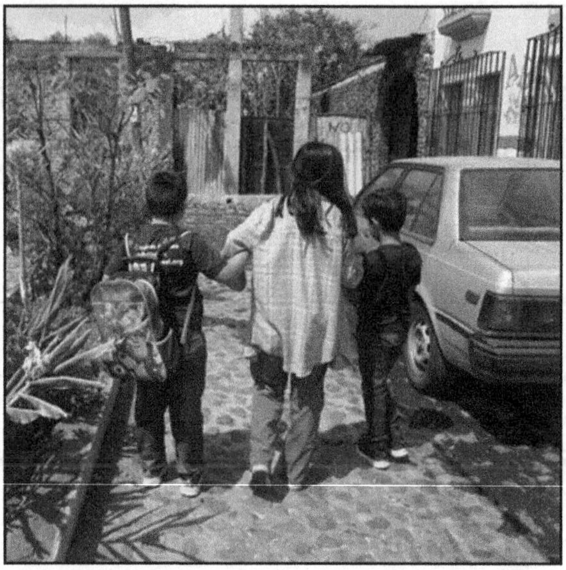

Figure 8-1. *Ayudando a una amiga* (helping a friend) scenario.

Coding Responses

The Brillo protocol instructs the examiner to write the child's entire response to each question or prompt. Taking into consideration the training and examiner qualifications of Guatemalan speech-language therapists, we chose grammaticality judgment ("Is the response grammatical?" Yes or No) as the method for coding the child's responses. Studies have established the construct validity of percent grammatical responses (PGR) as a measure of grammar and support the use of PGR as a measure to assess grammaticality (Eisenberg & Guo, 2018). Grammaticality judgment by native language listeners is intuitive and does not require specific training. The protocol provides the grammatical element and expected responses, aiding in the examiner's grammaticality judgment of the child's response.

The protocol also requires the examiner to code the clarity of pronunciation of each response ("Is the response pronounced clearly?" Yes or No), facilitating computation of the percentage of utterances produced correctly. Percent accuracy as an overall intelligibility measure can be used to determine whether further assessment of articulation and phonology is warranted. Figure 8-2 illustrates a sample page of the protocol for Scenario 12, Helping a Friend.

Interpreting Results

We considered how examiners would analyze the narrative responses. Given the current training received by Guatemalan speech-language therapists, we determined that morphosyntactic analysis would not be realistic for most examiners. Therefore, as with the phrase completion responses, the narrative responses are also coded for grammaticality (Yes or No) and clarity of pronunciation (Yes or No). Next, the number of words in each utterance is tallied. Number of words is separated into three categories: one to three words; four to seven words; and eight or more words. (The examiner circles the appropriate category of utterance length in words.) These utterance length categories are based on research indicating validity of the Grammaticality and Utterance Length Instrument in conjunction with grammaticality judgment (Castilla-Earls & Fulcher-Rood, 2018). It is important to

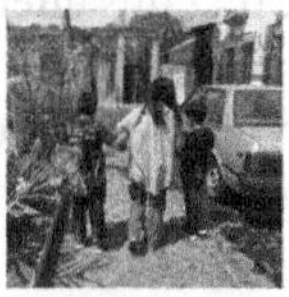

12. Ayudando a una amiga

	Pautas del examinador (*haga*, diga)	Escriba toda la respuesta del niño/a	¿Se pronunció claramente la oración?	¿La oración es gramática?	FUNCIONES y Ejemplos de respuestas
60	**Las niñas le ayudan a que ella...**		sí no	sí no	NARRATIVA **Subjuntivo O pretérito O presente progresivo O indicativo + persona correcta** <u>camine</u>
61	**¿Cómo está el clima? El día está...**		sí no	sí no	DESCRIBIR **Adjetivo + género + número correcto O adverbio** <u>asoleado</u> <u>caliente</u>
62	**¿Qué están haciendo ellas?**		sí no	sí no	DESCRIBIR **Gerundio** <u>Caminando</u> <u>Ayudando</u> <u>Llendo</u>
63	*Señale a la mochila* **Qué lleva en su espalda?**		sí no	sí no	NOMBRAR Artículo + género correcto en el sustantivo <u>Una mochila</u> <u>Su mochila</u> <u>La mochila</u>
64	**El carro es de su abuelo. La mochila es...**		sí no	sí no	DESCRIBIR Posesivo <u>De ella</u> / <u>De la niña</u>/ <u>Suya</u>
R12	**Cuéntame sobre una vez cuando le ayudaste a alguien, o cuando alguien te ayudó? ¿Cómo le ayudaste?**		sí no	sí no	Número de palabras en la oración 1-3 4-7 8+

Figure 8-2. Sample protocol scenario and stimulus items.

note that this utterance length instrument was validated in English. In Spanish, one word can contain more morphemes than its English equivalent word(s). For example, *Damelo* (one word) means "Give it to me" (four words). Even considering these linguistic differences, the three separate utterance length categories are indicative of distinct levels of language competence.

We explored mean length of utterance (MLU) as a potential component of the assessment. Guatemalan speech-language therapists confirmed that they did not find MLU time-efficient or useful commensurate with their level of training and experience. Given the ease of coding utterances for number of words rather than number of morphemes, Guatemalan speech-language therapists agreed that the approach was optimal for coding the narrative prompt responses.

Castilla-Earls and Fulcher-Rood's (2018) preliminary analysis of diagnostic accuracy suggests that grammaticality and utterance length have the potential to identify children with language impairment. Complete transcription and analysis of morphemes, such as SALT Software (Miller & Iglesias, 2008), provides a more detailed and comprehensive analysis of child language. The task completion time for determining grammaticality and utterance length in words is considerably shorter. Guatemalan speech-language therapists who have training in morphosyntax analysis methods could perform additional analysis as a supplement to the protocol.

Ensuring Important Knowledge, Skills, and Dispositions Among Participants and Acknowledging Important Limits in What Participants Will Be Permitted to Do

Focus Group

To guide development of our procedural manual, we conducted a focus group with 30 Guatemalan speech-language therapists to explore how the specific Guatemalan context shapes narrative production, development, and use. We developed our methodological approach by consulting experts and literature from across disciplines. We incorporated *grounded theory* to ensure our data collection and analysis were consistent with qualitative methods from social science and public health (Glaser & Strauss, 1967). Grounded theory begins with collection of qualitative data, which is then reviewed to determine which ideas or concepts emerge from the data. We incorporated *cultural domain analysis* (CDA) to learn more about how Guatemalan speech-language therapists view language and language sampling procedures. CDA is a viable method to collect and analyze data about cultural influences (Borgatti & Halgin, 2012). We explored narrative assessment relevant to the Guatemalan context through techniques described in the Angoff method (Frey, 2018) such as asking subject-matter experts to examine the content of test items and judge their predicted difficulty.

Following the focus group meeting, we reviewed the wording of instructions used in the Brillo for appropriateness in the local community in Guatemala. Participants suggested several wording changes on the protocol, such as using the term *señale* rather than *apunte* (for "point" to the pictures). We used qualitative and quantitative research methods to examine the internal validity and reliability of the individual stimulus items and to better characterize the perceptions and goals of the local partners. The resulting Brillo Assessment of Spanish Grammar and Personal Narratives is designed to identify grammatical morphemes and personal narrative skills that require further instruction and development. The overall aim of the tool is to characterize the children's grammatical and narrative skills, aid in developing language intervention goals, provide feedback to teachers regarding areas to target in classroom instruction, and ultimately improve children's language learning outcomes and our partners' ability to measure these outcomes. Refining the Brillo stimulus items and procedures required knowledge of child language development, local culture, school community needs, and application of appropriate research methods.

Field Testing

We assembled the photos taken in Guatemala along with our completed protocol and manual, and reviewed the materials with the director and the resource teacher at Collegio Brillo de Sol. We printed each photo as an 8-inch square image and laminated all 12 photos.

The director identified five children with typical expected overall language development representing various grade levels at the school. We reviewed the materials and procedures with these children. The purpose of this phase was not to analyze data obtained with the tool, but to assess the utility of the photographs as stimulus items and the children's ability to follow our instructions. While we had laminated the photos solely to protect them from damage, we noted that the children enjoyed holding each individual laminated photo while answering the elicitation prompts and questions. One child thanked us for the "fun activity," indicating the child was not aware it was a "test" or assessment. The children were attentive and cooperative throughout the assessment and were able to complete all 64 phrase completion questions and all narrative prompts. One prompt did not elicit the anticipated response (or grammatical form) from three of the children. We therefore changed that item to a different prompt appropriate for the picture stimulus.

Designing Formative and Summative Impact Assessments and Associated Steps for Responsiveness

Supplemental Assessor Manual

To support appropriate implementation of the *Brillo*, we created a Supplemental Assessor Guide to enhance the brief examiner instructions. This guide addresses the unique needs and training of the local assessors. Goals of the Supplemental Assessor Guide include:

- Overcome the barrier of lack of training in child language assessment tools appropriate for use in our partners' settings.
- Produce a tool that addresses the needs and goals of the local setting and students, including perceived relevance of the tool for assessors.
- Promote accurate implementation of the assessment procedures.

Cognitive Interviews

Cognitive interviewing, originally developed as a forensic method, has been adapted for social sciences as a data-gathering tool (Peterson et al., 2017). It is an approach, rather than a procedure, in which the interviewer does not interrupt the interviewee who is recalling and describing experiences. This method encourages interviewees to explain their experience in whatever way they choose, typically in a narrative, and provides significant details in comparison with more guided forms of interviewing (Waddington & Bull, 2007). We conducted cognitive interviews with six Guatemalan educators who have also completed technical degree programs in speech-language therapy and who work in a school setting with children with special needs.

We presented the assessment to the educators and asked them to provide feedback, exploring the process of administering and interpreting stimulus items. We recorded and later transcribed the cognitive interviews. As a result, we clarified and simplified instructions. Through cognitive interviews combined with mock assessment practice, these potential assessors participated in the development of the Supplemental Assessor Guide, ensuring appropriate cultural adaptation of the assessment tool. The final components include:

- Step-by-step administration instructions with descriptions of *why* the steps are important
- Glossary of terms (e.g., personal narrative)
- How to interpret results
- How assessment results may inform a child's educational program

Gathering input from end-users through cognitive interviewing can effectively inform the development of supplemental assessor guides and resulting implementation of culturally adapted tools.

Recognizing and Providing Appropriate Support for United States and Non–United States Participants

Eliciting Feedback

We conducted an interactive workshop with 25 Guatemalan speech-language therapists to review the final version of the entire procedure of the Brillo Assessment of Spanish Grammar and Personal Narratives, including the stimulus photos, protocol, instructions, and Supplemental Assessor Guide. We approached the feedback workshop as a bidirectional exchange of knowledge, skills, and perspectives, to ensure all materials effectively target grammatical and narrative language skills in a culturally and linguistically responsive manner.

We found that the Supplemental Assessor Guide was well received and useful for assessors who may have limited specialized training in clinical assessment methods. In addition to verbal discussion as we reviewed the materials, the participants were invited to edit the documents, and 16 of them returned their copies with suggested wording modifications. Changes were incorporated when suggested by more than one participant. For example, participants consistently preferred the term *terapista* (therapist) rather than *evaluador/a* (evaluator) and *objetivo* (objective) rather than *propósito* (purpose).

Ensuring Meaningful Reflection Throughout Each Step of Design and Implementation

Chapter Summary

Ethical international practice requires deliberate consideration of local partners, systems, services, programs, and needs. Our experience in communication disorders, bilingualism, cross-cultural service delivery, speech and language science, global health, and collaboration with colleagues in Guatemala led us to develop the Brillo Assessment of Spanish Grammar and Personal Narratives.

Our process of developing an authentic language assessment in Guatemala followed guidelines for effective, ethical global engagement. Partnering with practitioners from lower- and middle-resource countries to develop assessment tools can increase effectiveness, innovation, and capacity building. It is important to consider the knowledge and skills of the individuals who will implement the assessment procedures. Effective implementation of assessment tools includes training the individuals who will administer and score the procedures and interpret the assessment results. Our goal was to increase capacity for language assessment in a lower-resource setting, therefore improving the ability to accurately measure, intervene, track, and report child language and narrative outcomes. We continue to collaborate with our Guatemalan colleagues to ensure the Brillo materials are implemented in an effective and sustainable manner, through ongoing training, consultation, and feedback.

Here we provide examples summarizing how our development of an assessment measure of Spanish grammar and narrative language in Guatemala incorporated recommendations of the American Speech-Language-Hearing Association *Final Report by the Ad Hoc Committee to Develop Guidance for Members and Students Engaging Globally in Clinical, Scholarly, and Other Professional Activities* (Hallowell et al., 2021). The Committee suggests use of a checklist (see Appendix in this chapter) to guide collaboration with partners from various regions of the world, "to encourage meaningful, ethical decision making."

1. *Engaging host partners in program design and determination of the non–United States participants' needs and desires*

   Our project was conceptualized in response to the expressed need from our partner community for a procedure to assess children's language development. The partners had been using assessments developed in the United States that were outdated and inappropriate for the cultural context. Through community needs assessment, collaborating clinicians can focus on the host partner's goals and ensure that collaborative work is guided by the host partner.

2. *Ensuring reciprocity and mutuality*

   Our methods were designed for the purpose of creating opportunity for host colleagues to provide input into the design of the assessment measure and to ensure our final product would meet their needs. Use of cognitive interviewing and engaging with the stimulus items ensured these items function as intended. Cognitive interviewing with the instructions and assessor guide helped to ensure appropriate implementation. United States participants are bilingual in Spanish and English, while continuously learning Guatemala-specific terms and phrases. We rely on our partners to provide us with feedback regarding cultural and linguistic variation in the local area.

3. *Considering resource implications and addressing related ethical concerns (e.g., time, funding, personnel, transportation, meals, lodging, entertainment, tourism)*

   We conducted fundraising efforts to provide transportation and lodging for teachers from one partner school to visit another partner school for a joint workshop on the topic of personal narratives.

   In the development of the tool, we considered logistical issues. For example, we forewent color coding in the formatting of the tool so that it can be printed in black and white for use by the school.

   Most assessment batteries in higher-resource countries are designed for use by licensed professionals with advanced training, which becomes a barrier in many global settings. In developing the methodology, we considered the training of the personnel at the school who would be using the tool. We sought to address this barrier by aligning the tool with our colleagues' training and needs.
4. *Attending to sustainability and continuity*

   The sustainability of our work is ensured through the long-standing collaboration between our university and our partner organizations. The language assessment project has been an iterative process with many cycles of feedback and revisions.

   We also provide professional development lectures and workshops through the Guatemalan Association of Speech-Language Therapists (SomosTLgt) and the local university speech-hearing-language training program on topics they request.
5. *Thoughtfully representing the experience in advertisements and recruitment materials and in social media, photos, videos, and publications related to the experience*

   We do not share identifying information or personal information related to any child in our dissemination process, including presentations and publications. We acknowledge the roles we and our partners served in our work in all presentations and publications.
6. *Recruiting and preparing participants*

   We use consent scripts to clearly communicate to all host participants what their participation will entail so they know what to expect and that they can choose to stop participating at any time without consequence to them.

   When our university students participate in the process, they are briefed before and after their participation. They learn the principles of effective global engagement, set personal goals for developing competencies, and reflect on how they met these goals.
7. *Ensuring important knowledge, skills, and dispositions among participants and acknowledging important limits in what participants will be permitted to do*

   Our licensed clinicians, instructors, and graduate students acknowledge that they are bound by what their respective training and licensure permits them to do in their home state and country. They self-assess knowledge, skills, and dispositions to identify competencies for further development.
8. *Designing formative and summative impact assessments and associated steps for responsiveness*

   Currently underway, the implementation research phase includes a brief-interaction-debrief process, with Guatemalan speech-language therapists administering the assessment tool. Feedback addresses the specific assessment skills demonstrated.
9. *Recognizing and providing appropriate support for United States and non–United States participants*

   The assessment tool was designed to be low-cost to implement. Upon demonstration of skills in administration and interpretation of results, clinicians are provided a complete set of materials. They can print additional protocols as needed.

10. *Ensuring meaningful reflection throughout each step of design and implementation*

    Each phase of the project included dissemination of our findings and discussion with participants. We have sought input prior to workshops and feedback during and after workshops to ensure we are providing useful professional development. Our process has included informal check-ins before, during, and after project activities as part of the iterative process of development of our tool.

References

American Speech-Language-Hearing Association. (2021). Review of ASHA's current resources related to global engagement—And recommendations for enhancing them: Final report by the ad hoc committee to develop guidance for members and students engaging globally in clinical, scholarly, and other professional activities.

Borgatti, S., & Halgin, D. (2012). Elicitation techniques for cultural domain Analysis. In J. J. Schensul & M. D. LeCompte (Eds.), *Specialized ethnographic methods: A mixed methods approach*. https://ebookcentral-proquest-com.libproxy.lib.unc.edu

Castilla-Earls, A., & Fulcher-Rood, K. (2018). Convergent and divergent validity of the Grammaticality and Utterance Length Instrument. *Journal of Speech, Language, and Hearing Research, 61*, 120-129.

Durkin, M. S., Elsabbagh, M., Barbaro, J., Gladstone, M., Happe, F., Hoekstra, R. A., Lee, L.-C., Rattazzi, A., Stapel-Wax, J., Stone, W. L., Tager-Flusberg, H., Thurm, A., Tomlinson, M., & Shih, A. (2015). Autism screening and diagnosis in low resource settings: challenges and opportunities to enhance research and services worldwide. *Autism Research, 8*(5), 473-476. https://doi.org/10.1002/aur.1575.

Eisenberg, S. L., & Guo, L. (2018). Percent grammatical responses as a general outcome measure: Initial validity. *Language, Speech, and Hearing Services in Schools, 49*, 98-107.

Erskine, H. E., Baxter, A. J., Patton, G., Moffitt, T. E., Patel, V., Whiteford, H. A., & Scott, J. G. (2017). The global coverage of prevalence data for mental disorders in children and adolescents. *Epidemiology and Psychiatric Sciences, 26*(4), 395-402.

Frey, B. B. (2018). Angoff method. *The SAGE encyclopedia of educational research, measurement, and evaluation*. SAGE Publications.

Glaser, B. G., & Strauss, A. L. (1967). *The discovery of grounded theory: Strategies for qualitative research*. Aldine.

Grandin, G., Levenson, D., & Oglesby, E. (2011). The Maya: Before the Europeans. *The Guatemala Reader*. Duke University Press.

Hallowell, B., Hyter, Y. D., Watson, J. B., Combiths, P., Lansing, C. R., Ramkissoon, I., & Flynn, T. (2021). Final report by the ad hoc committee to develop guidance for members and students engaging globally in clinical, scholarly, and other professional activities. *American Speech-Language-Hearing Association*. https://www.asha.org/siteassets/reports/ahc-develop-guidance-for-engaging-globally.pdf

Hartley, S., & Newton, C. R. J. C. (2009). Children with developmental disabilities in the majority of the world. In M. Shevell (Ed.), *Neurodevelopmental disabilities: Clinical and scientific foundations* (pp. 70-84). Mac Keith Press.

Hyter, Y. D., Roman, R., Staley, B., & McPherson, B. (2017). Competencies for effective global engagement: A proposal for communication sciences and disorders. *Perspectives of the ASHA Special Interest Groups, SIG 17*(2), Part 1.

Hyter, Y. D., & Salas-Provance, M. (2019). Theoretical frameworks about culture and cultural responsiveness. In *Culturally responsive practices in speech, language, and hearing services*. Plural Publishing.

Langdon, H. (2012). *Spanish Structured Photographic Expressive Language Test, Third Edition*. Janelle Publications.

Maulik, P. K., & Darmstadt, G. L. (2007). Childhood disability in low- and middle-income countries: Overview of screening, prevention, services, legislation, and epidemiology. *Pediatrics, 120*(suppl 1), S1-S55. https://doi.org/10.1542/peds.2007-0043B.

Miller, J. F., & Iglesias, A. (2008). Systematic analysis of language transcripts (SALT), Bilingual SE Version 2008 [Computer software]. SALT Software, LLC.

Peterson, C. H., Peterson, N. A., & Powell, K. G. (2017). Cognitive interviewing for item development: Validity evidence based on content and response processes. *Measurement and Evaluation in Counseling and Development, 50*(4), 217-223. https://doi.org/10.1080/07481756.2017.1339564

Small, J. W., Hix, Small, H., Vargas, Baron, E., & Marks, K. P. (2019). Comparative use of the Ages and Stages Questionnaires in low- and middle-income countries. *Developmental Medicine & Child Neurology, 61*(4), 431-443.

Waddington, P. A. J., & Bull, R. (2007). Cognitive interviewing as a research tool. *Social Research Update*, 50. https://sru.soc.surrey.ac.uk/SRU50.html

Wallace, S., Fein, D., Rosanoff, M., Dawson, G., Hossain, S., Brennan, L., Hossain, S., Brennan, L., Como, A., & Shih, A. (2012). A global public health strategy for autism spectrum disorders. *Autism Research: Official Journal of the International Society for Autism Research, 5*(3), 211-217.

Westby, C., & Culatta, B. (2016). Telling tales: Personal event narratives and life stories. *Language, Speech, and Hearing Services in Schools, 47*, 260-282. https://doi.org/10.1044/2016_LSHSS-15-0073

Wickenden, M. (2013). Widening the SLP lens: How can we improve the wellbeing of people with communication disabilities globally? *International Journal of Speech-Language Pathology, 15*, 1.

APPENDIX

CHECKLIST

The American Speech-Language-Hearing Association *Final Report by the Ad Hoc Committee to Develop Guidance for Members and Students Engaging Globally in Clinical, Scholarly, and Other Professional Activities* (Hallowell et al., 2021) recommends use of a checklist to guide collaboration with partners from various regions of the world. They suggest addressing the following topics "to ensure recognition and discussion of ethical compromises and to encourage meaningful, ethical decision making."

	1. Engaging host partners in program design and determination of the non–United States participants' needs and desires
	2. Ensuring reciprocity and mutuality
	3. Considering resource implications and addressing related ethical concerns (e.g., time, funding, personnel, transportation, meals, lodging, entertainment, tourism)
	4. Attending to sustainability and continuity
	5. Thoughtfully representing the experience in advertisements and recruitment materials and in social media, photos, videos, and publications related to the experience
	6. Recruiting and preparing participants
	7. Ensuring important knowledge, skills, and dispositions among participants and acknowledging important limits in what participants will be permitted to do
	8. Designing formative and summative impact assessments and associated steps for responsiveness
	9. Recognizing and providing appropriate support for United States and non–United States participants
	10. Ensuring meaningful reflection throughout each step of design and implementation

Chapter 9

Drawing on Language Socialization Research to Improve Speech and Language Assessment

Keziah Conrad, PhD, MS, CCC-SLP

In studies of Indigenous Mexican children working together with family members or peers to carry out a common project, researchers have observed highly sophisticated forms of collaboration (Alcalá et al., 2018; Roberts & Rogoff, 2012). Children of Indigenous background in Mexico, as in many other parts of the world, are socialized to learn by watching intently and by participating in meaningful community endeavors (Gaskins & Paradise, 2010; Paradise & Rogoff, 2009). Given a complex task, they make extensive use of "fluid collaboration as an ensemble," ways of working together that build smoothly on the contributions of all participants, even those who are younger or less skilled; they often seem to anticipate one another's actions with little need of verbal dialogue (Alcalá et al., 2018). This cultural pattern contrasts with mainstream Euro-American models of learning or working together, which commonly involve extensive reliance on verbal explanation, negotiation, and solo engagement on individual components of the task.

These differences in cultural orientation influence the ways that Indigenous and Euro-American children behave, of course, but they also frame their perceptions of others' behavior. Roberts and Rogoff (2012) showed videos of Indigenous-heritage children collaborating and asked other children to comment on what was going on. They found that middle-class White children largely failed to recognize what was happening. Many of the Anglo children seemed uncertain as to how they might characterize what they saw, but their comments indicated an assumption that talking is necessary for collaborating, and if the children in the videos were not talking, they were not really helping each

Bortz, M. (Ed.). *A Guide to Global Language Assessment: A Lifespan Approach* (pp. 177-194).
DOI: 10.4324/9781003524472-12

other. Children from Euro-American, middle-class backgrounds articulated a belief that "working together" required partners to talk out loud, and this belief prevented them from appreciating the skillful interactions going on before their eyes (Roberts & Rogoff, 2012).

What do we miss, as clinical professionals who evaluate others' linguistic competence, when we fail to see beyond our own sociocultural frameworks for interpreting language use? One primary argument of this chapter is that we stand to miss a lot. Too often, we perceive differences as deficits and remain oblivious to strengths we do not think to look for. In a field where most of the professionals are White monolingual English speakers, much of the research base concerns White, middle-class monolingual English speakers, and intervention goals are explicitly about achieving normative success in monolingual English-speaking institutions (schools), clinicians urgently need to cultivate awareness of cultural and linguistic diversity. Furthermore, we need to do this not as "culture free" specialists standing apart from exotic others who "have" culture and "are" diverse, but as people cognizant of our own social and cultural positioning who bring curiosity, humility, and genuine appreciation to encounters with the people we serve.

This chapter reviews literature from anthropology, developmental psychology, and allied fields that falls within a paradigm known as *language socialization* research. Theorists of language socialization are concerned with the ways children and other novices become "socialized"—through interaction with others—into the norms of communication and comportment that characterize a particular community, gradually becoming competent members of that community. Research into language socialization is qualitative in nature and has typically brought together "microscopic" analysis of interactional moves, often recorded in videos, with "macroscopic" knowledge drawn from extended periods of *ethnographic* research and participant observation in a specific community. Scholars often present detailed analyses of language, gestures, and other embodied elements in conversational sequences, drawing from the tradition known as *conversation analysis* (Goodwin & Heritage, 1990; Sacks et al., 1974). While research drawing on these qualitative traditions is not unknown within the field of communication sciences and disorders (Crago, 1990; Damico et al., 1999, 2015; Duchan et al., 1999; Kovarsky et al., 1999; Simmons-Mackie & Damico, 2003; Wilkinson, 2010, 2020), it remains poorly integrated into clinical practice and underused as a resource for assessment.

The language socialization literature is large and constantly growing, but this chapter focuses on three areas of import to language development and disorders. The first section outlines major findings with regard to early language development and child-directed communication. Contrary to prevailing accounts of language acquisition based on research with Euro-American, middle-class children, language socialization research has documented the variation in childrearing practices worldwide and emphasized the cultural uniqueness of what we often take to be universal ways of being with children, arranging the environment, or accommodating to novices. The second section explores some of the implications of these differences for children from nondominant backgrounds within monolithic, measurement-driven educational systems. This literature condemns the widespread reliance on deficit discourses—such as the idea of a "word gap" currently in vogue in the United States—to explain the persistent struggles of students from stigmatized communities. Even for those who do not work in schools, this research is important because it highlights the role of racial, economic, and political disparities that shape assessments of linguistic and cognitive competence and place blame on individuals or their "culture." In the third section, this chapter turns to a smaller group of studies on language socialization and disabilities associated with autism, aphasia, and dementia. Here, the collaborative, contingent nature of communication is on full display as partners in an interaction reach toward intersubjective understanding despite language impairments. The last portion of the chapter explores implications for assessment.

Language Socialization in Early Childhood

Language socialization is an important theoretical focus that emerged in the 1980s within linguistic anthropology and allied fields as a push to broaden the scope of research on child language development to include cultural context (Sperry et al., 2020). Showing that it is not possible to separate language acquisition from the development of sociocultural competency, this work repositioned much of what researchers "know" about how children acquire language as an ethnocentric description of middle-class Western practices and ecologies of learning (Ochs & Schieffelin, 1984; Schieffelin & Ochs, 1986).

In an influential article, Ochs and Schieffelin (1984) analyzed examples of interactions between mother–child pairs presented in previous literature on child language development. In these transcripts, mothers appear to be alone with a single child. They use a baby-talk register with features such as exaggerated intonation, high pitch, diminutives, exclamations, and shorter sentences. They hold playful "proto-conversations" with very young infants. They actively monitor the child's possible communicative intentions and interpret these out loud. In sequences that the authors predict will feel "very familiar, desirable, even natural" to their college-educated, English-speaking readers, mothers work to clarify what their toddlers are trying to say, repeat and expand their utterances, and talk about child-centered topics (Ochs & Schieffelin, 1984, p. 283).

Ochs and Schieffelin (1984) then presented detailed observations and transcripts from their research in Kaluli (Papua New Guinea) and Samoan communities during the 1970s and 1980s. While these groups were quite different from one another—Kaluli society being egalitarian whereas Samoan society was highly stratified—both presented patterns of interaction between caregivers and young children that contrasted with middle-class norms seen in the United States and Europe. For one thing, neither Kaluli nor Samoan adults typically addressed babies or engaged them as conversational partners. Infants were rarely alone with a single caregiver but found themselves in a complex social environment with multiple participants visible and audible to them. They were generally held facing outward, so that their attention was directed toward others. The child's needs were satisfied in the flow of other household activities, but those activities did not center around the child's needs or interests. Older children and adults often talked (to each other, in the presence of the child) about the actions of a small child, but in both societies a generalized hesitancy to guess what another person thinks prevented people from interpreting or expanding what the baby might have been trying to say before the emergence of intelligible words. Instead, adults in the Kaluli community prompted toddlers to repeat fully formed phrases in triadic exchanges, often modeling assertive language to use with older children. In Samoa, adults also prompted toddlers to repeat statements verbatim, and children later took on the role of messengers for more mature family members.

Over the four decades since the inception of the language socialization paradigm, abundant global research has confirmed that childrearing practices typical in WEIRD societies—those that are Western, educated, industrialized, rich, and developed—are, in fact, "weird," and not the norm worldwide (Blum, 2017; de León & García-Sánchez, 2021; Henrich et al., 2010). In many communities, including some within the United States, babies appear to receive little input that is directed *at* them or simplified for them, and instead tend to be positioned as attentive observers and listeners in multi-party interactions (Brown, 2014; Casillas et al., 2020; Conrad, 2020; Crago, 1990; de León, 2014; Hauk, 2016; Heath, 1983; Takada, 2014). While practices vary from one setting to another, growing children in many communities may receive as much direct input from siblings and peers as from adults and are drawn into *triadic verbal routines* that include prompting, teasing, storytelling, arguing, gossiping, displays of politeness, and improvisational play (Briggs, 1999; de León, 2014; Duranti & Black, 2014; Fung et al., 2004; Goodwin, 1990; Miller & Sperry, 2012; Sperry et al., 2020).

Field (2001) illustrates the role of a triadic participation structure in socializing Navajo children into culturally appropriate notions of respect, autonomy, and relationship with others (*k'é*). "Triadic directives," in which an adult speaks to a target child through an intermediary, prompt children to take responsibility for their peers or younger siblings and see themselves as capable actors within a self-determining peer group. One example occurs in the following transcript (Field, 2001, p. 256):

(On the playground, Mara [age 3] falls down, skins her knee, and begins crying. The teacher [who is also her mother] is standing right next to her with another child, Kenny)

01→	*Teacher:* Kenny, help her. Help her up.
02	(Kenny goes over to Mara and gives her
03	a hand up. She is still crying)
04→	*Teacher:* Tell her "be tough."
05→	*Kenny:* Be tough.
	(Mara stops crying)

Rather than comfort her daughter herself, Mara's mother and teacher chooses to appoint another child to do so while she watches. She gives Kenny instructions on how to carry out his social role and provides a model of what he can say. In other transcripts, children are referred to by their clan names ("*Kinyaa'áanii* brother, go get *Tóbaazhní'ázhí* brother"; Field, 2001, p. 257) and are coached to stand up for themselves instead of looking to an adult authority figure. The triadic interactional pattern reinforces other cultural teachings about *k'é* and socializes children into a distinctively Navajo way of using language that also includes avoidance of direct eye gaze, appreciation of silence and slow or quiet speech, and a preference for indirection when making requests or telling others what to do (Field, 2001, pp. 253-254).

The language socialization literature shows rich diversity in the pathways to early language and social competency, as well as documenting how local practices can selectively amplify valued skills (Ochs & Schieffelin, 1995; Ochs et al., 2005). It also emphasizes how, despite this variation, all typically developing children do learn language and become competent members of their communities, reaching benchmarks such as joint attention, indexical pointing, and first words at similar points in time (Brown, 2014).

Language Socialization at School: "Gaps" and Their Repercussions

Beyond language acquisition in early childhood, language socialization research has focused on how children and other novices acquire competency in new communities of practice as they grow older, especially in institutional settings like school. Comparative ethnographic works, such as the multi-sited studies of preschool education in China, Japan, and the United States by Tobin and colleagues (Tobin et al., 1989, 2009), underline the cultural distinctiveness of school systems across the world and the key role of schools as sites where children encounter not just "knowledge" but core values of their society. Striking cultural differences and flash points of internal controversy emerge even in the most mundane practices such as bathroom routines. Whereas Chinese preschoolers in one recording enjoy communal time in an open, trough-style toilet, and a Japanese 5-year-old is filmed giving a lively lesson in how to use a urinal to a younger student, a United States teacher describes how she was disciplined for making direct observations of a 3-year-old's penis after he complained that it hurt (Tobin et al., 2009, pp. 45, 114, 201). Deeply held preferences for privacy, choice, individual self-expression, and a "mother-like" dyadic relationship between teacher and child characterize education in the United States preschools (Tobin et al., 2009, p. 245). In Japan, on the other hand, high student–teacher ratios and deliberate practices of nonintervention, even during emotionally intense conflicts, cultivate children's attention to peers and their abilities to function in groups "as a self-monitoring, self-controlling community" (Hayashi & Tobin, 2011, p. 153). These core sensibilities come to life in the school setting, so schools are key institutions involved in shaping young children into culturally competent members of their society.

Yet schools are also locations in which some children encounter barriers to competence or social practices that alienate rather than include them. Worldwide, the impetus toward schooling in high-prestige, colonialist languages means that many children end up "doubly disadvantaged," failing to access the curriculum because they have not properly learned the language of instruction (Bhattacharya, 2013, p. 15). Bhattacharya (2013) describes a school in an economically insecure community in India where official rhetoric strongly emphasizes the importance of English as an economic imperative, a prerequisite for economic mobility. However, she finds the school is not very successful at teaching English or conveying academic content, instead ultimately reinforcing global hierarchies. Moore (1999) similarly finds that in northern Cameroon, where local people speak 25 different languages, formal schooling is led by teachers from outside the community who insist on monolingual use of French in the classroom. Even though students are adept at using and acquiring multiple languages in the community, they are not allowed to apply these strategies in school. Not only do they develop little proficiency in French, but fewer than one-third of students manage to complete primary school (Moore, 1999, p. 331; cf. Higgins & Cole, 2016). Among Brazilian youth and adults enrolled in literacy programs, Bartlett (2007) documents widespread experiences of ridicule and shame associated with their use of nonstandard language varieties and a deeply internalized belief in a single "correct" Portuguese language. These cases are reminders that school is not merely a place where unformed novices are smoothly molded into fully-functioning members of their society; it is also a space in which students negotiate hierarchies, status, and various forms of exclusion (García-Sánchez, 2014).

An extensive literature, situated primarily in "multicultural" settings in the Global North, points to discontinuities between WEIRD institutional norms and the "ways with words" that children from minoritized communities bring to school. These discontinuities include not just use of other languages and nonstandard dialects, but subtler, more profound differences in interactional ecologies and rhetorical strategies that set up clashing expectations for how learning is organized, how knowledge is displayed, and who is rewarded or disciplined (Genishi & Dyson, 2009; Heath, 1983; Labov, 1972a; Moore, 2006). So, for instance, during ethnographic work in northern Quebec, Crago (1992) found that mainstream White teachers were confounded by Inuit students who did not participate verbally in the classroom in ways that the teachers could make sense of. The teachers depended on a form of classroom discourse known as an initiation-response-evaluation (IRE) routine, in which the teacher asks a question she knows the answer to, selects an individual student to respond, and publicly evaluates the answer. This is a discourse pattern at odds with norms guiding participation, child–adult interactions, and displays of competence in Inuit and many other Indigenous communities, where novices are socialized to learn through observation and collaboration (Crago, 1990; 1992; Eriks-Brophy & Crago, 2003; Paradise & Rogoff, 2009; Philips, 1983). Crago's work revealed that children experienced significant stress at school, whereas teachers believed Inuit students lacked knowledge and suspected that as many as 30% of the children in their classes might have language disabilities (Crago, 1992, p. 497).

In terms of educators' ability to assess language and communication, there is ample evidence that teachers and other professionals often fail to recognize what children can do. Processes of "systematic misrecognition" (Miller & Sperry, 2012) cut both ways, as children from middle-class, mainstream backgrounds appear to understand classroom genres and reasoning patterns without having to be taught—and are perceived as "smart"—while economically insecure and minority group children may display types of logic not easily apparent to teachers (Michaels, 2005). Rather than offering these children ways to build on their existing verbal repertoires, education systems privilege dominant practices, restrict stigmatized children's access to stimulating learning experiences, place blame on students for "unwillingness" to learn, and sometimes undercut their competency through cumulative patterns of oppositional relationship (Adair et al., 2017; Cekaite, 2012; Dudley-Marling & Lucas, 2009; Michaels, 1991; Romero-Little et al., 2007; Sperry et al., 2020; Wortham, 2004).

The major point of this body of literature has been that *schools* are systematically failing these children, underestimating the linguistic resources they bring to the classroom and delegitimating the communicative practices most closely tied to their identities and home communities (García-Sánchez & Orellana, 2019; Miller & Sperry, 2012; Zentella, 2005). Heath, who carefully documented home literacy and oral narrative practices in working-class South Carolina families during the period of racial desegregation, worked with teachers to develop creative pedagogies that cast children as "language detectives" and brought communicative practices from home into the school (Heath, 1983). Yet even as she wrote the epilogue to her book in the early 1980s, Heath noted that the climate of education was changing in ways that stifled teachers' autonomy and privileged a rigid, uniform curriculum.

As political and economic trends in the United States have only intensified the regimentation of schooling, findings about discontinuities between home and school practices tend to get taken up and distorted in *deficit discourses* that position families and individual children as the ones who need to fix their patterns of interaction (Avineri et al., 2015; Blum, 2017; de León & García-Sánchez, 2021; McCarty, 2015). Currently, the powerful "word gap" hypothesis dominates popular and scholarly discourses, accounting for persistent patterns of educational failure by focusing on a supposed gap of 30 million irretrievably lost words that seals the fate of toddlers from economically insecure families before they ever set off to school. Inspired by a single, flawed study by Hart and Risley (1995, 2003), the idea of a catastrophic word gap originating from parents' failure to talk to their children has been taken up enthusiastically by researchers, popular media, and funders eager for a silver bullet to eliminate educational inequality (Adair et al., 2017; Sperry et al., 2020).

Critiques of the word gap gospel center not just on methodological and ideological problems with Hart and Risley's study itself but on the observable repercussions of this discourse for minoritized children (Adair et al., 2017; Baugh, 2016; Johnson, 2019; Johnson et al., 2017; Paugh & Riley, 2019; Sperry et al., 2018, 2020). Adair, Colgrove, and McManus (2017), for example, found that teachers of low-income Latinx students pointed to lack of vocabulary as the primary reason why they could not use high-quality, agentic learning practices in their classrooms. Although educators watched videos of Latinx students successfully participating in a noisy, dynamic, agentic classroom and *praised* what they saw, they drew the (erroneous) conclusion that the students in the video differed from the ones in their schools and said that these students obviously had come to school with better vocabularies and more parental support (Adair et al., 2017, p. 319). Most teachers framed agentic learning as something their students should have access to only once they crossed a threshold of basic vocabulary knowledge. They transmitted to their students the idea that learning must be quiet, compliant, and independent, and that students should be punished for actions such as talking while working or getting out of their seat to help a peer (Adair et al., 2017, p. 325). Word gap discourses thus translate directly into discrimination, as the very children who could benefit most from high-quality pedagogy are denied opportunities for learning that are routinely available to more privileged children.

To avoid the persistent misinterpretation of research about educational discontinuities, language socialization scholars have called for increasing attention to the underlying similarities in the skills children build across contexts (de León & García-Sánchez, 2021; García-Sánchez & Orellana, 2019). Orellana and Reynolds (2008), for example, investigated Mexican-American children's experiences as "language brokers" for adult family members who have limited English, suggesting that the linguistic dexterity children develop in putting complex material into their own words could be directly leveraged in difficult school tasks such as paraphrasing and summarizing texts. Children's skillful incorporation of bi- or multilingual repertoires in codeswitching or *translanguaging* practices also demonstrates nuanced audience awareness (Martínez et al., 2019) as well as metalinguistic knowledge about morphology, semantics, and historical linguistic connections (García-Sánchez, 2019). Studies focused on hip hop and other counterhegemonic youth "ill-literacies" (Alim, 2011) reveal enormous linguistic and rhetorical sophistication in these styles and argue that they are valuable resources in a pluralistic society (Alim, 2003; Paris, 2011; Paris & Alim, 2014; Young, 2010). Yet others caution that all of this research proving the linguistic dexterity and creativity of stigmatized communities will never be enough as long as White supremacy and socioeconomic stratification continue to "orient the ears" of "listening subjects from whose perspectives 'language gaps' are perceived" (Rosa & Flores, 2015, p. 78). Like the middle-class White children watching Indigenous-heritage children collaborate in Roberts' and Rogoff's study (2012), we see what we are looking for and we hear what we listen for.

Language Socialization and Disability

What of children or adults who do, unquestionably, face challenges to communication due to neurodevelopmental or cognitive disabilities? Language socialization scholars have paid increasing attention to conditions like autism, aphasia, and dementia that shed light on human sociality and the nature of communicative competence precisely because they interrupt or "make strange" processes that ordinarily occur outside of our awareness (Maynard & Turowetz, 2022; Solomon & Bagatell, 2010; Sterponi, 2017). This work, too, highlights forms of misrecognition associated with supposedly objective, "culture-free" biomedical models that focus on what an individual cannot do in a laboratory setting. Close attention to people's participation across a range of home, community, and clinical interactions shows linguistic (in)competence to be deeply contextual and distributed among multiple participants—not simply an intrapsychic phenomenon. Once again, it matters what beliefs and ideologies participants bring to the situation, how bodies are arranged, what activities and semiotic modalities are centered, and exactly how partners try to accommodate to perceived deficits.

Given their interest in the social and cultural "practical logic" of situated communication (Ochs & Solomon, 2005), anthropologists have contributed nuance to the interpretation of deficits framed as properties of the individual. While impairments do not disappear, otherwise unseen aspects of competency come to the fore when analysts look carefully at interactions using video data and ethnographic observation. For example, in a series of articles analyzing his father's daily interactions in the years following a massive stroke, Goodwin (1995, 2000, 2004) raises the paradox of how a person could be "a competent speaker who cannot speak." Goodwin points out that in a clinical evaluation that required him to produce extended turns at talk in isolation, his father—who could speak only three words: *yes*, *no*, and *and*—would appear utterly inadequate as a speaker. In the context of ongoing activities and conversational structures, however, Goodwin was able to tie his speech to others' at finely tuned intervals within unfolding sequences, combining his words with resources such as nonsense syllables, prosodic intonation patterns, gestures, body orientation, and gaze in order to participate meaningfully in conversations, even position himself as the principal teller of a narrative (Goodwin, 2004). Similarly, Sterponi and her colleagues show that in the context of ongoing exchanges, autistic children with limited language can mobilize resources like echolalia or appender questions[1] to respond creatively to others' speech, express affiliation or challenge, and shift the trajectory of the interaction (Sterponi & Fasulo, 2010; Sterponi & Shankey, 2014).

[1]Like tag questions ("right?" "isn't it?"), appenders are questions syntactically affixed to a prior sentence. Examples in Sterponi and Fasulo's article include "because?" and "or else?" Both appender and tag questions generate a slot for the other speaker to say more, extending the conversation.

Attention to the structure of conversational sequences also shows how common practices used by conversational partners inadvertently conceal or even undermine competency. Ochs, Solomon, and Sterponi (2005) argue that the conventional types of simplification that are emphasized in Euro-American babytalk (e.g., face-to-face orientation, exaggerated eye contact, prosodic extremes, slowed or elongated speech, and profuse praise) form a *habitus* or default mode of interaction that may interfere with autistic children's ability to understand and participate in communication. These findings are mirrored in research on "elderspeak," which is experienced by many people as demeaning and has been associated with social isolation and cognitive decline (Corwin, 2018).

Other didactic moves that exert a high degree of control over conversation, including school-like questions, imply low faith in an interlocutor's capacities and may signal low interest in their unique human qualities, yet these are deeply engrained professional practices. Kovarsky, Kimbarow, and Kastner (1999), for example, analyze a group therapy session for adults with traumatic brain injury, during which the therapist was so focused on carrying out an abstract listing game that she failed to acknowledge authentic, relevant contributions if they violated the rules. Fasulo and Fiore (2007) describe how clinicians aiming to improve autistic children's conversational skills frustrated and shut down the children's communication by constantly evaluating their turns, censoring topics that the children found interesting, and insisting that the children produce explicit answers to obvious questions. Yet, Maynard (2019) shows how neurotypical adults fail to recognize how their own interactional moves create the conditions that children respond to, so that they often experience autistic children as behaving in atypical ways "out of the blue." Caught up in professional protocols and procedures, authority figures including police officers, school personnel, and clinicians describe incidents of problematic behavior as if they were initiated by the child, even when video recordings of the same event reveal the child to be *responding* to something the adult did.

On the other hand, literature from the language socialization paradigm also provides many examples of how interactional practices may be transformed to create a "prosthetic environment" that supports and empowers communicators (Maynard & Turkowetz, 2022). Some of these are practical changes, adjustments as simple as sitting side-by-side rather than face-to-face, orienting to a communication board rather than requiring speech, or toning down excessive positive affect (Ochs et al., 2005; Solomon, 2014). Other adjustments include arranging the environment to scaffold participation, grounding learning activities in the joint accomplishment of meaningful tasks (Conrad, 2020; Goodwin & Cekaite, 2018; Paradise & Rogoff, 2009). Even more importantly, what emerges from ethnographic observation is the critical difference made by conversational partners who bring an attitude of respect toward their interlocutor and trust in their capacities to communicate. These respectful conversational partners can include family members and therapists who ask authentic questions, following up on topics of interest or working laboriously and systematically to make sure they understand the desires of a person with impaired language (Fasulo & Fiore, 2007; Goodwin, 2000; Kremer-Sadlik, 2004; Solomon, 2014). They can be members of the community who continue using complex language around elder peers with dementia, bathing them in familiar genres such as blessings, jokes, and storytelling that invite open-ended participation without demanding any particular response (Corwin, 2018, 2021). They can be classmates who have been trusted with information about their peer's diagnosis and learn to respond generously to unexpected behavior (Ochs et al., 2001). They can be parents who co-narrate stories with their autistic children, centering them as capable, engaged, socially included protagonists (Sirota, 2010), or who accompany them on flights of verbal fancy, using language play to generate intense pleasure and new possibilities for intersubjectivity (Sterponi & Fasulo, 2010).

Implications for Assessment

The language socialization literature is not written by clinicians, nor is it aimed at a clinical audience. Most of it does not deal directly with clinical procedures or settings, instead exploring how communicative competence is achieved (or not) and how informal judgments about linguistic competence are made and acted on in everyday interactions. Language socialization researchers seek to illuminate the social world and contribute to broad social theory, not provide quick models, actionable tips, or tools for assessment. Differences in disciplinary expectations can make their messages difficult to absorb, especially for practitioners who have been socialized to value experimental techniques and quantitative statistics (Higginbotham & Engelke, 2013). Nevertheless, this research has clear relevance for clinicians and should be more familiar within our field. The remainder of the chapter identifies two major lessons emerging from language socialization literature and then traces their implications with regard to two primary goals that a clinician may have while conducting an assessment: (1) to determine whether a disability exists (and what kind) and (2) to plan for treatment by documenting current functioning.

First and foremost, language socialization research challenges us to rethink pat notions of culture and diversity. The field of communication sciences draws on a thin and outdated vision of "culture" as a set of static traits shared by people within an ethnic or racial group, and casts linguistic and cultural "diversity" as something belonging to *other people*, namely, people identified as ethnic or racial minority groups. Language socialization research, on the other hand, is part of anthropological and sociolinguistic traditions that have long grappled with these concepts and advance dynamic, experience-grounded, process-oriented conceptualizations of culture (Kirmayer, 2012; Lakes et al., 2006; Watson et al., 2016). In the writings of language socialization scholars, culture does have to do with deeply shared values, behavioral norms, and orientations, but the emphasis is on how these are communicated, taken up, performed, manipulated, challenged, and even changed within specific communities of practice. All people, by virtue of being human, are cultural beings socialized into particular socially defined ways of seeing and doing—whether they are highly specialized professionals, high school nerds in the United States, or Moroccan immigrants in Spain (Bucholtz, 1999; Gárcia-Sánchez, 2013; Goodwin, 1994). Diversity is an empirical phenomenon related to the variety in cultural forms and practices; it may also be seen as good and a challenge to life within pluralist societies. Language socialization research highlights the great diversity in human ways of communicating and of becoming competent actors.

Second, the studies reviewed here all insist that we understand linguistic competence in social context—or rather, as a fundamentally social accomplishment inseparable from what we typically consider "context" (Goodwin & Duranti, 1992; Ochs & Schieffelin, 1984). They destabilize commonly held intuitions about language as an intrapsychic phenomenon or even as a set of decodable messages that move in a linear fashion between a "sender" and a "receiver" (Shannon & Weaver, 1949). Instead, these studies of talk-in-interaction emphasize the ways participants in a conversation create meaning together in an intricate choreography of sound, movement, and physical space, responding to the demands of the situational context (e.g., when you run into someone you are expected to greet them) but also co-creating it (e.g., your greeting generates the expectation of a reciprocated greeting and sets the stage for further conversation). When discussing the communicative difficulties posed by cultural variance or disability, language socialization scholars prompt us to ask whether, or to what extent, (in)competence might be an artifact of interactional processes. Much like disability rights advocates, they therefore challenge a fundamental assumption of clinical practice that deficits *in an individual* should be the main focus of measurement and intervention (Montgomery, 2020; Van der Klift & Kunc, 2019). They also help us understand how, as clinicians, our attention can be systematically deflected away from what *we* do in interaction and drawn to faults that are imagined to lie within a child, home, or "culture."

Culture and Diversity: Difference Versus Disorder

One key message that emerges from language socialization research is that beyond certain benchmarks (e.g., the development of joint attention and first words), norms associated with the linear development of capabilities in a single language are not universal, nor are they neutral. Children may begin life exposed to one set of communicative norms, then be expected to function in a very different milieu when they start school (Crago, 1990; Miller & Sperry, 2012; Moore, 1999). Their skills in heritage language(s) may wax and wane over time depending on opportunities for practice and their own evolving affiliations (He, 2014). They may actively manipulate key features of phonology, lexicon, syntax, or pragmatics in order to demarcate identities, play with language, create art, or deliberately distance themselves from the norms of academic language (Alim, 2011; Eckert, 1989; Mendoza-Denton, 2008; Paris, 2011; Rampton, 1995; Rosa, 2019). Professionals—often monolingual members of the dominant social class with little training in parsing sociolinguistic differences—are ill-equipped to recognize these nuances and may be inclined to denigrate rather than celebrate them, perpetuating White supremacy and classism (Dudley-Marling & Lucas, 2009). And, standardized tests can tell us very little about such heterogeneous language skills.

This may be discouraging, but it is not news. We already know that no arbitrary cutoff score on a standardized test can reliably distinguish children with language impairments from those that are typically developing, no matter how normative a child's background (Spaulding et al., 2006). Especially when we are dealing with individuals from dual-language or nondominant communities, we know that it is not appropriate to rely on decontextualized, norm-referenced assessments that center on dominant practices (Solano-Flores et al., 2015) and intrapsychic processes (Wiig & Secord, 2006). Diagnosis of language impairments is rarely straightforward because of the complexity of communication, the connections between language disorders and a host of other conditions, and the varied ways language difficulties can be conceptualized or classified; diagnosis is instead "a contingent, interpretive, temporal process" (Maynard & Turowetz, 2017) that depends on building a case using multiple sources of evidence. The language socialization research reviewed here, therefore, adds to an already extensive evidence base supporting authentic, holistic, multi-faceted, and dynamic assessment practices (see Bishop et al., 2016; Henderson et al., 2018; Orellana et al., 2019; Paradis et al., 2011; Shipley & McAfee, 2021; Vining et al., 2017; Wiig, 2000). It reinforces calls to use qualitative methodologies like interviews, naturalistic observations, and conversation analysis, guided by principles that include an open stance to data collection and a commitment to representing the perspective of the person being assessed (Tetnowski & Franklin, 2003). It also provides a largely untapped source of data for speech-language pathologists to expand their awareness of sociolinguistic variation.

Diagnosing speech and language impairments often requires making judgments about whether presenting behavior represents a disability or a difference; that is, whether it truly indicates an impairment or whether it might be an artifact of a person's greater familiarity with some other dialect, language, or social context. Crowley et al. (2015) argue that specific knowledge of language variants is crucial for culturally competent practice and propose, above all, that speech-language pathologists improve their command of grammar so that they can systematically analyze language samples. This is excellent advice, but on its own it perpetuates an emphasis on linguistic *form* rather than use in social context. Ethnographically informed research suggests that differences in usage—norms for displaying politeness, asking and answering questions, choosing topics, organizing narratives, and so on—can be just as consequential as adults make judgments about children's competence or decide whether or not they need speech-language services. Unfortunately, speech-language pathologists often have even less knowledge about this dimension of sociolinguistic difference than they do about morphosyntactic variance.

The problems with this lack of empirical grounding are evident in a series of articles about incarcerated adolescent girls by Sanger and colleagues (Sanger et al., 1999, 2000, 2001, 2003). The authors call attention to the difficulty of diagnosing language disorders in this population, but nevertheless present estimates of language impairment based on the teenagers' performance on standardized measures. Although they employ qualitative methods to investigate the girls' communication, including interviews and observations in the detention center, the authors never abandon a rigid, scandalized, adult, White, middle-class attitude about what language *should* be like and how it should be used. They describe themselves as "professionals ... who adhere to the expectations of society as a whole" (Sanger et al., 1999, p. 290) and the girls as "delinquents" who may be *assumed* to have deficits in behavior and judgment "by virtue of the fact that [they] are incarcerated" (Sanger et al., 2001, p. 19). All of the authors' observations are cast in a negative light, emphasizing the girls' resistance to authority, self-centeredness, casual acceptance of violence, and even manipulativeness (in that many of the girls seem *able* to follow normative conversation expectations in structured settings or when they recognize a benefit to themselves, but *don't* in most situations). Sanger and colleagues cautiously suggest that perhaps the teenagers' language behaviors might be appropriate in some other (unspecified) speech community, but on the whole, they argue that these teenagers are either suffering from language deficits that need remediation or are simply deviants, committed to acting in defiance of social norms (Sanger et al., 1999).

Though motivated by the sweetest of intentions to help "delinquents" improve their lives, Sanger and colleagues' work is irresponsible in its ethnocentrism and in the fact that it apparently did not occur to any of the authors (or their peer reviewers) that there might exist other valid pragmatic norms, let alone some way of *finding out* about language practices used by anybody other than prim, professional adults. Their research stands in contrast to more deeply contextualized anthropological work such as Mendoza-Denton's (2008) account of the language practices of girls in Latina youth gangs. Many of the girls Mendoza-Denton worked with did poorly in school, were tracked into English Learner classes or special education, and certainly were surveilled by law enforcement. Mendoza-Denton encountered some of the same practices that Sanger and her colleagues found reprehensible—profanity, antagonistic threats and insults, an interest in topics such as violence and betrayal rather than displays of "world knowledge" (Sanger et al., 2000, p. 44). However, since Mendoza-Denton does not impose an attitude of knee-jerk moral judgment, she is able to show readers the sophisticated inner workings of a life-world in which teenage girls use language to demarcate identities, form coalitions, maintain face, tell jokes, write poetry, and self-consciously subvert the norms of polite, well-educated, wealthy society. Investigating this life-world on its own terms, Mendoza-Denton shows the coherence—and, indeed, the vibrancy—of their language within a particular community of practice.

Sanger and her fellow researchers would not have had access to Mendoza-Denton's study or allied work on youth language and identities published more recently (Alim, 2011; Paris, 2011; Rosa, 2019), but they missed an abundant literature dating back to the 1970s on the language practices of adolescents from many different cultural backgrounds (see Eckert, 1989; Goodwin, 1990; Kusserow, 1999; Labov, 1972b; Rampton, 1995; Smitherman, 1977; Zentella, 1997). Furthermore, they obviously were not acquainted with the research reviewed earlier in this chapter about deficit discourses, misrecognition, and the feedback loops through which some children come to be characterized as problematic (see Cekaite, 2012; Wortham, 2004). None of these ethnographic studies could have been used as an exact yardstick against which to measure the incarcerated teenagers' performance, yet even a passing familiarity with this literature might have guided these clinicians to ask better questions—questions that sought to understand the girls' language practices in a larger social context, rather than trying to make sense of them as enigmatic individual aberrancies.

Assessment and the Social Environment

Language socialization research encourages clinicians to attend to the social context(s) in which targets of evaluation display their strengths and weaknesses: the political and sociocultural context, but also the physical context, the situational context, and the microcontexts that emerge as an interactional sequence unfolds, each turn creating an invitation or closure of possibility for interlocutors. What would it mean to think more carefully about these social environments as we carry out an evaluation, or to look for strengths and weaknesses that might be located *in the interactional environment* instead of solely in the individual? We might start with the testing environment itself. Labov (1972a) long ago depicted the conundrum faced by an adult trying to elicit a language sample from a child. As part of a project on the language of Black children in South Central Harlem in the 1960s, a researcher named Clarence Robins—a man from the community who was familiar with the children—tried to record an interview with an 8-year-old named Leon, to no avail. Leon gave monosyllabic answers and seemed unable to answer the simplest question. After consideration of the social factors at play, Clarence returned for a second try. This time, he:

1. Brought along a supply of potato chips, changing the "interview" into something more in the nature of a party.
2. Brought along Leon's best friend, 8-year-old Gregory.
3. Reduced the height imbalance. When Clarence got down on the floor of Leon's room, he dropped from 6 feet, 2 inches to 3 feet, 6 inches.
4. Introduced taboo words and taboo topics, and proved to Leon's surprise that one can say anything into our microphone without any fear of retaliation. It did not hit or bite back. The result of these changes is a striking difference in the volume and style of speech (Labov, 1972a, p. 61).

Suddenly, Labov writes, Leon was competing with Gregory for the floor, making outrageous claims, and using complex language. Simple strategies allowed Clarence to establish a different relationship with Leon, one that made possible a very different display of his language competence.

The point is not that clinicians should imitate Clarence's strategies, but that during assessments we are (inevitably) arranging the environment in ways that powerfully influence speakers' abilities to demonstrate what they can do. In their research on an urban clinic for autism diagnosis, Maynard and Turowetz further point out that while assessment instruments and the actions of clinicians are both important influences on a child's performance, "these performances are, as a matter of course, attributed to the child alone" (2022, p. 26). Examining video footage of diagnostic encounters, they can see details such as the way one boy declined a task no fewer than 11 times before he got up from the table—an action that the clinician found notable and reported during follow-up conversations. In her evaluation report, she wrote, "When asked to demonstrate how he brushes his teeth during a particular activity, Dan walked away from the table and faced the wall in the corner of the room" (Maynard, 2019, p. 24). Dan's refusal to attempt this task is clearly atypical for a child of his age and may be consistent with autism; the issue in this case is not that the clinician arrived at the wrong diagnosis. However, the adult's role in pressing him over and over after he had quite politely declined is deleted from the picture, giving an impression of Dan as an even more erratic actor than he really was. In this evaluation, only Dan's behavior is under the microscope, but the clinician's elision of her own actions obscures information that could be useful in understanding this child, how he responds to demands, and how the social environment could be rearranged so that he might be more successful. It deprives the team of information that could be useful to planning interventions at school and in other contexts where Dan meets with similar challenges.

A speech-language pathologist may or may not have direct access to other domains within which the target of an assessment is expected to function—school, home, work—but can still ask deliberate questions to investigate the influence of the interactional ecology on the ways a person's competence is revealed or concealed. In a classroom, how is the physical environment laid out, and how are people and objects oriented within it? What participation frameworks or verbal routines are characteristic? How supportive are teachers and peers as communication partners, and what strategies are they using that facilitate or discourage communication? What happens at home, at the grocery store, or elsewhere in the community? Even in areas of practice that already emphasize training of communication partners, such as aphasiology, dementia care, or augmentative and alternative communication, nuanced information about other people and what they do to structure, facilitate, or interfere with interaction can be overlooked. In a review of the literature on communication partner training in aphasia, for example, Turner and Whitworth (2006) comment that while all the studies provided information about the characteristics of the person with aphasia, few mentioned anything about the partner other than minimal demographic information. Nevertheless, a growing research base suggests that using conversation analytic approaches to examine interactions, identify treatment goals, and train communication partners in open-ended interactional strategies can improve outcomes in people with a variety of conditions (Damico et al., 2015; Hengst & Duff, 2007; Kent-Walsh, 2015; Troche et al., 2019). These findings converge with those of language socialization researchers and suggest that one of the major issues at stake is helping communication partners (including clinicians) to approach interactions from an ethical orientation of respect, trust, and openness rather than tight control.

Competence in the interpretive work of diagnosis and planning intervention must be an iterative, lifelong process of engagement with clients, peers, and emerging research. In this chapter, I have argued that clinicians working to improve the communication and quality of life of people with language impairments can gain a lot by looking beyond the research base explicitly aimed at clinicians and exploring the language socialization literature. Despite the challenges posed by reading across disciplinary expectations and goals, speech-language pathologists need a richer, more complex sense of the connections that bind language and culture, a deeper appreciation for the ways power and inequality operate in our institutions and professional practices, and more nuanced ways of analyzing the details of social interactions. We benefit from ethnographic information about social and linguistic diversity as we try to identify appropriate candidates for therapy, and as we plan treatment goals. In turn, the people we serve gain stronger allies.

References

Adair, J. K., Colegrove, K. S., & McManus, M. E. (2017). How the word gap argument negatively impacts young children of Latinx immigrants' conceptualizations of learning. *Harvard Educational Review, 87*(3), 309-334.

Alcalá, L., Rogoff, B., & Fraire, A. L. (2018). Sophisticated collaboration is common among Mexican-heritage US children. *Proceedings of the National Academy of Sciences, 115*(45), 11377-11384. https://doi.org/10.1073/pnas.1805707115

Alim, S. (2003). On some serious next millennium rap ishhh: Pharoahe monch, hip hop poetics, and the internal rhymes of internal affairs. *Journal of English Linguistics, 31*(1), 60-84.

Alim, H. S. (2011). Global ill-literacies: Hip hop cultures, youth identities, and the politics of literacy. *Review of Research in Education, 35*(1), 120-146.

Avineri, N., Johnson, E., Brice-Heath, S., McCarty, T., Ochs, E., Kremer-Sadlik, T., Blum, S., Zentella, A. C., Rosa, J., Flores, N., Alim, H. S., & Paris, D. (2015). Invited forum: Bridging the "language gap." *Journal of Linguistic Anthropology, 25*(1), 66-86.

Baugh, J. (2016). Meaning-less differences: Exposing fallacies and flaws in "the word gap" hypothesis that conceal a dangerous "language trap" for low-income American families and their children. *International Multilingual Research Journal, 11*(1), 39-51.

Bartlett, L. (2007). Literacy, speech and shame: The cultural politics of literacy and language in Brazil. *International Journal of Qualitative Studies in Education, 20*(5), 547-563.

Bhattacharya, U. (2013). *"Globalization" and the English imperative: A study of language ideologies and literacy practices at an orphanage and village school in suburban New Delhi* [Doctoral dissertation]. UC Berkeley. https://escholarship.org/uc/item/862751z2

Bishop, D. V. M., Snowling, M. J., Thompson, P. A., Greenhalgh, T., & the CATALISE consortium. (2016). CATALISE: A multinational and multidisciplinary Delphi consensus study. Identifying language impairments in children. *PLoS ONE, 11*(7), e0158753. https://doi.org/10.1371/journal.pone.0158753

Blum, S. (2017). Unseen WEIRD assumptions: The so-called language gap discourse and ideologies of language, childhood, and learning. *International Multilingual Research Journal, 11*(1), 23-38.

Briggs, J. L. (1999). *Inuit morality play: The emotional education of a three-year-old.* Yale University Press.

Brown, P. (2014). The cultural organization of attention. In A. Duranti, E. Ochs, & B. B. Schieffelin (Eds.), *The handbook of language socialization* (pp. 29-55). Wiley Blackwell.

Bucholtz, M. (1999). "Why be normal?": Language and identity practices in a community of nerd girls. *Language in Society, 28*, 203-223.

Casillas, M., Brown, P., Levinson, S. C. (2020). Early language experience in a Tseltal Mayan village. *Child Development, 91*(5), 1819-1835.

Cekaite, A. (2012). Affective stances in teacher-novice student interactions: Language, embodiment, and willingness to learn. *Language in Society, 41*(5), 641-670.

Conrad, K. (2020). *A shared endeavor: Appropriate early intervention for speech and language in Navajo families* [Audio podcast episode]. SoundCloud. https://soundcloud.com/user-806134260/a-shared-endeavor-appropriate-early-intervention-for-speech-and-language-in-navajo-families

Corwin, A. (2018). Overcoming elderspeak: A qualitative study of three alternatives. *Gerontologist, 58*(4), 724-729.

Corwin, A. (2021). *Embracing age: How Catholic nuns became models of aging well.* Rutgers University Press.

Crago, M. B. (1990). Development of communicative competence in Inuit children: Implications for speech-language pathology. *Journal of Childhood Communication Disorders, 13*, 73-84.

Crago, M. B. (1992). Communicative interaction and second language acquisition: An Inuit example. *TESOL Quarterly, 26*(3), 487-505.

Crowley, C. J., Guest, K., & Sudler, K. (2015). Cultural competence needed to distinguish disorder from difference: Beyond Kumbaya. *Perspectives on Communication Disorders and Sciences in Culturally and Linguistically Diverse Populations, 22*, 64-76.

Damico, J. S., Simmons-Mackie, N. N., Oelschlaeger, M., Elman, R., & Armstrong, E. (1999). Qualitative methods in aphasia research: Basic issues. *Aphasiology, 13*, 651-666.

Damico, J., Tetnowski, J., Lynch, K., Hartwell, J., Weill, C., Heels, J., & Simmons-Mackie, N. (2015). Facilitating authentic communication: An intervention employing principles of constructivism and conversation analysis. *Aphasiology, 29*(3), 400-421.

de León, L. (2014). Language socialization and multiparty participation frameworks. In A. Duranti, E. Ochs, & B. B. Schieffelin (Eds.), *The handbook of language socialization* (pp. 81-111). Wiley Blackwell.

de León, L., & García-Sánchez, I. M. (2021). Language socialization at the intersection of the local and the global: The contested trajectories of input and communicative competence. *Annual Review of Linguistics, 7*, 421-48.

Dudley-Marling, C., & Lucas, K. (2009). Pathologizing the language and culture of poor children. *Language Arts, 86*(5), 362-370.

Duranti, A., & Black, S. P. (2014). Language socialization and verbal improvisation. In A. Duranti, E. Ochs, & B. B. Schieffelin (Eds.), *The handbook of language socialization* (pp. 443-463). Wiley Blackwell.

Eckert, P. (1989). *Jocks and burnouts: Social categories and identity in the high school.* Teachers College Press.

Eriks-Brophy, A., & Crago, M. B. (2003). Variation in instructional discourse features: cultural or linguistic? Evidence from Inuit and non-Inuit teachers of Nunavik. *Anthropology and Education Quarterly, 34*(4), 396-419.

Fasulo, A., & Fiore, F. (2007). A valid person: Non-competence as a conversational outcome. In A. Hepburn & S. Wiggins (Eds.), *Discursive research in practice: New approaches to psychology and interaction* (pp. 224–246). Cambridge University Press.

Field, M. (2001). Triadic directives in Navajo language socialization. *Language in Society, 30*, 249-263.

Fung, H., Miller, P. J., & Lin, L. (2004). Listening is active: Lessons from the narrative practices of Taiwanese families. In M. W. Pratt & B. H. Feise (Eds.), *Family stories and the life course: Across time and generations.* Lawrence Erlbaum and Associates, Publishers.

García-Sánchez, I. M. (2013). The everyday politics of "cultural citizenship" among North African immigrant school children in Spain. *Language & Communication. 33*(4), 481-499.

García-Sánchez, I. M. (2014). Language socialization and exclusion. In A. Duranti, E. Ochs, & B. B. Schieffelin (Eds.), *The handbook of language socialization* (pp. 391-419). Wiley Blackwell.

García-Sánchez, I. M. (2019). Centering shared linguistic heritage to build language and literacy resilience among immigrant students. In I. M. García-Sánchez & M. Faulstich Orellana (Eds.), *Language and cultural practices in communities and schools: Bridging learning for students from non-dominant groups* (pp. 139-160). Routledge.

García-Sánchez, I. M., & Orellana, M. F. (Eds.). (2019). *Language and cultural practices in communities and schools: Bridging learning for students from non-dominant groups.* Routledge.

Gaskins, S., & Paradise, R. (2010). Learning through observation. In D. F. Lancy, J. Bock, S. Gaskins (Eds.) *The anthropology of learning in childhood* (pp. 85-117). Alta Mira.

Genishi, C., & Dyson, A. H. (2009). *Children, language, and literacy: Diverse learners in diverse times.* Teachers College Press.

Goodwin, C. (1994). Professional vision. *American Anthropologist, 96,* 606-633.

Goodwin, C. (1995). Co-constructing meaning in conversations with an aphasic man. *Research on Language and Social Interaction, 28*(3), 233-260.

Goodwin, C. (2000). Gesture, aphasia, and interaction. In D. McNeill (Ed.), *Language and gesture* (pp. 84-98). Cambridge University Press.

Goodwin, C. (2004). A competent speaker who can't speak: The social life of aphasia. *Journal of Linguistic Anthropology, 14*(2), 151-170.

Goodwin, C., & Duranti, A. (1992). Introduction. In C. Goodwin & A. Duranti (Eds.), *Rethinking context: Language as an interactive phenomenon* (pp. 1-42). Cambridge University Press.

Goodwin, C., & Heritage, J. (1990). Conversation analysis. *Annual Review of Anthropology, 19,* 283-307.

Goodwin, M. H. (1990). *He-said-she-said: Talk as social organization among Black children.* Indiana University Press.

Goodwin, M. H., & Cekaite, A. (2018). Socializing enskilment. In *Embodied Family Choreography: Practices of control, care, and mundane creativity* (pp. 207-224). Routledge.

Hart, B., & Risley, T. R. (1995). *Meaningful differences in the everyday experience of young American children.* Brookes.

Hart, B., & Risley, T. R. (2003). The early catastrophe: The 30 million word gap by age 3. *American Educator, 27*(1), 4-9.

Hauk, J. (2016). *Making language: The ideological and interactional constitution of language in an indigenous Aché community in Eastern Paraguay* [Unpublished doctoral dissertation]. University of California, Los Angeles.

Hayashi, A., & Tobin, J. (2011). The Japanese preschool's pedagogy of peripheral participation. *Ethos, 38*(2), 139-164.

He, A. W. (2014). Heritage language socialization. In A. Duranti, E. Ochs, & B. B. Schieffelin (Eds.), *The handbook of language socialization* (pp. 587-609). Wiley Blackwell.

Heath, S. B. (1983). *Ways with words: Language, life, and work in communities and classrooms.* Cambridge University Press.

Henderson, D. E., Restrepo, M. A., & Aiken, L. S. (2018). Dynamic assessment of narratives among Navajo preschoolers. *Journal of Speech, Language, and Hearing Research, 61,* 2547-2560.

Hengst, J. A., & Duff, M. C. (2007). Clinicians as communication partners. *Topics in Language Disorders, 27*(1), 37-49.

Henrich, J., Heine, S. J., & Norenzayan, A. (2010). The weirdest people in the world? *The Behavioral and Brain Sciences, 33*(2-3), 61-83. https://doi.org/10.1017/s0140525x0999152x

Higginbotham, D. J., & Engelke, C. R. (2013). A primer for doing talk-in-interaction research in augmentative and alternative communication. *Augmentative and Alternative Communication, 29*(1), 3-19.

Higgins, N. (Producer), & Cole, A. (Director). (2016). *Colours of the Alphabet* [Film]. Documentary Educational Resources.

Johnson, E. J. (2019). A critical interrogation of the "language gap." In N. Avineri, L. R. Graham, E. J. Johnson, R. Conley Riner, & J. Rosa (Eds.), *Language and social justice in practice.* Routledge.

Johnson, E. J., Avineri, N., & Johnson, D. C. (2017). Exposing gaps in/between discourses of linguistic deficits. *International Multilingual Research Journal, 11*(1), 5-22.

Kent-Walsh, J., Murza, K. A., Malani, M. D., & Binger, C. (2015). Effects of communication partner instruction on the communication of individuals using AAC: A meta-analysis. *Augmentative and Alternative Communication, 31*(4), 271-284. https://doi.org/10.3109/07434618.2015.1052153

Kirmayer L. J. (2012). Rethinking cultural competence. *Transcultural Psychiatry, 49*, 149-64.

Kovarsky, D., Duchan, J., & Maxwell, M. (Eds.). (1999). *Constructing (in)competence: Disabling evaluations in clinical and social interaction.* Erlbaum.

Kovarsky, D., Kimbarow, M., & Kastner, D. (1999). The construction of incompetence during group therapy with traumatically brain injured adults. In D. Kovarsky, J. Duchan, & M. Maxwell (Eds.) *Constructing (in) competence: Disabling evaluations in clinical and social interaction* (pp. 291-311). Erlbaum.

Kremer-Sadlik, T. (2004). How children with autism and Asperger syndrome respond to questions: A 'naturalistic' theory of mind task. *Discourse Studies, 6*(2),185-206.

Kusserow, A. (1999). De-homogenizing American individualism: Socializing hard and soft individualism in Manhattan and Queens. *Ethos, 27*(2), 210-234.

Labov, W. (1972a). Academic ignorance and Black intelligence. *The Atlantic, 229*(6), 59-67.

Labov, W. (1972b). *Language in the inner city: Studies in the Black English vernacular.* University of Pennsylvania Press.

Lakes, K., López, S., & Garro, L. (2006). Cultural competence and psychotherapy: Applying anthropologically informed conceptions of culture. *Psychotherapy, 43*(4), 380-396.

Martínez, R. A., Durán, L., & Hikida, M. (2019). Where everyday translanguaging meets academic writing: Exploring the tensions and generative connections for bilingual Latino/a/x students. In I. M. García-Sánchez & M. Faulstich Orellana (Eds.), *Language and cultural practices in communities and schools: Bridging learning for students from non-dominant groups* (pp. 139-160). Routledge.

Maynard, D. W. (2019). Why social psychology needs autism and why autism needs social psychology: Forensic and clinical considerations. *Social Psychology Quarterly, 82*(1), 5-30.

Maynard, D.W., & Turowetz, J. (2017). Doing diagnosis: Autism, interaction order, and the use of narrative in clinical talk. *Social Psychology Quarterly, 80*(3), 245-275.

Maynard, D. W., & Turowetz, J. (2022). *Autistic intelligence: Interaction, individuality, and the challenges of diagnosis.* University of Chicago Press.

McCarty, T. L. (2015). How the logic of gap discourse perpetuates education inequality: A view from the ethnography of language policy. *Journal of Linguistic Anthropology, 25*(1), 70-72.

Mendoza-Denton, N. (2008). *Homegirls: Language and cultural practice among Latina youth gangs.* Blackwell Publishing.

Michaels, S. (1991). The dismantling of narrative. In A. McCabe & C. Peterson (Eds.), *Developing narrative structure.* Erlbaum.

Michaels, S. (2005). Can the intellectual affordances of working-class storytelling be leveraged in school? *Human Development, 48*(3), 136-145.

Miller, P. J., & Sperry, D. E. (2012). Déjà vu: The continuing misrecognition of low-income children's verbal abilities. In S. T. Fiske & H. R. Markus (Eds.), *Facing social class: How societal rank influences interaction* (pp. 109-130). Russell Sage.

Montgomery, C. (2020, October 23). Smart again. *Cal's blog: A blog about disability.* https://montgomerycal.wordpress.com/2020/10/23/smart-again/

Moore, L. C. (1999). Language socialization research and French language education in Africa: A Cameroonian case study. *The Canadian Modern Language Review, 56*(2), 329-350.

Moore, L. C. (2006). Learning by heart in Qur'anic and public schools in northern Cameroon. *Social Analysis, 50*(3), 109-126.

Ochs, E., Kremer-Sadlik, T., Solomon, O., & Sirota, K. G. (2001). Inclusion as social practice: Views of children with autism. *Social Development, 10*, 399-419.

Ochs, E., & Schieffelin, B. (1984). Language acquisition and socialization: Three developmental stories. In R. A. Shweder & R. A. LeVine (Eds.), *Culture theory: Essays on mind, self, and emotion* (pp. 276-320). Cambridge University Press.

Ochs, E., & Schieffelin, B. (1995). The impact of language socialization on grammatical development. In P. Fletcher & B. MacWhinney (Eds.), *The handbook of child language* (pp. 73-94). Blackwell.

Ochs, E., & Solomon, O. (2005). Practical logic and autism. In C. Casey & R. B. Edgerton (Eds.), *A companion to psychological anthropology.* Blackwell Publishing.

Ochs, E., Solomon, O., & Sterponi, L. (2005). Limitations and transformations of habitus in child-directed communication. *Discourse Studies, 7*(4-5), 547-583.

Orellana, C. I., Wada, R., & Gillam, R. B. (2019). The use of dynamic assessment for the diagnosis of language disorders in bilingual children: A meta-analysis. *American Journal of Speech-Language Pathology, 28,* 1298-1317.

Orellana, M. F., & Reynolds, J. F. (2008). Cultural modeling: Leveraging bilingual skills for school paraphrasing tasks. *Reading Research Quarterly, 43*(1), 48-65.

Paradis, J., Genesee, F., & Crago, M. B. (2011). *Dual language development and disorders: A handbook on bilingualism and second language learning, (2nd ed.).* Paul Brookes Publishing Co.

Paradise, R., & Rogoff, B. (2009). Side by side: Learning by observing and pitching in. *Ethos, 37*(1), 102-138. https://doi.org/10.1111/j.1548-1352.2009.01033.x.

Paris, D. (2011). *Language across difference: Ethnicity, communication, and youth identities in changing urban schools.* Cambridge University Press.

Paris, D., & Alim, S. (2014). What are we seeking to sustain through culturally sustaining pedagogy? A loving critique forward. *Harvard Educational Review, 84*(1), 85-100.

Paugh, A. L., & Riley, K. C. (2019). Poverty and children's language in anthropolitical perspective. *Annual Review of Anthropology, 48,* 297-315.

Philips, S. U. (1983). *The invisible culture: Communication in classroom and community on the Warm Springs Indian Reservation.* Longman.

Rampton, B. (1995). *Crossing: Language and ethnicity among adolescents.* Longman.

Roberts, A., & Rogoff, B. (2012). Children's reflections on two cultural ways of working together: "Talking with hands and eyes" or requiring words. *International Journal of Educational Psychology, 1*(2), 73-99. https://doi.org/10.4471/ijep.2012.06

Romero-Little, M. E., McCarty, T. L., Warhol, L., & Zepeda, O. (2007). Language policies in practice: Preliminary findings from a large-scale national study of Native American language shift. *TESOL Quarterly, 41*(3), 607-618.

Rosa, J. (2019). *Looking like a language, sounding like a race: Raciolinguistic ideologies and the learning of Latinidad.* Oxford University Press.

Rosa, J., & Flores, N. (2015). Hearing language gaps and reproducing social inequality. *Journal of Linguistic Anthropology, 25*(1), 77-79.

Sacks, H., Schegloff, E. A., & Jefferson, G. (1974). A simplest systematics for the organization of turn-taking for conversation. *Language, 50,* 696-735.

Sanger, D., Coufal, K. L., Scheffler, M., & Searcey, R. (2003). Implications of the personal perceptions of incarcerated adolescents concerning their own communicative competence. *Communication Disorders Quarterly, 24*(2), 64-77.

Sanger, D. D., Cresswell, J. W., Dworak, J., & Schultz, L. (2000). Cultural analysis of communication behaviors among juveniles in a correctional facility. *Journal of Communication Disorders, 33,* 31-57.

Sanger, D. D., Hux, K., & Ritzman, M. (1999). Female juvenile delinquents' pragmatic awareness of conversational interactions. *Journal of Communication Disorders, 32,* 281-295.

Sanger, D. D., Moore-Brown, B. J., Magnuson, G., & Svoboda, N. (2001). Prevalence of language problems among adolescent delinquents: A closer look. *Communication Disorders Quarterly, 23*(1), 17-26.

Schieffelin, B. B., & Ochs, E. (Eds.). (1986). *Language socialization across cultures.* Cambridge University Press.

Shannon, C., & Weaver, W. (1949). *The mathematical theory of communication.* University of Illinois Press.

Shipley, K. G., & McAfee, J. G. (2021). *Assessment in speech-language pathology: A resource manual* (6th ed.). Plural Publishing.

Simmons-Mackie, N., & Damico, J. (2003). Contributions of qualitative research to the knowledge base of normal communication. *American Journal of Speech-Language Pathology, 12,* 144-154.

Sirota, K. G. (2010). Narratives of distinction: Personal life narrative as a technology of the self in the everyday lives and relational worlds of children with autism. *Ethos, 38*(1), 93-115.

Smitherman, G. (1977). *Talkin and testifyin: The language of Black America.* Houghton Mifflin.

Solano-Flores, G., Backhoff, E., Contreras-Niño, L. A., & Vásquez-Muñoz, M. (2015). Language shift and the inclusion of indigenous populations in large-scale assessment programs. *International Journal of Testing, 15,* 136-152.

Solomon, O. (2014). Rethinking babytalk. In A. Duranti, E. Ochs, & B. B. Schieffelin (Eds.), *The handbook of language socialization* (pp. 121-149). Wiley Blackwell.

Solomon, O., & Bagatell, N. (2010). Introduction: Autism: Rethinking the possibilities. *Ethos, 38*(1), 1-7.

Spaulding, T. J., Plante, E., & Farinella, K. A. (2006). Eligibility criteria for language impairment: Is the low end of normal always appropriate? *Language, Speech, and Hearing Services in Schools, 37*, 61-72.

Sperry, D. E., Miller, P. J., & Sperry, L. L. (2020). Hazardous intersections: Crossing disciplinary lines in developmental psychology. *European Journal of Social Theory, 23*(1), 93-112.

Sperry, D. E., Sperry, L. L., & Miller, P. J. (2018) Re-examining the verbal environments of children from different socioeconomic backgrounds. *Child Development, 90*(4), 1303-1318.

Sterponi, L. (2017). *Language socialization and autism*. In P. A. Duff & S. May (eds.) *Language socialization*. Encyclopedia of Language and Education. https://doi.org/10.1007/978-3-319-02327-4_28-1

Sterponi, L., & Fasulo, A. (2010). "How to go on": Intersubjectivity and progressivity in the communication of a child with autism. *Ethos, 38*(1), 116-142.

Sterponi, L., & Shankey, J. (2014). Rethinking echolalia: Repetition as interactional resource in the communication of a child with autism. *Journal of Child Language, 41*(2), 275-304.

Takada, A. (2014). Preverbal infant-caregiver interaction. In A. Duranti, E. Ochs, & B. B. Schieffelin (Eds.), *The handbook of language socialization* (pp. 56-80). Wiley Blackwell.

Tetnowski, J. A., & Franklin, T. C. (2003). Qualitative research: Implications for description and assessment. *American Journal of Speech-Language Pathology, 12*, 155-164.

Tobin, J., Hsueh, Y., & Karasawa, M. (2009). *Preschool in three cultures revisited: China, Japan, and the United States*. University of Chicago Press.

Tobin, J., Wu, D., & Davidson, D. (1989). *Preschool in three cultures: Japan, China, and the United States*. Yale University Press.

Troche, J., Willis, A., & Whiteside, J. (2019). Exploring supported conversation with familial caregivers of persons with dementia: A pilot study. *Pilot and Feasibility Studies, 5*, 10. https://doi.org/10.1186/s40814-019-0398-5

Turner, S., & Whitworth, A. (2006). Conversational partner training programmes in aphasia: A review of key themes and participants' roles. *Aphasiology, 20*(6), 483-510.

Van Der Klift, E., & Kunc, N. (2019). *Being realistic isn't realistic: Collected essays on disability, identity, inclusion, and innovation*. Tellwell Talent.

Vining, C., Long, E., Inglebret, E., & Brendal, M. (2017). Speech-language assessment considerations for American Indian and Alaska Native children who are dual language learners. Perspectives of the ASHA Special Interest Groups: SIG 14. *Cultural and Linguistic Diversity, 2*(14), 29-40.

Watson, P., Raju, P., & Soklaridis, S. (2017). Teaching not-knowing: Strategies for cultural competence in psychotherapy supervision. *Academic Psychiatry, 41*, 55-61.

Wiig, E. H. (2000). Authentic and other assessments of language disabilities: When is fair fair? *Reading & Writing Quarterly, 16*(3), 179-210. https://doi.org/10.1080/105735600406715

Wiig, E. H., & Secord, W. A. (2006). Clinical measurement and assessment: A 25-year retrospective. *ASHA Leader, 11*(2). https://doi.org/10.1044/leader.FTR4.11022006.10

Wilkinson, R. (2010). Interaction-focused intervention: A conversation analytic approach to aphasia therapy. *Journal of Interactional Research in Communication Disorders, 1*, 45-68. https://doi.org/10.1558/ jircd.v1i1.45

Wilkinson, R. (2020) Commentary: Developing the comparative perspective in atypical interaction research. *Clinical Linguistics & Phonetics, 34*(10-11), 1045-1054. https://doi.org/10.1080/02699206.2020.1786604

Wortham, S. (2004). From good student to outcast: The emergence of a classroom identity. *Ethos, 32*(2), 164-187.

Young, V. A. (2010). Should writers use they own English? *Iowa Journal of Cultural Studies, 12*(1), 110-118.

Zentella, A. C. (1997). *Growing up bilingual: Puerto Rican children in New York*. Wiley.

Zentella, A. C. (2005). *Building on strength: Language and literacy in Latino families and communities*. Teachers College Press.

Chapter 10

Identifying Developmental Communication Milestones in Western Kenya

A Community-Based Approach

Monika Molnar, PhD; David K. Rochus; Rachael Gibson; Florence Omolo; and Lynn Ellwood, MHSc, S-LP(C), Reg. CASLPO

The project presented in this chapter was designed to build the capacity of frontline practitioners and education professionals to identify communication and/or language disabilities in children in Western Kenya. According to the most recent 2019 census, almost 70% of Kenya's population live in rural areas, and in these rural areas there is a high concentration of school-aged children (i.e., less than 15 years of age; Kenya Population and Housing Census, 2019). Rural areas of Kenya are typically associated with less access to medical and health services compared to urban areas (Lewis et al., 2013). In these areas, children with communication disorders often do not receive appropriate care, partially due to the scarcity of speech-language pathologists/professionals in the country and a lack of understanding about communication development/disorders.

The context for identifying communication developmental norms and related disabilities in Kenya is complex due to the many languages spoken. The two official languages of Kenya are Kiswahili and English (Githoria, 2006). More than 40 tribal languages are also spoken across the country. The current research focuses on the rural areas of Kisumu, Siaya, Vihiga, and Kakamega located in the western part of Kenya where the predominant tribal languages are Kiswahili, Wanga, and Dholuo. The structure of these languages is very different from English or most European languages. Kiswahili and Wanga are both agglutinative. This means that word bases and affixes come together to form words what in English would be called phrases. Instead of gender that is typical to many languages (e.g., French), these languages use "classes" that are based on culturally-bound classifications and bear little resemblance to the categorization systems we are familiar with in Western languages. Dholuo is a tonal language with tones affecting both word meanings and grammar (more

Bortz, M. (Ed.). *A Guide to Global Language Assessment: A Lifespan Approach* (pp. 195-221).
DOI: 10.4324/9781003524472-13

information on these languages can be found in Chapter 3). Many children also learn English in addition to their tribal languages or learn more than one tribal language. Multilingualism is a common occurrence in Western Kenya. Moreover, Kiswahili serves as lingua franca for much of Eastern Africa, consequently it has a lot of second language speakers, increasing the number of multilinguals in the region.

The goal of this chapter is to describe and reflect on the first steps of establishing our community-based research (CBR) supporting speech-language pathology and related health promotion services in this area in order to provide guidance to others seeking to accomplish similar aims. An important context for this type of work is the fact that local speech-language pathology and health promotion services play a general role in the community as they cater to clients with a wide range of communication disabilities and swallowing difficulties. Frontline practitioners within these services include community health workers, community-based rehabilitation workers, volunteers, education staff, and health professionals, all of whom can participate in this research model. Given that CBR is scarce in most African regions (Appiah, 2020), and it is a rather time-consuming process without a one-size-fits-all approach (Israel et al., 1998), our description could serve as a starting point for those considering CBR within communication disorders in regions similar to Western Kenya.

In addition, throughout this chapter, links will be made to the World Health Organization's *International Classification of Functioning, Disability and Health* (WHO-ICF; 2001) as it is paramount to take many factors into account when assessing multilingual children, like those in Western Kenya. This project links all five classifications, and based on the CBR model it encompasses, it is also an integrated approach to the social and medical models of disability. By ensuring there are norms and assessment tools that are applicable to the context, services will be able to map their provision successfully against the WHO-ICF. For individuals, the norms will support an understanding of their level of functioning and what interventions will maximise their functioning. At an institutional level (schools), the norms will support their training, school placement of children, resource planning and quality improvement (of serving their students). Finally, at a social level, it will support the eligibility for social security benefits, legislation and ensuring an accessible environment.

In recent years, as the first phase of our plans, we have established the research infrastructure necessary for our long-term goals (i.e., building collaborations, piloting participant recruitment, and some elements of data collection). Our reflections focus on this first phase of the CBR. In the following sections, we (1) present our project goals, synthesize relevant language-related research that has already emerged in the region, and present the conceptual framework guiding our project; (2) describe and illustrate how to develop and implement a CBR approach; (3) present methodology and iterative modifications for our CBR project that targets establishing local communication developmental norms; and (4) provide further guidance based on challenges and lessons learned thus far. The chapter concludes with guidelines for setting up a CBR project in communication disorders, and additional resources are included in the chapter's appendices.

Project Description

Context

In recent years, due to increased access to education, the number of students enrolled in schools has dramatically increased in Kenya (Oburu & Mbagaya, 2019). This positive change in the Kenyan education system, however, also led to some challenges. Oburu and Mbagaya (2019) reported high drop-out rates at the primary school level. This high drop-out rate can be explained by various factors, including financial difficulties (Oburu & Mbagaya, 2019; Sekiya & Ashida, 2017). However, learning disabilities are also often a cause for children not being able to complete their education (Wagner, 1991).

In Kenya, due to lack of developmental norms, it is difficult to identify children with mild disabilities. These children often end up in mainstream schools without any support and are constantly repeating years and being classed as "slow learners" without any understanding of their needs (Bruce & Venkatesh, 2014).

Project Goals

The overarching goal of the research project is to provide tools for Kenyan educators and frontline practitioners to identify young children with communication disabilities and special education needs. This will be addressed through the two main objectives of the proposed project:

- *Objective 1:* Determine the typical developmental milestones associated with language and communication development in multilingual children in Western Kenya learning Wanga, Dholuo, or Kiswahili (often in addition to English) between the ages of 2 and 5.
- *Objective 2:* Build the capacity of local frontline practitioners, teachers, and other education professionals by sharing with them the typical language and communication developmental milestones of children growing up in Western Kenya, and train them to recognize the signs of communication and language disorders.

Prior Non–Community-Based Research

There has been minimal research conducted thus far on developmental communication norms in Kenyan children. As of now, studies related to language development in Kenya have focused mainly on some aspects of typical language use, policy, and assessment methods. While the literature has yet to provide clear milestones with respect to various aspects of language development, there are several studies that can be examined to provide a backdrop for incoming research into this subfield (see Abdulaziz, 1982; Alcock, 2006; Alcock & Alibhai, 2013; Mohochi, 2003; Mule, 1999).

In 2015, Alcock et al. looked at the validity and reliability of communicative development inventories (CDIs) to assess language in Kenyan children aged 8 months to 2 years 4 months. The CDIs measured vocabulary, gestures, and grammatical construction through interviews with caregivers. Their research found that CDIs are a reliable and acceptable way to determine language development when caregivers have low literacy levels. This work focused on the tribal languages spoken on the coastal region of Kenya (e.g., Kilifi).

A more recent study by Knauer et al. (2020) found that parent training paired with culturally appropriate children's books increased reading frequency and story-specific expressive vocabulary in children aged 24 to 83 months. This training helped improve young children's language acquisition. Knauer et al. (2020) also completed vocabulary tests in rural communities in Western Kenya in three languages: Luo, Swahili, and English on multilingual children aged 2 to 6. They found that when measuring children's vocabulary in various languages, the assessment of mother tongue receptive vocabulary is a strong indicator of overall language ability, whereas the second language (English) does not provide a good overview of vocabulary development. This is an important consideration that will inform assessment methods for incoming developmental language research.

With regards to literacy development in Kenyan children, Piper et al. (2014) examined the relationship between oral reading fluency and reading comprehension in four languages (English, Kiswahili, Dholuo, and Gikuyu). They found that while children in third grade could recognize

English words more easily compared to words in Kiswahili or their mother tongue, their reading comprehension was significantly lower in English. Therefore, the authors concluded that using English as an instructional route to gain reading comprehension in early grades is ineffective and should be discouraged from practice. Such studies highlight the importance of multilingual testing and between-language analysis of language development in multilingual/bilingual speakers. Overall, while there have been important steps taken toward the description of typical language and communication development in Kenya (see Alcock, 2006; Alcock & Alibhai, 2013; Knauer et al., 2020; Piper et al, 2014), currently no sufficient information is available for health care practitioners to identify young children with potential language and communication disorders.

Conceptual Framework Guiding the Project

This project is in line with local government initiatives. Kenya's 2030 vision includes the goal to have special provisions for Kenyans with various disabilities and previously marginalized communities (Kenyan Ministry of Education, 2018).

The project will contribute towards these priorities by:

1. *Increasing children's access to quality and relevant education in Western Kenya by providing tools for assessment and early intervention:* Our work alongside Kenyan Educational Assessment and Resource Centres (EARCs) will build educators' capacity in early identification of children with communication disabilities, and they will be able to provide functional strategies that can be easily implemented.
2. *Advocacy and awareness creation:* Our team works in the community to raise awareness about communication disabilities. Further data on norms will increase our ability to advocate at a national and county level for services for young children with communication disabilities.

How to Develop and Implement a Community-Based Research Approach: Our Experience

CBR is different from traditional academic research. It is a collaborative approach that engages community members and members outside of the given community (e.g., academic partners, students). It always addresses a community-identified need and often encompasses teaching, research, and service simultaneously. One of its main goals is to democratize knowledge by acknowledging the importance of a given community's experiences and priorities (Strand et al., 2003). First, we describe the composition of our CBR team, then we describe how we followed the main principles of CBR.

Establishing a Community-Based Research Team

Success with CBR depends on identifying or establishing a well-supported research team with essential members who are embedded in the community of focus. Our research team grew out of a long-standing partnership that had an initial focus on clinical education based on best practices for international clinical internships. Yellow House Health and Outreach Services (Yellow House), a nonprofit health and outreach service with speech and language services in Western Kenya, is a clinical education partner site with a clinical professional speech-language pathology master's degree program in Canada (University of Toronto), providing a 10-week advanced clinical placement for a pair of MHSc students each year. When the organization identified the critical need for communication developmental milestones, the focus of the partnership expanded and a closer collaboration with the university was built to meet the gap. The collaborator list grew to include a researcher with the requisite knowledge. In 2019 this research project was launched, guided by the community needs identified by the organization based on their expertise.

Community Partners

Yellow House is a nonprofit health and outreach service with locations in Kenya and the United Kingdom. Yellow House works with existing education infrastructure in Kenya, including schools and EARCs across Western Kenya. Yellow House partners with three EARCs in Western Kenya. EARCs are where children with disabilities are brought for assessment to determine what school placement will be most appropriate for them. Referrals are also made to other professionals, including occupational therapy, audiology, and optometry. Yellow House speech-language pathologists work within the EARCs to provide support in the assessments and therapy provided to children who have communication disabilities.

Within the organization of Yellow House, R. G. is a speech-language pathologist based in the United Kingdom with over 10 years of experience of working in Kenya and is the director of Yellow House. D. R. is a speech-language pathologist and clinical lead, and F. O. is a parent liaison officer (PLO) for Yellow House in Kenya. Yellow House speech-language pathologists work with a PLO who plays a key role in advising on family and community engagement and highlights subtle cultural factors that may influence the individual and social impact of the services. The PLO, who is also a member of the community that Yellow House works with, works directly with parents and families, promoting family involvement in the therapy process and taking a lead in community-based empowerment activities.

Academic Partners

The two academic partners (M. M. and L. E.) are from the Department of Speech-Language Pathology at the University of Toronto (U of T) in Canada. M. M. is an assistant professor whose research focuses on multilingual development. She is primarily responsible for designing the studies the proposed research is based on, in collaboration with the community partners. L. E. is an associate professor (teaching stream), whose role includes developing and managing high-quality international clinical internships. Clinical speech-language pathology master's students from the U of T also participated in literature searches, grant proposal writing, training of frontline staff during initial piloting stages, and facilitated data collection and analysis. The academic partners are guided by the vision, mission, and values of U of T's International Centre for Disability and Rehabilitation (ICDR), which focuses on improving the lives of people with disabilities globally through education and research that is founded on values including authentic partnerships, rights-based approach, inclusion, and sustainability.

Follow Principles of Community-Based Research

We followed the eight principles of CBR as defined by Israel et al. (1998):

1. *Recognize community as a unit of identity.* "Community-based approaches to research attempt to identify and to work with existing communities of identity, and/or to strengthen a sense of community through collective engagement" (Israel et al., 1998). We recognized the community of Western Kenya as a unit of identity. Collective engagement was facilitated through Yellow House. We built collaborations with the local EARCs and its main employees and with key persons in the community, such as religious leaders.
2. *Build on strengths and resources within the community.* "Community-based research explicitly recognizes and seeks to support or expand social structures and social processes that contribute to the ability of community members to work together to improve health" (Israel et al., 1998). First, the research team identified the already existing strengths and resources within community (e.g., EARCs, Yellow House), then we built our collaboration and research proposal on these to address the community's health concerns. The main community partner, Yellow House, has been operating in Western Kenya for over 10 years. Yellow House has developed partnerships with different interested parties that enable them to embed their services within the community to create awareness about communication disorders and speech-language pathology and outreach services they provide.
3. *Facilitate collaborative partnerships in all phases of the research.* The project facilitates collaborative partnership with entities that may not be members of the community of identity, including human service organizations, academia, and community-based organizations. In the current partnership, the academic entity is the U of T (Department of Speech-Language Pathology), and Yellow House UK is the oversight organization for Yellow House Kenya. All members of the partnership contribute to each stage of research and the collaboration focuses on health issues identified by the community itself. Throughout the decade Yellow House has been working in Western Kenya, an ongoing gap in clinical knowledge continued to be recognized; due to the lack of communication development norms, clinicians were basing their observations/assessments on UK/US norms. These norms do not take into account any of the multilingual and cultural aspects of language acquisition in Kenya that results in milder communication disorders not being identified. Speech-language pathology is not yet recognized as a profession in Kenya, which contributes to the lack of services and awareness. The Yellow House team uses their data to support the lobbying for the recognition of the profession and understanding the norms of communication development will aid that process.
4. *Integrate knowledge and action for mutual benefit of all partners.* "Community-based research seeks to build a broad body of knowledge related to health and well-being while also integrating that knowledge with community and social change efforts that address the concerns of the communities involved" (Israel et al., 1998). In line with this principle, our project was designed with the goal in mind that once results are obtained, our team will work in the community to raise awareness about the potential signs of communication disorders. Further, this project will increase the team's ability to advocate at a national and county level for services for people with communication disabilities in Kenya.
5. *Promote a co-learning and empowering process that attends to social inequalities.* "Community-based research is a co-learning and empowering process that facilitates the reciprocal transfer of knowledge, skills, capacity, and power" (Israel et al., 1998). As described in more detail in a following section, the academic research team has greatly relied on the experience and knowledge

of the community of identity. In every step of designing our study, we benefitted from the expertise of the local community members and always acknowledged that learning from the community of identity is just as important, or even more important, than what the noncommunity partners can teach to the community.

6. *Apply a cyclical and iterative process.* We developed and maintained a "cyclical and iterative" research process involving all the partners. The definition of our goals and all stages of the research (including data collection, analyses, and interpretation) are done in consultation with all partners. The cyclical and iterative process is maintained by regular online meetings and email correspondence. The schedule of meetings is driven in part by the annual clinical internship schedule. Annual debriefing and planning meetings between U of T and Yellow House are scheduled virtually, and address both clinical internship planning and research project next steps. Additional ad hoc meetings are arranged as needed.
7. *Address health from both positive and ecological perspectives.* "Community-based research addresses the concept of health from a positive model that emphasizes physical, mental, and social well-being" (Israel et al., 1998). Our project is in line with Kenya's 2030 government initiatives which emphasize the well-being of children with disabilities and marginalized communities.
8. *Disseminate findings and knowledge gained to all partners.* "Community-based research seeks to disseminate findings and knowledge gained to all partners involved, in language that is understandable and respectful, and where ownership of knowledge is acknowledged" (Israel et al., 1998). Following this principle, our primary objective is to share our research outcome with the community of identity (e.g., frontline practitioners, educators, teachers) by creating educational material in the local languages. Dissemination in academic platforms (e.g., international journals and conferences) is secondary, as these outlets are less accessible to the community of identity. For all academic and nonacademic communications about the project, to acknowledge the intellectual ownership of everyone involved, authorship to all community members is offered; further, all those with authorship contribute to the given communication.

Our Methodological Approach and Pilot Efforts

In this section, we describe the steps toward our long-term goals and the pilot results we have obtained so far, followed by the lessons learned at this stage of the project.

Development of Culturally Appropriate Questionnaires

Our first step was to develop a culturally appropriate questionnaire that collects information about the child participant's demographic information and language background. We also designed this questionnaire in such way that it provides us information about the child's language and speech development, and provides us with an opportunity to evaluate whether the child likely follows a typical pattern of communication development. The questionnaire was developed in consultation with staff at Yellow House Kenya and speech-language pathologists who had visited the Kenyan site and are familiar with the local cultural context.

The themes covered in this questionnaire are similar to those used in most North American research labs to collect demographic and socioeconomic information about participants. The questions that address communication development cover themes commonly assessed by speech-language pathologists. First, researchers and speech-language pathologists from U of T (this also included speech-language pathologists in training, for instance, the students who completed a clinical placement at the Kenyan site) compiled a set of questions that they deemed relevant from the research project's perspective. Then, the researcher from U of T organized these questions into themes. Finally, these questions were shared with the staff of Yellow House Kenya who provided feedback and the questions were adjusted in such way that they are meaningful in a Western Kenyan context. Importantly, this questionnaire was designed to work in an interview setting; caregivers do not fill in the questionnaires independently. During the pilot phase, a Yellow House staff member always conducted interviews with a caregiver and provided clarification and follow-up questions whenever it was necessary.

The questionnaire was developed in both Dholuo (Appendix A) and English (Appendix B). Themes A to D cover demographic and socioeconomic information, in addition to language background. It is common to grow up learning more than one language in Western Kenya. For this reason, it was important to evaluate the monolingual versus bilingual/multilingual status of each child. Based on the language background questions, it is also possible to estimate the dominant language of each child. Themes E through G cover information related to communication (e.g., language and gesture use). These questions were designed to fulfill two goals: evaluate whether the child follows a typical developmental pattern and to collect preliminary information about the details of typical communication development in Western Kenya (e.g., type and onset of first words, word combinations, and phrases and gestures used by young children growing up in Western Kenya). It is important to note here that while developmental research generally assumes that children across all cultures reach the typical milestones of communication development at the same pace (e.g., canonical babbling appears around 7 months of age, first words appear around 12 months of age, etc.), there is no sufficient empirical evidence to support such assumption. Most research on child development takes place in Western countries (i.e., the Global North), yet developmental variance across cultures is very much a possibility (Keller, 2017; Pendergast et al., 2018).

In addition to the development of the questionnaire described previously, we piloted a vocabulary checklist. As alluded to in other parts of this chapter, our original goal was to develop a vocabulary inventory for the tribal languages of Western Kenya, following the guidelines and structure of the MacArthur-Bates Communicative Development Inventories (MB-CDIs; Alcock et al., 2015; Fenson et al., 2000). However, after consulting the local community, based on the principles of community-based research, we decided that developing a CDI would not meet the needs of the local community. CDIs are ideal for estimating the receptive and expressive vocabulary size of children up to 3 years of age, and it is also somewhat suitable to assess whether age-appropriate gestures and phrases are produced by children up to this age. While this tool can be indeed useful for speech-language pathologists in certain contexts, the community-based research team decided that the focus of the CDI would be too narrow and limited in age; instead, a more general approach to describing the communication development of children would be more beneficial to the community (which is described in our long-term goals following). Nevertheless, before this decision was made, a Dholuo version of the vocabulary checklist was considered. Culturally appropriate Dholuo target words for piloting the vocabulary checklist were created by two native Dholuo speakers for the following semantic categories: animal sounds, animal names, food and drink, toys, vehicles, clothing, body parts, furniture, rooms, household items, outside things, people, games, action words, and descriptive words.

Piloting Data Acquisition Flow

The administration of the above-described questionnaire provided us with the opportunity of piloting the data acquisition chain, including the steps of (1) identifying the community contact person who can assist with the recruitment of participants; (2) gauge if the greater community shows interest in our project; (3) training Yellow House staff on administering the questionnaire; (4) verifying if administering the questionnaire via an interview process is feasible (i.e., Do we obtain desired information? Are caregivers comfortable?); (5) gauge whether/how participants are comfortable with having their caregiver-child interactions recorded; and (6) finding an ecologically valid way to record spontaneous caregiver-child interactions.

Through our pilot efforts, we were able to identify a local contact who helped us with participant recruitment. This person worked as a driver for Yellow House Kenya and was also closely involved with the local community through various church activities. He was able to explain to our participants the goal of our research and connect those participants who showed interest in the pilot study with Yellow House Kenya. Further, we were able to confirm that the interview style data collection worked well, and the questionnaire did not need major adjustments. It was also our plan to ask caregivers to play with their child on a mat with some toys while we recorded their spontaneous interactions with their child. This idea was based on research that collected data in Western cultures. However, we soon realized that this style of data collection is not culturally appropriate. The caregivers were not comfortable with playing with their children in this setting and did not like that the camera was in a static position. We realized that we can record spontaneous interactions if we opt for a smaller camera (e.g., GoPro) and follow the child-caregiver interactions as they move around in their home settings.

Preliminary Results

Using our questionnaire and preliminary vocabulary checklist, we were able to collect data from 29 caregivers with children between the ages of 10 months and 4.5 years. Participants were recruited from the Nyakach, Nyabondo, and Nyando regions of Western Kenya where Dholuo was commonly spoken. While this preliminary data set is not suitable for analyses (e.g., we do not have sufficient data points per age group), we share some preliminary patterns that we were able to extract from this pilot data set. However, it should all be interpreted with caution. In English, for instance, two-word phrases are quite common in children ages 2 years and up, and they often include various types of constructions (e.g., possessives, actor/action, locatives; Braine & Bowerman, 1976). Our limited sample in Dholuo does not reflect this trend: children's most frequent two-word phrases follow the "I want something" construction and we found no evidence for possessives or actor/action relationships in the two-word phrases. This could be explained by general syntactic differences between the two languages. Most children in our sample, however, produced a variety of prepositions by 2 years of age (e.g., inside, outside, on, under), while English-learning children's prepositions at the same age seem to be more limited. The most frequently known words, not surprisingly, reflect clear differences from words that children in Western countries learn first. Some of these examples are listed in Table 10-1.

Table 10-1
Contrasting Dholuo Frequently Known Words and English Equivalent

CATEGORY	DHOLUO	ENGLISH EQUIVALENT
Animal sound	meeh	goat sound
Animal name	rombo	sheep
Vehicle	apiko	motorcycle
Toy	toto	dolly
Food	chai	tea
Things around the house	yien	tree
Outside places	chiro	market
Action words	luoko	washing
Descriptive words	ng'ich	cold
Common two-word phrases	aduaro chai	I want tea
Copied actions	moto	collecting firewood

Long-Term Plans

Participants

To meet Objective 1, we will collect communication and language samples from 90 children within each of these age groups: ages 1 to 2, ages 2 to 3, ages 3 to 4, and ages 4 to 5 years (360 children in total). At least 90 children per age group is necessary because we expect that children will be exposed to various languages or the combination of these languages: Wanga, Dholuo, Kiswahili, and English. A relatively large sample size will enable us to collect sufficient data for each language context. Data collection will take place in four counties in Kenya: Kisumu, Siaya, Vihiga, and Kakamega, as Yellow House has already established networks in these regions. Families will be recruited from various socioeconomic backgrounds, from both rural and urban areas.

Procedure

We will video record each child interacting with their primary caregiver. To increase the reliability of our measurement, each child will be recorded twice within a 2-week period (360 children in total, 720 video recordings in total). The video recordings will be approximately 15 minutes long. Video recordings of similar length and context has been shown to be efficient for identifying communication and language behavior in young children (Tait et al., 2001).

Our pilot study showed that we will be able to record the most culturally appropriate parent–child interactions if a research assistant will conduct the video recording using one small camera (e.g., GoPro) in a home setting following the parent and the child if needed (ensuring that the child's face is visible most of the time). Video recording contexts commonly used in Western cultures (e.g., recording children playing with their caregiver on a mat while multiple cameras are facing at them) did not yield good quality recordings in our pilot experiment, as these kind of interaction contexts are uncommon in Western Kenya.

Before each testing session, we will explain to the caregiver the purpose of our study and will obtain consent. After the first recording session, via an interview with a research assistant, the primary caregiver will fill out a (1) language background questionnaire adapted for use in Western Kenya (will be developed based on Marian et al., 2007), (2) a demographic questionnaire, and (3) a socioeconomic survey. Based on the language background questionnaire, the children will be assigned to the group of each language under investigation, as monolingual or bilingual.

Analyses

To extract the typical language patterns for each age and language group, each video will be transcribed. Based on the transcriptions, we will identify the following linguistic characteristics for each age group: typical syntactic and morphosyntactic structures, typical receptive vocabulary, typical expressive vocabulary, and speech sounds typically produced correctly. To extract the typical communication patterns for each age and language group, each video will be coded using the ELAN software. The coding will identify the typical patterns of turn-taking, eye-contact, and gesture use (e.g., pointing, referential) within each group.

Developing Educational Material

Based on the outcome of Objective 1, we will develop the following educational material: (1) description of typical communication development between 1 and 5 years of age for children learning Wanga, Dholuo, Kiswahili, and English (or the combination of these languages); and (2) in relation to the description of typical development, we will highlight the potential signs of disorders in language (including speech sound production, vocabulary deficit, and deficit in syntactic/morphosyntactic development) and in broader communication (including gesture use, intentionality to communicate, and turn-taking). This material will be developed in online, booklet, and pamphlet formats. Collaborating with Kenyan Yellow House staff and speech-language pathologists will be critical in order to formulate the material in a way that is culturally appropriate and accessible to Kenyan teachers, education practitioners, and parents.

Training Teachers and Education Professionals in Western Kenya

Relying on the already established local network of Yellow House, we will be able to train teachers, education practitioners, community health volunteers, and parents. The primary focus of the training will be on primary school teachers and education practitioners in four counties in Kenya: Kisumu, Siaya, Vihiga, and Kakamega. In close collaboration with Yellow House staff, we will organize workshops and training sessions in these counties, relying on the educational material developed based on this study. In addition, capitalizing on the already established Yellow House network, we will have the opportunity to organize workshops for community health volunteers and parents in the regions mentioned earlier. The educational materials will be shared with student teachers still in training, optimizing their position of being fresh into their field.

Challenges and Lessons Learned

Community-Based Research Is a Time-Consuming Process

CBR is not something that can be done in a timely fashion. From a research perspective this might be a frustrating element, as the current dominant research model is "fast science" with very specific expectations about time, budget, and dissemination. CBR can be classified as "slow science" (Owens, 2013; Stengers, 2018). The goals of CBR are to empower communities and to do research that responds to a given community's need(s). This takes time and cannot be done within the principles of "fast science."

Time is a major consideration within CBR from various perspectives. First, it has been a long process to establish the current collaboration between the community and academic partners. The U of T Department of Speech-Language Pathology commits to no "one-off" international clinical internships and instead focuses on a small number of long-term sustainable partnerships (Ahluwalia et al., 2014). Yellow House stepped into the relationship cautiously, accepting its first pair of MHSc students in 2014, appreciating the considerable amount of advance preparation these students receive from U of T and the collaborative placement planning approach undertaken (Crump et al., 2010). Over subsequent years, annual debriefing meetings lead to iterative improvements in preparation of students and design of the clinical internship. Yellow House invests considerable time and resources in hosting and managing an annual clinical internship for a pair of MHSc students. They typically establish a working relationship with the students almost 1 year ahead of the assigned placement. U of T invests time and resources in carefully selecting the students and preparing them for a clinical placement with Yellow House. This process ensures both Yellow House and the students are best prepared for working together and adapting to cultural differences and methods of practice. This careful planning also ensures the impact of the student placement lasts beyond the 10 weeks.

U of T and Yellow House collaborate to enrich the partnership and ensure ongoing mutual benefit and service development. Joint professional activities have included copresentations at international forums, delivery of a regional communication disabilities conference in Kenya, coaching and staff development workshops at Yellow House, and development of virtual case-based teaching modules on the topic of global speech-language pathology service best practices, as examples. Close collaborations of these types lead to a deeper level of understanding and trust. A recent multi-stakeholder review of the clinical placement partnership experience revealed that the substantial investment in the partnership mitigated many of the commonly recognized risks, costs, and unintended harm frequently associated with clinical internships in global settings (Staley et al., 2019). This enduring partnership laid the foundation for establishing a CBR team committed to a "slow science" approach to research.

Second, active involvement from all partners is expected at all stages of the research project (Appiah, 2020; Israel et al., 1998; Smithies & Adams, 1993). Feedback is important from all the collaborators not only when it comes to the analyses and interpretation of the data but when the basic elements of research are designed (e.g., questionnaires, forms, testing material). For instance, in our case, it took about 6 months to develop an initial vocabulary list that we could pilot with families in the community. The initial development of this pilot tool, such as determining the main lexical components that should be covered, was done by the academic partners, and the community partners in Kenya played the important role in determining the actual lexical items that the pilot tool should include. Further, all aspects of research (e.g., participant recruitment, data collection, data entry, analyses) took much longer than it would have in the "fast science" non-CBR settings of a research laboratory where there are already well-established protocols for all the steps of data collection.

Research Methods

Defining Goals

In non-CBR, research goals are typically defined by relying on theoretical frameworks determined by previous studies and the actual goal is always set before the research begins. In our CBR project, some specific goals of the research underwent iterations several times, as the specific needs of the community became more visible throughout discussions among the partners. One example is that our initial plan was to focus on lexical development only in the given pediatric populations. This decision was made from a "fast science" perspective, as there are already lexical norms available in some tribal languages in Kenya (Alcock et al., 2015), and following in the footsteps of these previous efforts would have let to the most efficient research and dissemination outcomes. However, as the research developed, it became apparent that the community itself would not benefit from such a tool alone, as the frontline practitioners in Western Kenya cannot rely on lexical norms alone to diagnose communication disorders. For this reason, we made important adjustments to our design that enable the collection of data that is suitable for establishing other types of communication norms as well. This of course means that the research will take longer and will take us to some uncharted territories, which will likely result in more future challenges and adjustments in our research design.

Participant Recruitment and Incentives

There is no one-size-fits-all approach in CBR to create a participant recruitment channel. How participant recruitment is done greatly depends on the structure, culture, and beliefs of the given community (Appiah, 2020). To identify the appropriate contact person for participant recruitment, Yellow House Kenya contacted several people in their local network who play different roles in their communities. The criteria for the contact person were that they live in the local community and use at least one of the target languages. In our case, a driver of Yellow House Kenya ended up being the main community recruiter of those families who are interested in participating in the project. Given the limited public transportation options in Kenya, drivers are often employed by different organizations. This driver knew many members of the local community by being involved in local church activities.

Also, determining the thank-you gift for participation in the research was not straightforward, either. By consulting community members and considering recommendations from the ethics board on previous research done, it was determined that each participating family would be given a pack that included laundry soap, sugar, and tea leaves. Our community network had a good understanding of the needs of the families and advised that soap, tea leaves, and sugar would be of great use to the families. The latter two items are used to make chai, which is a valued drink for the families—it is a main part of their breakfast.

Equipment, Transportation, and Phone Communication Costs

The described phase of the project utilized the equipment that was already in use by the community partner, which included a printer, video camera, laptop, mobile phone, storage cabins, and office space. The next phase of the project will require most of that equipment plus additional such as a color printer, laptops, smart phones with videoing capabilities, an external microphone for the phone cameras, and an external hard drive for the data storage, most of which will need to be acquired from funds dedicated to the research project along with updating or replacing existing resources. The currently available equipment on the Kenyan site is limited.

Being a community-based project, the research team went to the participants, some of whom were remotely situated and inaccessible by public transportation. A car (taxi) would be hired to take the research team to each participant's home, the visits having been prior arranged through a community contact person. Most of the prior communications were done through phone.

Funding

The initial phase of the project that is described in the chapter (establishing collaborations and piloting research infrastructures) was mainly funded by a private donation by a long-term volunteer of Yellow House who has played a significant part in the development of the pilot project. Appropriate funding agencies are limited for international CBR projects. For instance, few agencies would fund a collaboration between international partners and even fewer agencies would be open to CBR projects, as the timelines and deliverables are harder to define in these sorts of projects. Moreover, because the main outcome of the project is not science-to-science dissemination of the findings, but to meet the given needs of the community (which hardly comes in the form of scientific articles), researchers might not find CBR as a "productive" way of doing research. The primary productivity indicator in science is the number of peer-reviewed scientific articles published by a given research group. CBR outcomes are rarely considered as a productivity indicator. While Knowledge Translation (KT) activities can obtain funding (which mostly covers science-to-public communications), we would like to note that the CBR approach has very different structure and goals than those of KT. For the reasons described previously, our team decided to break down the project into smaller parts and apply for smaller funding opportunities mostly provided within the local university context; our team has also submitted an application to the Spencer Foundation, which supports international, education-based research.

Ethics

Before starting the data collection phase, ethics approval will be obtained from the Ethics & Scientific Review Committee (ESRC), in addition to the National Commission for Science, Technology and Innovation (NACOSTI) research license. We will apply to the Jaramogi Oginga Odinga Teaching and Referral Hospital Ethics Review Committee. Unlike applying for an ethics approval in academic settings, there is cost associated with applying to these ethics boards. The basic fee is 30,050 Kenyan Shilling (Shs), which is approximately $280 USD. To expedite the review, an additional Shs 20,000 (about $180 USD in 2021) is required. The ethics committee meets once a month, and the review process may take 6 to 8 weeks. This timeline is similar to the ones of academic ethics boards.

Guidelines for Developing Community-Based Research in Communication Disorders

In this chapter, we have described our process for developing a CBR project to address a local need for communication developmental norms in Western Kenya. To develop similar projects in other global settings such as this, we offer the following guidelines, based on Israel et al. (1998).

Early Stages

Before the research project begins, or at the very beginning of the project, we found that the answers to the following questions should be clear. In our experience, it can take up to 2 years to be able to respond with actions to these questions and set up the initial stages of CBR.

- Are you able to build a CBR team with enough representatives from the community, a research lab, and other relevant parties?
- Does the focus of your research address the needs identified by those embedded in a local community?
- How can you facilitate collective engagement and strengthen a sense of community?
- How does your proposed project enable community members to work together to improve health?

Once Project Is Underway

Once the research project has begun (e.g., data acquisition is underway), the following questions should be revisited. The data acquisition phase will largely depend on the question to be answered. We anticipate that our data collection phase, and parallel analyses of the data, will last at least 4 years.

- Do all parties participate as equal members and share control over all phases of the research process?
- How are research results integrated with community change efforts?
- How do researchers acknowledge and address the inequalities between themselves and community participants?
- Does the research process involve a cyclical and iterative process from establishing and enriching partnerships to creation of sustainable implementation of outcomes?
- How does the project emphasize physical, mental, and social well-being?
- How does the project consider biomedical, social, economic, cultural, historical, and political factors as determinants of health and disease?

Late-Stage Considerations

Once the data collection and analyses are nearing their end, the following questions should be considered:

- How will findings and knowledge gained be disseminated to all partners involved, in language that is understandable and respectful?
- How will researchers consult with participants prior to submission of any materials for publication and acknowledge the contributions of participants?

In this chapter, we have described and illustrated how to identify communication milestones in a local setting. Having a set of local communication developmental norms is fundamental to assessing and providing service to young children with communication disorders. We believe the CBR approach is essential to the successful accomplishment of this goal and hope to see more CBR projects of this nature in the coming years.

Acknowledgments

The authors would like to gratefully acknowledge Maggie Macaulay, graduate of the U of T MHSc program, for her review of the chapter manuscript.

References

Abdulaziz, M. H. (1982). Patterns of language acquisition and use in Kenya: Rural-urban differences. *International Journal of the Sociology of Language, 1982*(34), 95-120.

Ahluwalia, P., Nixon, S., Cameron, D., Cockburn, L., Ellwood, L., & Mori, B. (2014). Analyzing international clinical education practices for Canadian rehabilitation students. *BMC Medical Education, 14*, 187.

Alcock, K. J. (2006). Literacy in Kiswahili. *Handbook of orthography and literacy* (pp. 405-419). Routledge.

Alcock, K., & Alibhai, N. (2013). Language development in sub-Saharan Africa. In M. Boivin & B. Giordani (Eds.), *Neuropsychology of children in Africa* (pp. 155-180). Springer.

Alcock, K., Rimba, K., Holding, P., Kitsao-Wekulo, P., Abubakar, A., & Newton, C. (2015). Developmental inventories using illiterate parents as informants: Communicative development inventory (CDI) adaptation for two Kenyan languages. *Journal of Child Language, 42*(04), 763-785.

Appiah, R. (2020). Community-based participatory research in rural African contexts: Ethico-cultural considerations and lessons from Ghana. *Public Health Reviews, 41*(1), 1-13.

Braine, M. D., & Bowerman, M. (1976). Children's first word combinations. *Monographs of the Society for Research in Child Development*, 1-104.

Brown, K. (2005). *Encyclopedia of language and linguistics* (Vol. 1). Elsevier.

Bruce, S. M., & Venkatesh, K. (2014). Special education disproportionality in the United States, Germany, Kenya, and India. *Disability & Society, 29*(6), 908-921.

Crump, J., A., Sugarman, J., & the Working Group on Ethics Guidelines for Global Health Training (WEIGHT). (2010). Ethics and best practice guidelines for training experiences in global health. *American Journal of Tropical Medicine and Hygiene, 83*(6), 1178-1182.

Fenson, L., Pethick, S., Renda, C., Cox, J. L., Dale, P. S., & Reznick, J. S. (2000). Short-form versions of the MacArthur communicative development inventories. *Applied Psycholinguistics, 21*(1), 95-116.

Githoria, C. (2006). Countries and languages of the world: Kenya. In K. Brown (Ed.), *Encyclopedia of language and linguistics* (2nd ed., pp. 18-182). Elsevier.

Israel, B. A., Schulz, A. J., Parker, E. A., & Becker, A. B. (1998). Review of community-based research: Assessing partnership approaches to improve public health. *Annual Review of Public Health, 19*(1), 173-202.

Keller, H. (2017). Culture and development: A systematic relationship. *Perspectives on Psychological Science, 12*(5), 833-840.

Kenya Population and Housing Census (2019). *Kenya National Bureau of Statistics.* https://www.knbs.or.ke/2019-kenya-population-and-housing-census-reports/

Kenyan Ministry of Education. (2018). *Implementation guidelines: Sector policy for learners and trainees with disabilities, May 2018.* Kenya National Bureau of Statistics. http://housingfinanceafrica.org/app/uploads/VOLUME-I-KPHC-2019.pdf

Knauer, H. A., Jakiela, P., Ozier, O., Aboud, F., & Fernald, L. C. (2020). Enhancing young children's language acquisition through parent–child book-sharing: A randomized trial in rural Kenya. *Early Childhood Research Quarterly, 50*, 179-190.

Lewis, M. L., Scott, D. L., & Calfee, C. (2013). Rural social service disparities and creative social work solutions for rural families across the life span. *Journal of Family Social Work, 16*(1), 101-115.

Marian, V., Blumenfeld, H. K., & Kaushanskaya, M. (2007). The Language Experience and Proficiency Questionnaire (LEAP-Q): Assessing language profiles in bilinguals and multilinguals. *Journal of Speech, Language, and Hearing Research, 50*(4), 940-967.

Mohochi, E. S. (2003). Language choice for development: The case for Swahili in Kenya. *Journal of African Cultural Studies, 16*(1), 85-94.

Mule, L. (1999). Indigenous languages in the school curriculum: What happened to Kiswahili in Kenya (pp. 227-242). In L. M. Semali & J. L. Kincheloe (Eds.), *What is indigenous knowledge*. Routledge.

Oburu, P., & Mbagaya, C. (2019). Education and parenting in Kenya. In E. Sorbring & J. E. Lansford (Eds.), *School systems, parent behavior, and academic achievement* (pp. 67-78). Springer.

Owens, B. (2013). Long-term research: Slow science. *Nature News, 495*(7441), 300.

Pendergast, L. L., Schaefer, B. A., Murray-Kolb, L. E., Svensen, E., Shrestha, R., Rasheed, M. A., ... & Seidman, J. C. (2018). Assessing development across cultures: Invariance of the Bayley-III scales across seven international MAL-ED sites. *School Psychology Quarterly, 33*(4), 604.

Piper, B., Zuilkowski, S. S., & Mugenda, A. (2014). Improving reading outcomes in Kenya: First-year effects of the PRIMR initiative. *International Journal of Educational Development, 37*, 11-21.

Sekiya, T., & Ashida, A. (2017). An analysis of primary school dropout patterns in Honduras. *Journal of Latinos and Education, 16*(1), 65-73.

Smithies, J., & Adams, L. (1993). Walking the tightrope: Issues in evaluation and community participation for health for all. *Healthy Cities: Research and Practice* (pp. 55-70). Routledge.

Staley, B., Ellwood, L., Rochus, D., Gibson, R., Hong, D., & Kwan, K. (2019). Looking through the kaleidoscope: Stakeholder perspectives on an international speech-language pathology placement. *Perspectives of the ASHA Special Interest Groups, Research Article 4*, 1-6. 10.1044/2019_PERS-SIG17-2019-0007

Stengers, I. (2018). *Another science is possible: A manifesto for slow science.* John Wiley & Sons.

Strand, K., Marullo, S., Cutforth, N. J., Stoecker, R., & Donohue, P. (2003). Principles of best practice for community-based research. *Michigan Journal of Community Service Learning, 9*(3), 5-15.

Tait, M., Lutman, M. E., & Nikolopoulos, T. P. (2001). Communication development in young deaf children: Review of the video analysis method. *International Journal of Pediatric Otorhinolaryngology, 61*(2), 105-112.

Wagner, M. (1991). *Dropouts with disabilities: What do we know? What can we do?* SRI International.

World Health Organization. (2001). *International classification of functioning, disability and health.* https://apps.who.int/iris/handle/10665/42407

Appendix A

Caregiver Questionnaire—Dholuo

NAMBA: ______________________ TARIK: ______________________

PENJO KUOM DONGRUOK E WECHE MAG TUDRUOK

A. KWAN MAR OGANDA (Demographic)

1. Nying nyathini mar batiso ______________________ Kido? Nyako/Wuoyi (Chwo tick)
2. En ja higni adi? ______________
3. Udak Kanye? County maru ____________ SubCounty maru ____________
   Gweng`u ____________
4. Nyingi mar batiso ______________________
5. In gi higni adi sani? ______________________
6. Tudruok mane mantie e kindu gi nyathini?

   ____

   ____

B. KAKA OGANDA ODAK (Socioeconomic)

1. Yori mar yuto en mane?

   ____

   ____

2. Ichopo Kanye gi sombi?

   ____

   ____

C. ANYUOLA (Family)

1. Nyithindo adi mantie e odi kae?

   ____

   ____

2. Gin johigni adi?

   ____

   ____

3. Nga maritoni nyithindo?

   ____

   ____

4. Udak ji adi e oduka?

   ____

   ____

D. YORE MAG TUDRUOK (Languages)

1. Dhok mage gini mutiyo godo e dalau ka?

 ____

 ____

2. Nga gini matiyo gi dhok go?

 ____

 ____

3. Dhok mage muwuoyo godo gi nyathini?

 ____

 ____

4. Dhok mane mutiyo godo ahinya gi nyathini? __________ Mane kendo ma utiyogo kode? __________ To mane ma otiyo godo mana ka dichiel dichiel? __________
5. Dhok mane ma nyathini nokuongo tiyogodo? __________, mar ariyo to mane? __________, to mar adek? __________

E. LALRUOK (Interactions)

1. Mbaka aila mage mugoyoga gi nyathi pile kapile

 ____

 ____

 ____

 ____

2. Gin ango gini mutimo ga gi nyathi odiechieng kodiechieng?

 ____

 ____

 ____

 ____

F. OKENGE MAG DONGO (Milestones)

Parane ka nyathini ne ja higni adek kapok ochako dhi sikul

Be ne okonyi timo tije mag ot? To be nongeyo dhi e choo kende? To be nohero ringo? To idho gik moko eyi ot? To be nonyalo rwakore kata lonyore kende ma ok okonye?

Kiparo ka nyathi ja higni adek, agombo penji penjo moko kaluwore gi kaka nyathi no puonjore mongeyo lalruok gi ji nyaka kama kawuono odongo ochopoe ni…..

1. Nyathini nochako golo duol (kaka kudho lake) ka orom nade?

 ____

 ____

2. Nyathini ne rom nade ka owacho wach mokwongo?

 ____

 ____

3. Wach mane ma nyathini nokwongo luongo?

 ____

 ____

4. E kind dweche auchiel gi higni adek, weche aila mage gini mane nyathini ohero tiyo godo? (Reminder: *And what is the English translation of the category?)

 ____

 ____

 ____

 ____

5. Gin weche mage maneifuenyo ni nyathini nyalo ngeyo eyo makare ikind dueche auchiel kod higni adek? (Reminder: *And what is the English translation of the category?)

____

____

6. Ere kaka nifwenyo ni ongeyo wechego?

____

____

____

____

Koro watem ane wuoyo matin kuom weche mane nyathi ohero wacho kapok ochopo higni adek …

1. Dibed ni noluongo nyinge mag lee/jamni? __________ Kaka lee/jamni mage gini?

   ____

   ____

2. Nokopo yuak mag lee/jamni? __________ Kaka yuak mag lee mage? (which sounds?)

   ____

   ____

3. Be noluongo nyinge mag nyamburko? __________ Nyamburko mane?

   ____

   ____

4. Be ne ohero kopo kaka nyamburko mor kapok nochopo higni adek? __________ Kaka mor mage? (which sounds?)

   ____

   ____

5. Be ne ohero luongo nying nyadoli? __________ Kaka nyadoli mage gini? (which toy names?)

   ____

   ____

6. Be ne ojaluongo nyinge chiemo kaa gik mimadho kapok ne oromo ja higni adek? __________ Kaka chiemo/math aila mage?

   ____

   ____

7. Be ne ojaluongo nyinge lewni? __________ Lewni mage gini?

   ____

   ____

8. Be ne onyalo luongo fuondni mad del? __________ Kaka fuonni mage gini?

   ____

   ____

9. Be ne onyalo luongo nyinge mg kombe gi gige ot mamoko? __________ Ango gini mane onyalo luongo?

   ____

   ____

10. Bende ne oluongo ga nying rooms mantiere e ot? __________ Room mane mane ojaluongo?

    ____

    ____

11. Bende ne oluongo nying gik mantie aluora mar ot? __________ Ango gini mane ojaluongo?

    ____

    ____

12. Be ne oluongo nying kuonde mantie e gwengu (Ok nyinge mag delni) [not homes of people])? __________ Nying kuonde mage mane ohero luongo?

    ____

    ____

13. Be ne oluongoga nyinge mag ji? __________ Nying nga gini ma ne ojaluongoga?

    ____

    ____

14. Be ne oluongo nyinge mag joot? __________ Kaka nying nga gini?

    ____

    ____

15. Be ne onyalo wuoyo kuom gik matimore odiechieng ka ondiechieng? (metho gokinyi, potty, dhi oko maduong) __________ Kaka gik mage gini?

    ____

    ____

16. Be ne onyalo luongo tije mitimo e dala? __________ Kaka tije mage?

    ____

    ____

17. Be ne onyalo lero chal mar gik moko (maduong`, mang`ich) kapok ne oromo ja higni adek? __________ Weche mage mane otiyogo kuom lerogi?

    ____

    ____

18. Be ne onyalo wacho rangi mag gik moko? __________ Kaka mage?

    ____

    ____

19. Be ne onyalo wacho seche mag odiechieng? __________ Kaka seche mage?

    ____

    ____

20. Be ne onyalo penjo wach? __________ Kaka penjo ila mage?

    ____

    ____

21. Be ne onyalo wacho kuonde ma gik moko nitie kotiyo gi (kaka iye, oko, wiye, buoye)? __________ Kaka mage gini?

    ____

    ____

22. Be ne onyalo tiyo gi weche mamedo dhadhu seche mowacho weche mamoko? __________ Kaka mage gini?

    ____

    ____

23. Be ne onyalo wacho weche man gi wach matudogi? __________ Kaka mage gini?

    ____

    ____

24. Be ne onyalo wacho weche ariyo kata mokalo kanyo kane pok oromo ja higni adek? ____________ Kaka weche mage? (dog ane chien e mbaka mag gik matimore kata weche ma jaritne ne opimoni kuom mbak magigoyoga kode)? (*And translate into English.)

____

____

G. RANYISI (Gestures)

1. Nyathini ne ja higni addi ka ne ochako tiyo gi ranyisi e yor tudruok? ____________ Ranyisi mage maneokwongo tiyogo?

____

____

____

____

2. Gin ranyisi mage gini meno nyathi tiyo godo e kind dweche auchiel gi higni adek?

____

____

3. Kopogore gi ranyisi mane nyathi tiyogo, mage kendo mane onyalo winjo tiende?

____

____

4. Ere kaka ninyalo fwenyo ni ne owinjo tiend ranyisi mitiyo godo?

____

____

5. Be ne ohero wuondore ni otimo gimoro? (gi gi moro koso gi gik moko) ____________ Ne onyalo wuondore eyore mage?

____

____

____

____

6. Be ne owuondore ni en baba/mama? ____________ Nowuondore e yore mage?

____

____

____

____

7. Be ne okopo timo gik ma jok madongo timo (kaka luoko sande, ywecho)? ____________ Tije mage mane otimoga?

____

____

____

____

TEM MATEK IRUCH NYING NYATHI GI JARITNE BANG` PENJOGO TO KARGI ITII GI NAMBNI MA OMIGI E NYANONRO …

Appendix B

Caregiver Questionnaire—English

ID# ____________ Date ____________

Language Development Questionnaire

A. Demographic

1. What is the child's first name? ____________
2. How old are they? ____________
3. Where do they live? County ____________ Sub-County ____________
   Village ____________
4. What is your first name? ____________
5. What is your age? ____________
6. What is your relationship to the child? ____________

B. Socioeconomic

1. What do you do for a living? ____________
2. What is your educational background? ____________

C. Family

1. How many children are there in your family? ____________
2. What are their ages? ____________
3. Who cares for/interacts with the children? ____________
4. How many people live in your home? ____________

D. Languages

1. What languages are spoken in your home? ____________
2. Who speaks those languages? ____________
3. What languages do you use with your child? ____________
4. Which language do you speak most often with your child? Which language do you use second-most often? Which one do you use the least?
   ____
   ____
5. What are the child's first, second, third, etc. languages?
   ____

E. Interactions

1. What are some examples of conversations you have with your child on a regular basis?
   ____
   ____
   ____
   ____

2. What are some activities that you do together with your child on a regular basis?

____

____

____

____

F. Milestones

I'd like you to try to remember (your child) at the age of 3 years—just before they started school. Did they help you around the house? Were they toilet trained yet? Were they running, climbing on things, dressing or undressing without help?

Now that you are remembering (your child) at the age of 3, I'd like to ask you some questions about their speech/language development up to that point.

1. How old was your child when they began babbling (playing with speech sounds)? ________

2. How old was your child when they spoke their first words? ________

3. What were their first words?

____

____

4. What kinds of words (category) did your child use between the ages of 6 months and 3 years?

____

____

____

5. What kinds of words did your child understand between the ages of 6 months and 3 years?

____

____

____

6. How could you tell that they understood those kinds of words?

____

____

____

____

Let's talk a little more about the words your child spoke before the age of 3 ...

1. Did they use animal names? ________ Which ones?

____

____

____

2. Did they use animal sounds? ________ Which ones?

____

____

____

3. Did they use vehicle names? ________ Which ones?

____

____

____

4. Did they use vehicle sounds or other sound effects before the age of 3? ________
   Which ones?
   ____
   ____
   ____

5. Did they use toy names? ________ Which ones?
   ____
   ____
   ____

6. Did they use food and drink words before the age of 3? ________ Which ones?
   ____
   ____

7. Did they use clothing words? ________ Which ones?
   ____
   ____
   ____

8. Did they use names of body parts? ________ Which ones?
   ____
   ____
   ____

9. Did they use furniture names or names of other household items? ________
   Which ones?
   ____
   ____
   ____

10. Did they use names of rooms in the house? ________ Which ones?
    ____
    ____
    ____

11. Did they use names of things outside of the house or in nature? ________
    Which ones?
    ____
    ____
    ____

12. Did they use names of places in the community? ________ Which ones?
    ____
    ____
    ____

13. Did they use names of people? ________ Which ones?
    ____
    ____
    ____

14. Does the child use names of people in the family? ________ Which ones?
    ____
    ____
    ____

15. Did they use names of daily activities (breakfast, potty)? ____________
    Which ones?
    ____
    ____
    ____

16. Did they use action words? ____________ Which ones?
    ____
    ____
    ____

17. Did they use describing words (big, wet) before the age of 3? ____________
    Which ones?
    ____
    ____
    ____

18. Did they use color words? ____________ Which ones?
    ____
    ____
    ____

19. Did they use words about time? ____________ Which ones?
    ____
    ____
    ____

20. Did they use question words? ____________ Which ones?
    ____
    ____
    ____

21. Did they use prepositions (in, out, over, under)? ____________ Which ones?
    ____
    ____
    ____

22. Did they use qualifiers in their sentences, phrase, or on their own? ____________
    Which ones?
    ____
    ____
    ____

23. Did they use connecting words in their sentences or phrases? ____________
    Which ones?
    ____
    ____
    ____

24. Did they use phrases (two or more words) before the age of 3? ____________
    Which ones? (Refer back to the conversations/activities the caregiver reported in the Interactions section previously.)
    ____
    ____
    ____

G. Gestures

1. How old was your child when they began using gestures? ____________
   What were their first gestures?

   ____
   ____
   ____

2. What other kinds of gestures did your child use between the ages of 6 months and 3 years?

   ____
   ____
   ____

3. What kinds of gestures did your child understand between the ages of 6 months and 3 years?

   ____
   ____
   ____

4. How could you tell that they understood those gestures?

   ____
   ____
   ____

5. Did they use pretend actions (with or without objects)? ____________ Which ones?

   ____
   ____
   ____

6. Did they pretend to be "Mommy?" ____________ Which pretend actions did they use?

   ____
   ____
   ____

7. Did they imitate other adult actions (wash dishes, sweep)? ____________ Which ones?

   ____
   ____
   ____

BE SURE TO MARK OUT NAMES OF CHILD AND CAREGIVER AFTER INTERVIEW AND ONLY USE ID# FOR REFERENCE GOING FORWARD.

Chapter 11

Assessment of Creole Languages in the Absence of Norms
A Case Study on Guyanese Creole

Sulare Telford Rose, PhD, CCC-SLP;
Tamirand Nnena De Lisser, PhD;
and Anna Monina M. Vanta, MS, CCC-SLP

Introduction

This chapter seeks to provide a background on creole languages, particularly those that emerged out of the colonial context, with implications for assessing children in the field of speech-language pathology. In the absence of developmental normatives, it is challenging to evaluate the linguistic competencies of children who speak creole languages. However, this chapter provides a framework for assessing the morphosyntactic features of creole languages in children with Guyanese Creole (GC; a Caribbean Creole with English as its lexifier) as a case study. In the absence of norms, clinicians must be able to identify language disorders in children and avoid misdiagnosis by learning about the linguistic rules of the language and by borrowing the framework used for assessing languages where normatives or assessment tools do not exist. While this is not ideal, it can lend to the reduction of misdiagnosis. Since culture and language are so intricately related and one informs the other, the chapter also provides a cursory background on Guyanese cultural norms.

As a child of the Caribbean sun (S. T. R.), I grew up believing that my native tongue was inferior, substandard, and repulsive. As a daughter of schoolteachers trained in this postcolonial context, I was encouraged to speak "properly" using the "Queen's English." Decades later, I was introduced to scholars like Kay Payne, Linda Bland-Stewart, John Rickford, Orlando Taylor, Shondel Nero, Yvette Hyter, and Walt Wolfram, sociolinguists who attested through their work and teaching that creole languages were legitimate, rule-governed languages with their content, use, and form. These languages were

Bortz, M. (Ed.). *A Guide to Global Language Assessment: A Lifespan Approach* (pp. 223-245).
DOI: 10.4324/9781003524472-14

worthy of study, use, and celebration. And so began my unlearning and my passion for learning and studying Caribbean English Creoles. I begin this chapter with my personal narrative to give you context around the importance and relevance of this chapter and the work of undoing and retraining that is necessary to evoke change in a world bent toward White and Eurocentric superiority.

In a sense, believing that my native language, GC (the language spoken by people in Guyana, South America, and its diaspora around the globe), was inferior and akin to believing that I was inferior. Our language is so closely connected with our identity, culture, expression, and worldview that suppressing it is like hiding oneself. This notion was true for many native creole language speakers and me. It is, therefore, the work of the speech-language pathologist, teacher, and greater society to rewrite the narrative and widespread fallacy that creole languages are "inferior, haphazard, broken, and bastardized versions of older, longer-established languages" (Todd, 1990). Moreover, and just as important, is the issue of misdiagnosis. Because the semantics, syntax, morphology, and phonology of creole languages and their apparent resemblance to longer-established languages have not been studied as much as European languages, the creole languages may be diagnosed inappropriately as a disordered form of the European (or lexifier) language; therefore, it is pertinent to know about the unique linguistic features of creole languages. So the question thus arises, what are creole languages?

Background on Pidgins and Creoles

Pidgins and creoles are found in every continent across the globe; however, our focus will be on Caribbean Creoles. From the early 1500s to the 1600s, the Portuguese, followed by other European countries, began sponsoring travels to find new frontiers (Todd, 1990). Once these discoveries were made, the Europeans began colonizing the natives living in the lands to gain political control over them. To expand their authority, wealth, and power, the Europeans captured and enslaved West Africans to work as forced laborers on their plantations. In the colonial contexts, for fear of a revolt, the enslaved people were strategically separated so that they did not speak one common language. However, in order to work on the plantations, enslaved people and the colonists had to communicate. This gave rise to the formation of what is known as a "pidgin." A pidgin may be defined as "a simple form of a language used for limited communication between people with no common language" (Todd, 1990). Pidgins emerge in multilingual contexts when groups of people who do not speak the same language need to communicate, and extensive vocabulary or detailed ideas do not need to be exchanged. Pidgins typically draw vocabulary explicitly from one language, and in the colonial plantation society, this is usually the European language. The grammatical structures of the pidgin are simplified and tend to mirror the languages of the enslaved. In cases where the communicative needs of the pidgin are no longer required, the language dies. However, in other cases, the pidgin develops into a creole language. This happens when children are born in the pidgin situation and learn the pidgin as their first language. Todd (1990) asserts that a creole language is a language which "develops when a pidgin becomes the mother tongue capable of fulfilling all the linguistic needs of its speakers." The process by which the pidgin changes to become more complex over time, and the vocabulary expands to suit the new, more complex communication needs of the new generation of native speakers, is known as *creolization*.

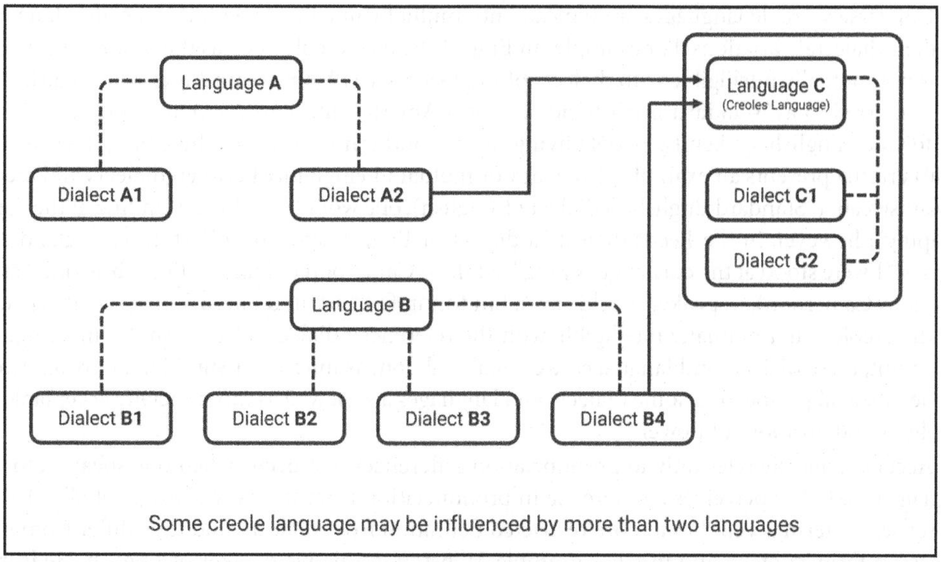

Figure 11-1. A simplified schema of the relationship between language, dialects, and creoles.

It is from this context that Haitian Creole (a French-based Creole), Papiamento and Cape Verdean Creoles (Portuguese-based Creoles), Berbice-Dutch Creole (an extinct Dutch-based Creole), and English-based Creoles such as Jamaican (also known as Patois), Sranan Tongo, and Guyanese Creole (also known as Creolese) developed. In the field of speech-language pathology, work has been done to a lesser extent than mainstream Englishes, on creoles such as Jamaican Creole (Karem & Washington, 2021; Malcolm, 2021; Washington et al., 2021) and Haitian Creole (Elie et al., 2018).

Differences Between Languages, Creoles, Dialects, and Accents

You may now be wondering how the terms *languages, dialects, creoles,* and *accents* differ? The answer is not simple, but the authors attempt to explain it so that the fundamental differences are apparent. Creoles and dialects are both legitimate language systems. A language is a system of communication that has rules. Languages consist of form (syntax/grammar), content (vocabulary), and use (form and content in different communication contexts). The term *creole* describes how a particular language system is formed. As seen in Figure 11-1, creoles are types of languages formed solely from multilingual contexts where two or more languages/dialects (Dialect A2 and Dialect B4) merge to form a new language (Language C).

As demonstrated in Figure 11-1, Language A, like Languages B and C, has dialects. The term dialect is used to highlight variations or differences within a specific language system (Adger et al., 2014; Todd, 1990). For example, the English language has different dialects like British English, Southern American English, African American English, Appalachian American English, Australian English, Guyanese English, etc. Everyone that speaks a language speaks a dialect of that language, as dialects are variations of one language due to regional, cultural, or social differences, including sex, gender, age, race, etc. Furthermore, some dialects, particularly English dialects, are mutually intelligible.

Conversely, creole languages are typically not mutually intelligible with their lexifier languages and their dialectal variations. For example, an English-lexified creole, such as the basilectal variety of GC, is not mutually intelligible with dialects of English such as Mainstream American English (popularly referred to as "standard English" across Latin America and East Asia) and southern English (the form of English spoken by people living in the southern portions of the United States). Todd (1990) craftily presents an example of the lack of mutual intelligibility between dialects and creoles: In Mainstream ("Standard English," a dialect of English), one would say, "I was standing at the corner gossiping"; however, in the Leeds dialect (a dialect of English spoken in Yorkshire, England), one may say, "I were stood at the corner gossiping"; while in Cameroon pidgin (an English-lexified creole spoken in Cameroon), a speaker would say "a bin tɑnɑp fɔ kɔnɑ ɑn ɑ bin di kɔnggɔsa." It is evident that the creole is not mutually intelligible with the referenced dialects of English. From a linguistic standpoint, these dialects and languages are equal and none is inferior or superior. However, from a broader societal perspective, some dialects and languages are viewed as more socially acceptable due to politics and positions of power.

Accents typically refer only to pronunciation differences that occur when one speaks a foreign language or another perceives a difference in pronunciation from their own (Adger et al., 2010). In this sense, the term accent has a more restricted definition from dialects, and they differ from other dialects in form, content, and use. For example, Winston is a native speaker of English. He learned French in college and knows the language pretty well. However, whenever Winston speaks to native French speakers, although they understand him, it is evident that French is not his first language because he sounds different from native French speakers when he speaks (Adger et al., 2010). This is because his accent is different.

Creoles and Linguistic Discrimination

Morgan and Alleyne (1994) and Degraff (2005) argue that creoles, particularly Caribbean Creoles, are "the most stigmatized of the world's languages" for reasons that can be traced back to now-defunct race theories of the colonial era. Degraff (2005) asserts that European enslavers view enslaved people as subhuman or monstrous; therefore the language of the monster was considered as a "linguistic monstrosity." This notion seems to permeate, albeit to a lesser degree, in the postcolonial era. He postulates that this form of racism exists in a new form he coins as "European scientific racism."

Language became a tool for the oppressors to maintain power and control. They spread the propaganda that anything, including language systems not typical of their European ideals, was substandard and unworthy. The more non-European something was, the more unwanted it became. So people of darker complexions were deemed less desirable than those whose complexions approximated Whiteness like that of the Europeans. This was no different for creole languages, which became the first language of most oppressed enslaved people and indentured laborers who worked the fields. These attitudes toward creoles still exist today. In many cases, those who spoke a creole language as their first or second language also began taking up the same attitudes towards their languages and self-expression. With language being so closely aligned with self-identity, this notion became a form of self-hatred.

In classrooms, children from creole-speaking backgrounds who speak creole as their first language are expected to abandon their languages in place of the European languages like English, French, and Portuguese (a language that resembles their own but is too distant to access). Some teachers who speak primarily in creole themselves have little command of the European languages like English and are expected to speak and teach a language that is foreign to their own. Students are assessed in their second language that they have not fully mastered and were never explicitly taught.

They never fully develop competencies in either language, as the first language was not positively promoted in the early years, and the second language was not modeled or taught adequately. Many of these children living outside of the creole context who move or migrate to other countries but learn a creole as their first language from parents are often viewed as having language disorders when they do not, thus perpetuating the fallacy of linguistic and hence racial inferiority.

It is therefore against this background that this chapter aims to explore some of the morphosyntactic features of GC that are potentially misdiagnosed as language disorders in children. Additionally, we propose a framework for assessing GC as normatives or assessment tools do not currently exist for this language or in this cultural context. More specifically, we aim to answer the following research question:

How should speakers of Guyanese Creole be assessed in order to not be misdiagnosed by speech-language pathologists as having a language disorder?

The chapter utilizes a descriptive research design and is organized as follows: First we present a brief overview of the development and current context of speech-language pathology in Guyana, followed by a description of the country and people. We zoom in on the linguistic situation in Guyana, highlighting the dominant language of Guyana, Guyanese Creole, and the creole continuum. Some general cultural norms, values, and beliefs are discussed that may have implications on linguistic behavior. The chapter then provides a description of education and literacy in Guyana, followed by details of the integral morphosyntactic features of GC that may contribute to misdiagnosis. The subsequent section documents the assessment considerations that are to be explored. A succinct conclusion and a case study task wraps up the chapter.

Overview and Context of Speech-Language Pathology in Guyana

Speech-language pathology is an emerging field in the Caribbean context, with Guyana as no exception. Before 2015, there were no speech-language pathologists in Guyana. However, in 2015, the Guyanese Ministry of Health (GMH), in conjunction with the Pan-American Health Organization (PAHO); a branch of the World Health Organization (WHO); the University of Guyana; and the American Speech-Language-Hearing Association (ASHA) launched the first Speech-Language Therapy and Audiology Program at the University of Guyana. The GMH-ASHA-PAHO collaboration led to the training of five speech-language therapists who graduated and began providing services in 2018. These pioneers, Gordonieka DeFreitas, Kerrianne Richards, Lisa Sam, Michelle Jackman, and Sonia Fredericks, paved the way for the development of the field in Guyana.

However, the study of language development among Guyanese children is in its infancy. Apart from work in progress by Caesar (2023), there are no speech or language developmental normatives for children in this context who speak GC or Standard Guyanese English. As such, there are no criterion-referenced or standardized tests specifically designed to assess the linguistic competencies of children. In the absence of developmental normatives, criterion-referenced, or standardized tests specifically designed for this population, the authors of this chapter seek to provide foundational knowledge on Guyanese culture and language with implications for language assessment (Figure 11-2).

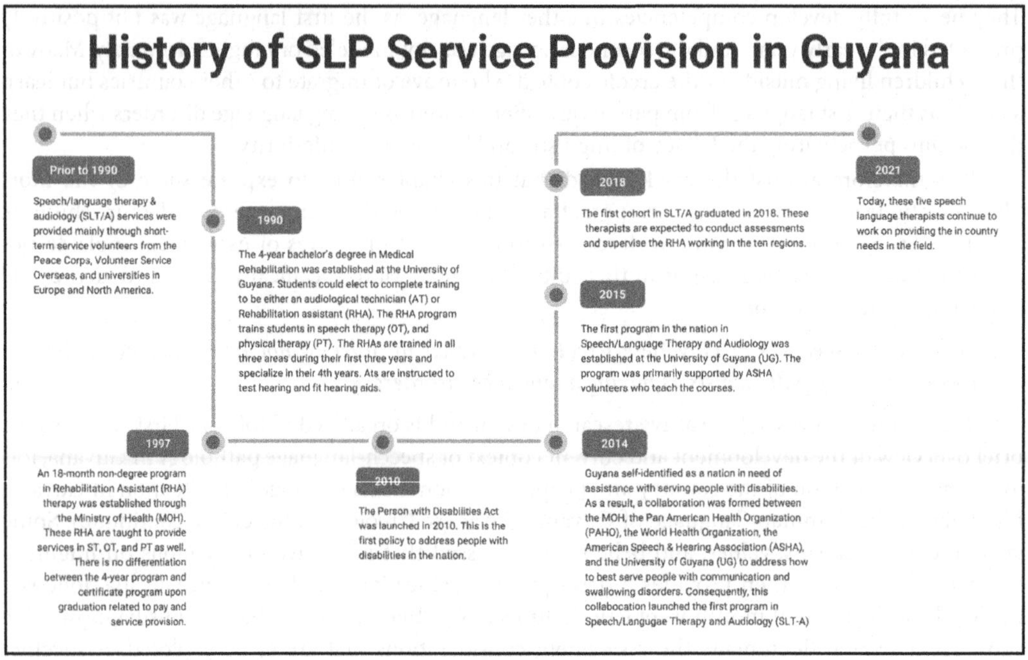

Figure 11-2. The history of speech-language pathology service provision in Guyana.

Description of the Country and People

Located on the northern coast of South America, Guyana boasts a population of just under 800,000 people, with most of its inhabitants on the coastlines (World Population Review, 2023). It has a landmass of 83,000 square miles and is bordered by the Atlantic Ocean to the north, Venezuela to its west, Suriname to its east, and Brazil to its south and southwest. While Guyana is located in South America, its language and culture are more closely aligned with that of the Caribbean.

While Guyana has long been described as one of the most economically insecure countries in South America, the discovery of crude oil has led to its rising gross domestic product (GDP) of 5.4 billion dollars (Guyana Ministry of Education and Cultural Development Planning Unit, 1995). The country is also rich in other natural resources, including gold and bauxite.

The original inhabitants of Guyana were the Amerindians. However, a variety of ethnic immigrant groups arrived in Guyana between the early 1600s to the end of the 1800s (Rickford, 1987). These groups included colonists from major European nations (Gibson, 2001). The Dutch were the first recorded European settlers to Guyana in 1581 (Gibson, 2001). The British in 1831 seized control of the three Dutch colonies, forming British Guiana, and did not relinquish their rule until Guyana gained its independence in 1966 (Gibson, 2001; Rickford, 1987). The European settlers brought forced laborers, who included African slaves and East Indian and Chinese indentured laborers, to work on coffee, cotton, and sugar plantations (Gibson, 2001). These groups of people who spoke a plethora of languages were forced to intermingle amongst themselves and the European landowners, which caused them to communicate using a mix of their languages. This language mix is known as pidgin. When a new generation spoke the pidgin as their first language, Guyanese Creole was born.

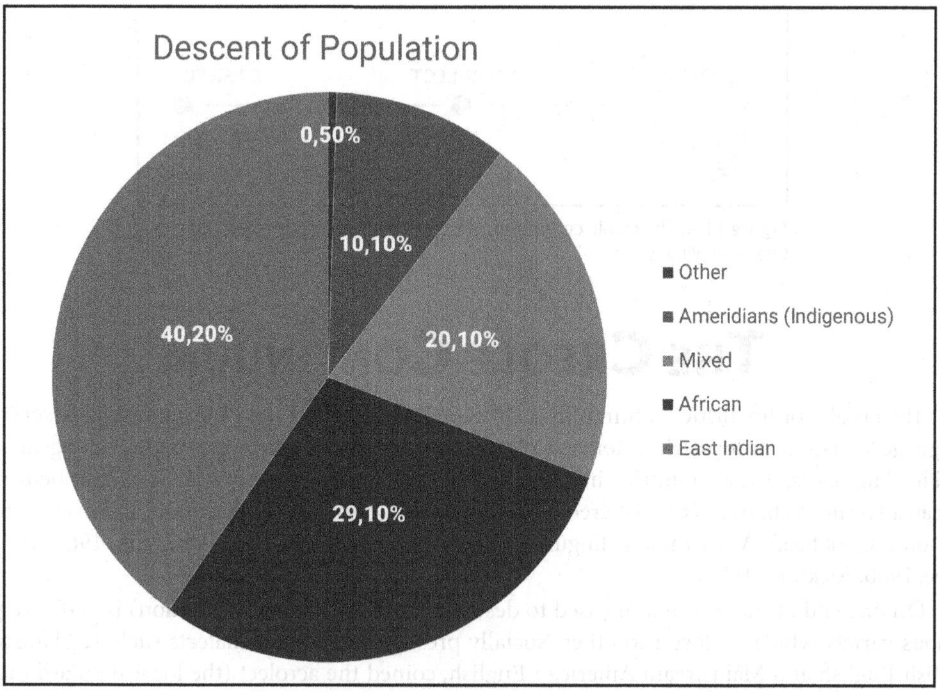

Figure 11-3. Ethnic groups in Guyana. (Data source: World Population Review [2023].)

People of East Indian descent represent the largest ethnic population in Guyana (40%). The second-largest ethnic group includes people of African descent (29%), followed by mixed-race people (20%). The Amerindians (Indigenous Guyanese) now only make up 10% of the population, and the remaining 0.5% fall under the "Other" category, which includes Chinese and European Guyanese (World Population Review, 2023). Figure 11-3 provides an illustration of the Guyanese ethnic group breakdown.

Guyanese Creole

According to Telford Rose et al. (2020), GC native speakers may speak language varieties anywhere along a creole continuum between Standard Guyanese English (SGE) and GC. Allsopp and Allsopp (1996) illustrates this by contending that there are not merely two discrete ways of saying "I told him" in GC, but at least nine, ranging from the most standard (the acrolect) to the least standard (the basilect). Intermediate or mesolectal versions include "a tel im" and "a tel ii." The most basilect or distinctly creole version is "mi tel am" (Rickford, 1987). The term *lect* refers to any variety along the creole continuum from acrolect to basilect. Banwarie and Wilkinson (2013) illustrate the creole continuum in Figure 11-4.

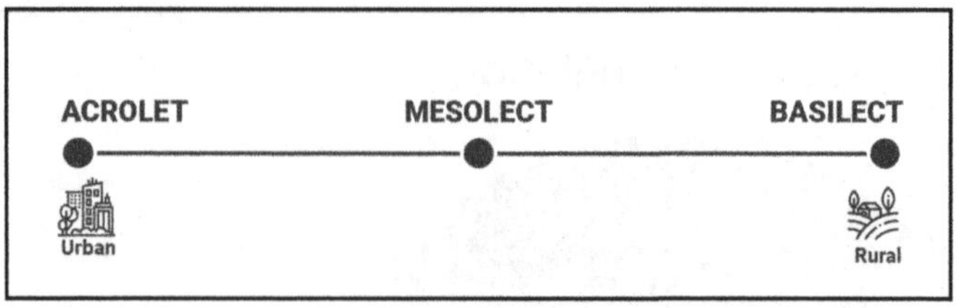

Figure 11-4. The creole continuum. (Reproduced with permission from Charlene Wilkinson.)

The Creole Continuum

The creole (or linguistic) continuum is a theoretical construct used by linguists to describe the language variation in formerly colonized societies where creole languages operate alongside their lexifier languages. These countries include, but are not limited to, Guyana, Trinidad, Belize, and Jamaica (Ivrine-Sobers, 2018). The creole continuum has been widely discussed and even "refuted" by some Caribbean (West Indian) linguists (Alleyne, 1980; Bailey, 1971; DeCamp, 1961, 1971; Le Page, 1960; Rickford, 1987).

On one end of the continuum (used to describe Guyana's linguistic situation) is SGE, the prestigious variety which is closest to other "socially prestigious" English dialects such as Mainstream British English and Mainstream American English, coined the acrolect (the local standard dialect) by W. A. Stewart (1965). On the other end of the creole continuum is the basilect. The basilect most resembles the communication patterns of its original speakers and is qualitatively and decidedly different from that of the acrolect. The basilect often maintains the West African grammatical structure. Still, it borrows vocabulary from its European (lexifier) language and the original West African languages of the enslaved/indentured people. However, the pronunciation is starkly different from the European language. Intermediate varieties (mesolect) also exist. Some linguists argue that the description of the continuum is misleading and situating a speaker along the continuum may be difficult or even impossible. Other issues surround the notion that the continuum is fluid and speakers may control different aspects of the continuum, or the entire continuum. Additionally, there are no ways of defining where on the continuum one language variety ends and the other begins (Irvine-Sobers, 2018).

Stewart (1965) depicted the acrolect as the utmost prestigious dialect on the creole continuum (likely because it most closely approximates the European languages of the colonizers and that of people in the society from the upper social strata). Stewart (1965) saw the acrolect to fall at the top and basilect to be at the bottom, hence the use of the term "acro" from "apex" and "basi" to mean "bottom" (Irvine-Sobers, 2018). DeCamp (1961) differentiates the "lects" on the continuum by describing (quite offensively, we may add, although acceptable at his time), the type of person who may use the acrolect versus the basilect. He states the acrolect may be used by the "well-educated," and the basilect would most likely be used by "the most backward peasant or labourer." The offense lies in using the word "backward," which indicates a lack of intelligence.

Both Stewart and DeCamp's depictions of the continuum reveal the sentiment of the time that the language used most aligned with that of the European Colonizers; the acrolect was more valuable or admirable. Those views are flawed and deeply steeped in racism and linguistic imperialism. Sociolinguistics like John Rickford and Shondel Nero, among others, view these dialects as having equal linguistic value and importance. The view of the linguists, however, may be in opposition to society's general opinion. While not initially depicted in Stewart's work, a wide range of intermediate varieties, or the mesolect, are in between the acrolect and basilect on the creole continuum. Rickford (1987) states that there is no clear cleavage between one variety to the next.

Some speakers of the creole languages may be able to use varieties anywhere across the continuum, intentionally or not, while others may need more flexibility in their linguistic abilities. For example, Winston is asked by a supervisor at work who recently migrated from the United Kingdom, "Did you tell Andrew that you will arrive early today?" He may respond, "Yes, I told him," using the acrolect. If asked the same question by his Guyanese peer or colleague he may say, "a tel ii," using the mesolect. When asked the same question by his wife, his response may be, "mi tel am," using the basilect (Rickford, 1987).

Irvine-Sobers (2018, p. 1) in her text *The Acrolect in Jamaica: The Architecture of Phonological Variation* provides possible rationale for the existence of the of the varieties outlined on the creole continuum:

1. The intermediate varieties have been "attributed" to decreolization (Bickerton, 1973; DeCamp, 1971), due to the "targeting of English by Creole speakers with varying levels of access to the prestige or high variety."
2. The "basilectalization brought about by increasing numbers of West Africans arriving over time and acquiring approximations of approximations of English" (Mufwene, 1996, 2001).
3. The "social stratification of plantation communities from the earliest stages of language contact" (Alleyne, 1980).

In addition to considerations of the creole continuum, which may impact the variety of language produced, general cultural norms, values, and beliefs are also contributing factors to the linguistic choices employed. These will be explored in the subsequent section.

General Cultural Norms/Values/Beliefs

Language and cultural norms, values, and beliefs are intertwined. Generally, cultural norms, values, and beliefs are expressed through language, and one's linguistic behavior reflects their culture. Cultural norms, beliefs, and values may affect stereotypes and attitudes toward language and language varieties and the general interaction among people. An understanding of the cultural norms, values, and beliefs strongly upheld in the Guyanese society is therefore crucial in understanding the Guyanese linguistic situation. It should be noted, however, that not every Guyanese adheres to these norms and care should be taken when making assumptions about the language. Table 11-1 illustrates some of the common verbal inflections in Guyanese and some potential implications for language.

Education and Literacy

The Guyanese school system is modeled after the British school system and consists of four parts: (1) early childhood education/nursery school, which is not compulsory and lasts for 2 years starting at 3.5 years old; afterward (2) primary school for 6 years with compulsory attendance; next is (3) secondary school, in which students take an exam to determine placements in secondary school; and finally (4) technical and vocational (London, 2018). Secondary school is structured in three parts:

- General/Prestigious Secondary Schools (GSS)
- Community High Schools (CHS)
- Primary Tops (Secondary Department of the Primary School)

Table 11-1
Examples of Verbal Inflections in Guyanese Creole

MORPHOSYNTACTIC FEATURE		EXAMPLES	
		Guyanese Creole	*English*
Tense	Bare non-stative verb	Shi go in shi seef plees.	She went to her safe place.
	"bin" + non-stative verb	Shi jraa aal a di ting dem wa dem bin larn wen dem bina go aal bout di plees.	She drew everything they had learned on their adventure.
	Bare stative verb	Awii noo da, Seera.	We know, Sara.
	"bin" + stative verb	Liila bin noo shi nyuu matii dem bin keer bout shi nof nof.	Leila knew her new friends cared a lot about her.
Modal	Ability/permission	Awii kyan fait am.	We can fight it.
	Obligatory	Awii gafu kiip dem seef.	We have to keep them safe.
	Necessity	Ayo mos laisn ayo chransileeshan.	You need to license your translation.
Aspect	Progressive	Na aal badii a staan hoom.	Not everybody is staying home.
	Prospective	Dat gon help tu.	That is going to help too.
	Habitual	Piipl wa sik doz get fiiva.	People who are sick get a fever.
Infinitive	Marked	Ariyo aks dem fu lak dem ai.	Ario asked them to close their eyes.
	Bare	Ayo waahn chrai du da wid mi?	Would you like to try this with me?

GSS consists of 5 to 6 years with the highest quality education, CHS which when completed can gain access to GSS through high scores on an Secondary School Proficiency Exam (SSPE), whilst Primary Tops programs are oriented toward the acquisition of prevocational skills (London, 2018). Top scoring students are placed in GSS, lower scoring students in CHS, and the lowest scoring students in Primary Tops. Placement in GSS is limited and is available to ~45% of students taking the SSPE. Additionally, rural areas are disadvantaged due to lack of available seats in GSS (Holbrook & Holbrook, 2001). Students who are not placed in GSS are perceived as academically inferior and are allowed only "specialized, lower-level post secondary programmes [which] do not provide credentials that are recognized in the labour market" (Guyana Ministry of Education and Cultural Development Planning Unit, 1995). Only ~8% of students qualify for GSS and only students that attend GSS have the opportunity to take the Caribbean Examination Council (CXC), which is a necessity for tertiary education (Guyana Ministry of Education and Cultural Development Planning Unit, 1995).

Guyana has declined in quality of education (since their independence) due to supply shortages; water, electrical, and sewage problems; poor resources; and low morale for teachers. Specifically, there are inadequate teacher wages, lack of textbooks/teaching materials, as well as poor teaching-learning environments from budget cuts due to structural adjustment programs (Holbrook & Holbrook, 2001). Guyana's educational system and labor force have struggled with "brain drain," where roughly half of the population that have tertiary education migrate out while 39% reside abroad. Thus, this limits Guyana's ability to progress in fields such as education, medicine, and engineering (World Bank, n.d.).

Roughly 11% of the Guyanese youth population had a high level of functional literacy, with females having higher functional literacy as compared to males. Furthermore, most of the low level literacy population never attended beyond primary school or low status secondary school, thus typically prompting unemployment or semi/unskilled jobs (Jennings, 2000). Although literacy is reported at 97% (UNESCO Institute for Statistics, 2021), a study on literacy of young Guyanese adults suggested this percentage to be closer to 70% (Jennings, 2000). GC is discouraged from use in school systems as it is viewed as negative and as a substandard form of English that requires consistent correction (Semple-McBean, 2007). GC is not officially recognized in the school system (along with many other settings), even though many students use GC outside of school. Additionally, in earlier grades some students only understand GC when being taught (Holbrook & Holbrook, 2001).

Assessment of Morphosyntactic Features

Morphosyntactic Features of Guyanese

As previously mentioned, GC (or Creolese, as amicably called by its speakers) is an English-lexified creole language, spoken natively by the vast majority of the population (Devonish & Thompson, 2010) and the Guyanese diaspora. Though most of its lexical items are English-based, semantically, words are not always used in the same manner as they are used in English. Morphosyntactically, GC is quite distinct from English. As both languages operate side-by-side due to the continuum situation in Guyana, there tend to be overlapping features of the varieties. It is therefore integral that examples of the GC structures that are distinct from English structures be provided, as these will help speech-language pathologists understand how the language systems differ, what is the grammatical structure for a GC speaker, whether the Guyanese speaker with whom the speech-language pathologists are working are producing grammatical structures or not, and where areas of misdiagnosis can be corrected or avoided. For the purposes of this analysis, we will focus on five morphosyntactic features of the most conservative (or basilectal) varieties of GC:

- Tense, mode, and aspect
- Pronouns
- Plural markings
- Serial verb constructions
- Prepositions

Note that these are not the only areas of difference, but space requirements for the current chapter will not allow a comprehensive analysis of all relevant features. Additionally, space requirements will not allow us to explore other types of creoles except for English-lexified creoles. The primary data in the description of the language, unless otherwise specified, are taken from De Lisser and Fraser's (2020) translation of *My Hero Is You: How Kids Can Fight COVID-19!* This book is a 6455-word resource of authentic GC sentences.

Tense, Mode, and Aspect

Based on De Lisser and Telford Rose (in press) tense, mode, and aspect may be expressed using free preverbal morphemes in GC, which require no subject-verb agreement. When non-stative GC verbs are unmarked, they are interpreted as simple past (Example 1); however, unmarked stative verbs have a default non-past reading (Example 2):

1. **Jan kik hii** (De Lisser & Telford Rose, in press)
   John kick 3SG
   "John kicked him/her."
2. **Jan laik hii** (De Lisser & Telford Rose, in press)
   John like 3SG
   "John likes him/her."

Conversely, to mark past tense on stative verbs requires the preverbal morpheme *bin* (as exemplified in 3). Where *bin* is used with non-stative verbs, it is normally interpreted with a pluperfect meaning, as demonstrated in 4.

3. **Jan bin laik hii** (De Lisser & Telford Rose, in press)
   John TNS like 3SG
   "John liked him/her."
4. **Jan bin kik hii** (De Lisser & Telford Rose, in press)
   John TNS kick 3SG
   "John had kicked him/her."

Progressive aspect is marked with *a*, prospective aspect with *go/gon*, and habitual aspect is marked with *doz,* as exemplified in Table 11-2. Also in Table 11-2, we see that ability/permission, obligatory, and necessity modals are marked with *kyan, gafu,* and *mos*, respectively.

As demonstrated in Table 11-1, infinitives can be marked or unmarked.

The difference in marking verbal inflections in GC may affect interpretations and meanings in English. If these differences should be ignored in an assessment, then speech-language pathologists may misdiagnose a GC speaker.

Table 11-2

Examples of Invariability of Case on Pronouns in Guyanese Creole

MORPHOSYNTACTIC FEATURE		**EXAMPLES**	
		Guyanese Creole	*English*
Invariable Pronouns	Nominative case	Hii flai kraas di tong.	He flew across the city.
	Accusative case	Mi neva stap keer bout hii.	I never stopped caring about him.
	Genitive case	Hii a staan a hii bejruum.	He's staying in his bedroom.

Pronouns

In GC, unlike in English, pronouns are invariable for nominative, accusative, and genitive cases as exemplified in Table 11-2. GC will therefore grammatically produce the same pronoun *hii,* where English is required to alternate between "he," "him," or "his." Not recognizing this difference when assessing a GC speaker may lead to incorrect assessment and possible misdiagnosis.

Plural Marking

In GC, plurals in definite noun phrases are generally marked by *dem*. However, it is not necessary that *dem* is always used to express plurality, as there are other ways as detailed in Table 11-3. Also, *dem* does not always encode plurality as in the English plural marker, but may be inclusivity based on association (in line with Stewart, 2006). The assessment of the use of plurals for a GC speaker will therefore be distinct from how plural marking is applied in English, and cases where the plural morpheme is obligatory in English does not require an obligatory marker in GC. Understanding these differences is therefore integral for accurate assessment of a GC speaker.

Serial Verb Construction

Serial verb constructions, as defined by Adone (2012, p. 144) are "complex predicates containing at least two verbs within a single clause." These structures are common in GC, and are attested as different types, as detailed in Table 11-4. Serial verb constructions are, however, not a feature of English, and as such a GC speaker producing these structures may be easily seen as producing ungrammatical structures by a speech-language pathologist who is not cognizant of the features of GC. It is therefore important that the various forms of serial verb constructions in GC be understood and applied to any assessment of GC speakers.

Prepositions

Prepositions in GC, for the most part, are similar to prepositions in the lexifier language. Importantly, however, is the use of preposition *a* or a null preposition instead of English forms such as "to" or "at."

5. Jan a go (a) skuul (De Lisser and Telford Rose, in press)
   John PROG go (to) school
   "John is going to school."
6. Jan de (a) skuul (De Lisser and Telford Rose, in press)
   John LOC (at) school
   "John is at school."

Additional prepositions used differently in GC when compared to English are detailed in Table 11-5. The use of these prepositions are different from the prepositions in English, and as such, it is pertinent that speech-language pathologists understand these differences so as to correctly apply them in their assessment of GC speakers.

Table 11-3
Examples of Pluralization and Inclusion in Guyanese Creole

MORPHOSYNTACTIC FEATURE		EXAMPLES	
		Guyanese Creole	*English*
Pluralization and Inclusivity	Postnominal dem	Mi kyan kaal mi matii dem.	I can call my friends.
	Plural demonstrative dem	Dem Staar Gyal ga majik pouwa.	Those heroes have super powers.
	Inclusive dem	Ariyo dem.*	Ario and the children.
	Unmarked, context determined, or generic nouns	Awii doz riid buk.	We read books.
	Numeral or quantifier	Awii gafu staan moo dan chrii fut fram ayo.	We have to stay at least 3 feet away.

*This example was not taken from the main source.

Table 11-4
Serial Verb Constructions in Guyanese Creole

MORPHOSYNTACTIC FEATURE		EXAMPLES	
		Guyanese Creole	*English*
Serial Verb Construction	Directional	Shi ron go shoo shi moda wa shi jraa.	She ran to her mum with her drawing.
	Causative	Bot yu mek mi memba.	But you remind me.
	Dative	So mi a go staan op hee an fling wahn hog gi ayo.	So I will throw you a hug.
	Intentional	Som piipl in awii eerya bin kom an help out a awii hous.	People in our community helped us at home.

Table 11-5
Examples of Prepositions in Guyanese Creole

MORPHOSYNTACTIC FEATURE		EXAMPLES	
		Guyanese Creole	*English*
Prepositions	A used as "at"	Yu a staan a yu hous.	You are staying at home.
	Pon used as "to"; in used as "by"	Dem flai dong pon ort an lan in wahn lil vilij.	They soared down to earth and landed by a small village.
	Pon used as "at"	Di piipl dem (ina di pleen) luk pon dem.	The passengers looked out at them.
	A used as "to"	Awii gramaa an grafaada dem bin gafu go a di haspital.	Our grandparents had to go to the hospital.
	Null preposition	Shi waahn fu go skuul bot shi skuul klooz.	She wanted to go to school but her school was closed.

The data presented in Table 11-5 provide examples of the structures of GC that are essential for any speech-language pathologist to understand when assessing GC speakers, or otherwise run the risk of continuing the practice of misdiagnosing GC children. The structures are similar to other English-lexified creoles and as such the considerations applied in the subsequent section can be applied to other English-lexified creoles of the Caribbean for example Jamaican, Trinidad English Creole, Antiguan and Barbudan Creole, Limonese Creole, among others.

Assessment Considerations

According to the *Resource Guide for the Education of New York State Students From Caribbean Countries Where English Is the Medium of Instruction* (Ruiz et al., n.d., p. 5), when assessing children from Caribbean English Creole contexts, the assessor should note that English-lexified creole-speaking children from the Caribbean:

- Speak English and a local Caribbean Creole or a language other than English
- Manifest varying degrees of understanding and proficiency in both the Standard Caribbean English spoken in their country, as well as in Standard American English
- May be bilingual, speaking English and one of the varieties of other languages spoken in the Caribbean
- Are from cultures and traditions different from those of the United States
- May be unfamiliar with the sociocultural features of American society
- May have strong academic skills commensurate with their age and grade level

There are no speech or language developmental normatives currently available for Guyanese children, and this is true for many creole languages. Additionally, no widely published or validated standardized or criterion-referenced assessments have been developed specifically with consideration for Guyanese children (Telford Rose et al., 2020). Speech-language pathologists working with Guyanese children should first familiarize themselves with the linguistic features of GC as outlined in the previous section. Some salient grammatical features of Guyanese features are presented in this chapter; however, Devonish and Thompson (2010) provide a detailed account of other GC grammatical features in their book *A Concise Grammar of Guyanese Creole (Creolese)*. The *Dictionary of Caribbean English Usage* is also a great source for lexical features and definitions of GC and other Caribbean English Creoles (Allsopp, 2013). Grannum-Solomon (2008) provides an in-depth analysis and explanation of many common Guyanese proverbs. Telford Rose et al. (2020) provide critical phonological features of GC.

After reviewing and familiarizing oneself with the language system, the speech-language pathologist is then recommended to conduct a language sample. Any features found that are consistent with GC should be marked as correct. However one should take caution when features that vary from the data are found, as there are not developmental norms. In this case it is pertinent for speech-language pathologists to work closely with cultural and linguistic brokers, ones who are familiar with both the creole language and the mainstream culture and language. Cultural and linguistic brokers can advise the clinician during the evaluation process. These cultural and linguistic brokers can also assist with differentiating typical and atypical productions. Utilizing a cultural or linguistic broker who works with or spends time with children will provide further insights.

Parents are experts in the child's language. So, trusting them in the diagnostic process is critical. Ask for their opinions on the child's communication development. The parent is usually the first to identify when children are not developing typically (like people within their community). While parents may not be able to express fully where the areas of difficulty are, they may be the first to know that something is different (McLeod & Baker, 2017). Be careful to note that many people, including parents in creole contexts, may view their own language as disordered. So be careful to ask if they believe that the child speaks like themselves or others in their environment who are the same age, rather than only ask if they believe their child has a language disorder. Parents may not fully understand the role of speech-language pathologists and therefore expect clinicians to teach their children the "standard" or the mainstream language of the country, which is outside our scope of proactive as the difference does not mean disorder (Hyter & Salas-Provance, 2023).

Dynamic assessment rather than static assessment is suggested for assessing the linguistic competencies of creole speakers as it allows the clinician to assess whether a client simply hasn't been taught a specific concept or if they indeed have a language pathology that requires more in-depth intervention. If the use of standardized tests is mandated for insurance or other purposes, using it without modifications to directives, stimuli, and scoring is not recommended and could lead to misidentification. "While scoring modifications, such as extending acceptable responses for GC-speaking children, may be a viable strategy for ensuring more appropriate scoring ... clinicians must do so with extreme caution so as not to mask true language disorders" (Telford Rose et al., 2020). If standardized tests are mandated by a governing entity, consider reporting scores in the standardized format then report scores based on the modifications to the assessment. Hyter and Salas-Provance (2023) provide a framework and guidelines for testing modification.

Alternatives to Standardized Tests

The use of language samples is the gold standard for assessing children from multicultural populations where no normative information is available. Both Language samples and dynamic assessment have been widely recommended in the literature for assessing speakers of nonmainstream language (Johnson & Gatlin-Nash, 2020). Chapters 6, 7, and 16 in this text provides details on alternatives to standardized testing.

Language Samples

When selecting stimuli for language samples, be sure to use culturally appropriate stimuli. Consider using children's books written by and for Caribbean children as stimuli for language samples. For example, stimuli that prompt children to discuss snow or a mailbox may not be appropriate due to Guyanese children being unfamiliar with these concepts. When appropriate, use oral and written literature from the Caribbean (Winer, 2009). With consideration to the cultural norm that children should be seen not heard, one should consider that some Guyanese children may need more prompting and familiarity with the examiner before feeling comfortable engaging in a one-to-one conversation with an adult. When collecting language samples from Guyanese children consider:

1. Selecting culturally appropriate stimuli for collecting one's language sample.
2. Building rapport with the child before collecting data.
3. Fostering an environment where the child feels comfortable expressing themselves in the language most comfortable for them.
4. Collecting a language sample between the child and a familiar communication partner such as a sibling, cousin, or friend during play.
5. Remember that many Guyanese children may be bilingual or multilingual and may be using the linguistic patterns found in GC, SGE, and the country in which the assessment is being conducted. Consider each language in your analysis.

6. Caesar (2023) provided language samples of Guyanese children on the Systematic Analysis of Language Transcripts (SALT) transcription analysis software, therefore, using this software to analyze the speech of Guyanese children may be very useful.
7. Enlist linguistic brokers in the analysis of the speech sample who know and understand GC to answer or provide insight on utterances that are not included in the tables of this chapter. Cultural and linguistic brokers can help advise during the evaluation process. These cultural and linguistic brokers can assist with differentiating typical and atypical productions.
8. Do not penalize or cite as errors any linguistic patterns that are typical to GC speakers.

Regardless of the mode of assessment chosen, speech-language pathologists must remember that Guyanese children exist in a dual language context to varying degrees. It is essential to look at both language systems when assessing language skills, even if the children and families themselves do not consider themselves bilingual. While socially this is not the popular view, the linguistic dexterity of this complex language system should be celebrated.

Conclusion

In the absence of norms, speech-language pathologists must be able to correctly assess speakers of GC and other English-lexified creoles in order to avoid misdiagnosis. In order to do this, a great understanding of the morphosyntactic features of GC that are distinct from English is required. Adopting the framework we proposed for assessing GC is therefore integral for the accurate assessment of GC and other English-lexified creole languages. The chapter established the basis of how speakers of GC should be assessed in order to not be misdiagnosed by speech-language pathologists as having a language disorder. Key considerations to take away include the need for comprehensive knowledge of the morphosyntactic structures of the language and how they differ from English structures; an appreciation for cultural differences; the application of dynamic assessment strategies; and considerations of alternatives to standardized tests.

Case Study

Client Background

Hiya Mohabeer is a 9-year-old female who is currently enrolled at P. S. #51 in the New York City (NYC) public school system. Hiya moved to NYC 6 months ago from Guyana. She has no reported history of developmental delays or disorders, and no visual or sensory impairments (e.g., hearing loss, blindness, autism spectrum disorder). She is currently enrolled in the third grade; when she moved to the United States she was required to repeat the third grade. She was referred for a speech-language assessment by her classroom teacher. Hiya's teacher (Ms. Slooth) expressed that Hiya has difficulties forming grammatically correct sentences, following complex directions, and has poor writing skills (her writing includes many grammatical errors). Ms. Slooth also noted that Hiya does not participate in class discussions and is often reluctant to speak. When she does attempt to communicate, Hiya is only about 60% intelligible to her teacher and peers. When asked if they had any concerns about Hiya's speech or language skills, Hiya's dad responded "Mi een noo. If somting rong, di tiicha mos noo na."

Language Sample

Fors a went tu di biich wit mai mom, mai broder an mai an mii antii, an wii went tu di biich wii swim an soo. Wen ai swim ai put aan a dok an xx- an den ai go an ai sidong, jringkin an soo. Ai fel api an soo.

Den mii an ma kozn went a di bakdam tu plee tu plee a krikit. An mii an mii ge onjred, an mii win di geem. An ai fiil api an xx- an mi waahn plee ageen.

1. What other questions should you ask about Hiya regarding her culture and language?
   Suggested Responses:
   - Which part of Guyana is she from? (See section …)
   - Are her parents able to understand her?
   - Do her parents believe that she speaks, uses words, forms sentences, etc., like other Guyanese children her age?
   - Do they believe that she can follow their directions?
   - Does Hiya communicate with siblings and peers from her community?
2. Based on the language sample, what grammatical features of GC do you observe?
   Suggested Responses:
   - First person singular "mii" (with phonological variant /ma/) used invariably in nominative case and genitive case
     - No overt marking of past tense
     - Serial verb construction
     - Use of preposition "a" instead to "to"
     - Use of bare infinitive (e.g., "plee" instead of "to play")
3. Based on the language sample, do you observe any grammatical differences that are not consistent with GC or other forms of English? If so, do you suspect that Hiya may have a language disorder?
   - Answers: No

References

Adger, C. T., Wolfram, W., & Christian, D. (2010). *Dialects in schools and communities.* Routledge.

Adger, C. T., Wolfram, W., & Christian, D. (2014). *Dialects in schools and communities.* Taylor and Francis.

Adone, D. (2012). *The acquisition of Creole languages: How children surpass their input.* Cambridge University Press.

Alleyne, M. C. (1980). *Comparative Afro-American: An historical-comparative study of English-based Afro-American dialects of the New World.* Karoma Publishers.

Allsopp, J., & Allsopp, R. (1996). *Dictionary of Caribbean English usage.* Oxford University Press.

Allsopp, R. (2013). *Dictionary of Caribbean English usage: The proposed.* Caribbean Lexicography Project.

Bailey, B. (1971). Jamaican Creole: Can dialect boundaries be defined? In D. Hymes (Ed.), *Pidginization and creolization of languages* (pp. 341-348). Cambridge University Press.

Banwarie, K., & Wilkinson, C. (2013, Jul 15). *Language awareness [PowerPoint].* https://www.slideserve.com/chadrick/introduction-to-the-use-of-english

Bickerton, D. (1973). The nature of a creole continuum. *Language, 49*(3), 640. https://doi.org/10.2307/412355

Caesar, L. (2023). *A tale of two continents: Comparing African American and Guyanese children's oral narratives.* https://plan.core-apps.com/asha2023/event/519b79a2279abf51f2a245ec7a75b2de

DeCamp, D. (1961). Social and geographic factors in Jamaican dialects. In R. B. Le Page (Ed.), *Creole language studies* (pp. 61-84). Macmillan.

DeCamp, D. (1971). Toward a generative analysis of a post-creole speech continuum. In D. Hymes (Ed.), *Pidginization and Creolization of languages* (pp. 349-370). Cambridge University Press.

Degraff, M. (2005). Linguists' most dangerous myth: The fallacy of Creole exceptionalism. *Language in Society, 34*(4), 533-591. http://www.jstor.org/stable/4169447

De Lisser, T., & Fraser, C. (2020). 'Mi Staar Gyal a Yu: Hou piknii kyan fait Kovid-19!' Translation of Helen Patuck, My Hero Is You: How Kids Can Fight COVID-19! In Guyanese Creole. Inter-Agency Standing Committee Reference Group on Mental Health and Psychosocial Support in Emergency Settings (IASC MHPSS RG) https://interagencystandingcommittee.org/system/files/2020-05/My%20Hero%20is%20You%2C%20Storybook%20for%20Children%20on%20COVID-19%20%28Guyanese%20Creole~Creolese%29.pdf

De Lisser, T., & Telford Rose, S. (in press). *A descriptive analysis of the performance of Guyanese Creole-speaking children on the DELV-NR test.*

Devonish, H., & Thompson, D. (2010). *A concise grammar of Guyanese Creole (Creolese).* Lincom Europa Academic Publications, LINCOM GmbH.

Elie, M., Lucker, J., Martinez, S., & Wright-Harp, W. (2018). *Use of the Preschool Language Scale-4th Edition with Haitian Creole speakers: Does dialect scoring make a difference?* EHEARSAY. https://www.ohioslha.org/wp-content/uploads/2018/07/eHearsayCLD.pdf

Gibson, K. (2001). *COMFA religion and Creole language in a caribbean community.* State University of New York Press.

Grannum-Solomon, V. (2008). *Proverbial wisdom from Guyana.* BookSurge Publishing.

Guyana Ministry of Education and Cultural Development Planning Unit. (1995). *Guyana: Mid-decade review of progress toward education for all.* UNESDOC Digital Library.

Holbrook, D. J., & Holbrook, H. A. (2001). Guyanese creole survey report. *Semantic Scholar.* https://www.semanticscholar.org/paper/Guyanese-Creole-Survey-Report-Holbrook-Holbrook/8b4d62092ccd786e60b1c69dbce4698919bb7ff4

Hyter, Y. D., & Salas-Provance, M. B. (2023). *Culturally responsive practices in speech, language and hearing sciences* (2nd ed.). Plural Publishing.

Irvine-Sobers, G. A. (2018). *The acrolect in Jamaica: The architecture of phonological variation.* Language Science Press.

Jennings, Z. (2000). Functional literacy of young Guyanese adults. *International Review of Education, 46*(1/2), 93-116. https://doi.org/10.1023/a:1003926406978

Johnson, L. C., & Gatlin-Nash, B. (2020). Evidence-based practices in the assessment and intervention of language-based reading difficulties among African American learners. *Perspectives on Language and Literacy, 46*(2), 19-23.

Karem, R. W., & Washington, K. N. (2021). The cultural and diagnostic appropriateness of standardized assessments for dual language learners: A focus on Jamaican preschoolers. *Language, Speech, and Hearing Services in Schools, 52*(3), 807-826. https://doi.org/10.1044/2021_lshss-20-00106

LePage, R. B. (1960). *Jamaican Creole: An historical introduction to Jamaican Creole.* Macmillan.

London, T. (2018). Assessing competing perspectives: A critical analysis of Guyana's national grade six assessment. *Africology: The Journal of Pan-African Studies, 11*(4).

Malcolm, T. R. (2021). *Cross-linguistic morphosyntactic influence in bilingual speakers of Jamaican Creole and Jamaican English.* CUNY Academic Works. https://academicworks.cuny.edu/gc_etds/4455

McLeod, S., & Baker, E. (2017). *Children's speech: An evidence-based approach to assessment and intervention.* Pearson.

Morgan, M. H., & Alleyne, M. C. (1994). *Language & the social construction of identity in Creole situations.* Center for Afro-American Studies, University of California, Los Angeles.

Mufwene, S. S. (1996). The founder principle in creole genesis. *Diachronica, 13*(1), 83-134. https://doi.org/10.1075/dia.13.1.05muf

Mufwene, S. (2001). *The ecology of language evolution.* Cambridge University Press. https://doi.org/10.1017/CBO9780511612862

Rickford, J. R. (1987). *Dimensions of a creole continuum: History, texts, and linguistic analysis of Guyanese creole.* Stanford University Press.

Ruiz, P., Latortue, R., & Rosefoot, N. (n.d.). *Resource guide for the education of New York State students from Caribbean countries where English is the medium of instruction* [Gray Manuscript on working with students from the Caribbean]. The New York State Education Department, The University of the State of New York. https://docs.steinhardt.nyu.edu/pdfs/metrocenter/nbm3/english_caribbean_students.pdf

Semple-McBean, M. (2007, January). Teachers' attitudinal ambivalence to mother tongue use in … *Research Gate.* https://www.researchgate.net/publication/307771353_Teachers'_Attitudinal_Ambivalence_to_Mother_Tongue_Use_in_Classroom_Instruction_in_Guyana.

Stewart, L. (2006). *Quantification in Jamaican Creole. The syntax and semantics of evri ("every") in interaction with indefinites.* Doctoral Thesis, University of the West Indies.

Stewart, W. A. (1965). Urban Negro speech: Sociolinguistic factors affecting English teaching. In R. Shuy, A. Davis & R. Hogan (Eds.), *Social dialects and language learning: Proceedings of the Bloomington, Indiana conference* 1964, 10-19. National Council of Teachers of English.

Telford Rose, S., Payne, K. T., De, Lisser, T. N., Humanities, F. O., Harris, O. L., & Elie, M. (2020). *A comparative phonological analysis of Guyanese Creole and Standard American English: A guide for speech-language pathologists.* https://pubs.asha.org/doi/full/10.1044/2020_PERSP-20-00173

Todd, L. (1990). *Pidgins and creoles.* Routledge.

UNESCO Institute for Statistics. (2021, September). *Literacy rate, youth total (% of people ages 15-24) - Guyana.* World Bank. https://data.worldbank.org/indicator/SE.ADT.1524.LT.ZS?locations=GY

Washington, K. N., Westby, C., Fritz, K., Crowe, K., Karem, R. W., & Basinger, M. (2021). The narrative competence of bilingual Jamaican creole- and English-speaking preschoolers. *Language, Speech, and Hearing Services in Schools, 52*(1), 317-334. https://doi.org/10.1044/2020_lshss-20-00013

Winer, L. (Ed.). (2009). *Dictionary of the English/Creole of Trinidad and Tobago: On historical principles.* McGill-Queen's University Press.

World Bank. (n.d.). *Country overview.* https://www.worldbank.org/en/country/guyana/overview

World Population Review. (2023). *Guyana population 2023 (live).* https://worldpopulationreview.com/countries/guyana-population

Chapter 12

The Development of Standardized Language Assessments and Screeners for Mandarin-Speaking Children in China

Lessons for Global Practice

Xueman Lucy Liu, AuD/CCC-A/FAAA, MS/CCC-SLP;
Wendy Lee, MS, CCC-SLP; Teresa Hutchings, MEd, CCC-SLP;
Jill de Villiers, PhD; and Eric Rolfhus, PhD

Introduction and Overview

This chapter describes some more general lessons learned by the research team and their clinical associates as they sought to make available new standardized language assessments and screeners for children in Mainland China. This work extends over the last decade and has resulted in the development of two assessments and two screeners for infants and children in the age range of 0 to 7 years 11 months. We begin with a short discussion of the special problems encountered in China. Then we turn to an overview of the process used to develop and validate the tests in the absence of existing instruments, and how the team adapted the tests to the unique situations and training needs of available personnel in China.

The Special Circumstances of China

We assume that early language impairment or developmental language disorder (DLD) is a worldwide phenomenon, with some significant genetic components (Rice, 2013). If one applies the U.S. prevalence rate to the 2010 Chinese census (China Data Center, 2012) it would suggest approximately 7,185,276 children in China just between 4 and 8 years of age are currently in need of

Bortz, M. (Ed.). *A Guide to Global Language Assessment: A Lifespan Approach* (pp. 247-262).
DOI: 10.4324/9781003524472-15

identification and rehabilitation service for DLD. There are few trained clinical professionals with the linguistic knowledge to assess a child with language impairments, and departments that teach the information are only now being established. There were past attempts by pioneering pediatricians and some linguists to develop language screeners and assessments for early identification of a possible language disorder among Mainland Chinese children, but until recently there were no formal standardized and comprehensive language assessment tools normed in Mainland China that meet psychometric standards (Friberg, 2010) to assist in diagnosing whether children have a language impairment if an overt medical diagnosis, such as hearing impairment, is not present.

Due to the shortages in the profession of speech-language pathology and trained clinicians in China, people administering the assessments need to be trained to present material in a standard way, to ensure the validation of the instrument. They also need to be trained to score the results, and furthermore be trained to interpret the language assessment's results together with the child's comprehensive medical results into a clinical diagnosis. Without training, it will also be difficult for the testers to convert test results into a straightforward description of the functional issues that families can understand and relate to. Finally, such individuals may lack the skills to design intervention procedures contingent on the problems that children exhibit. In the United States and Europe, these tasks are difficult even for skilled practitioners, but there is a well-established profession: speech-language pathology, with many services and continuing education practices to assist. Furthermore, parents and families are becoming more educated about children's development and potential disabilities. Unfortunately, these conditions are not yet met in China. For these reasons, making an assessment to help identify language difficulties is merely the first step in a cascade of supports that must be put in place to scaffold the process effectively. We offer this account in the hope that it will provide lessons for practitioners around the globe facing some of the same issues.

General Lessons Learned

Collaboration Among Experts

Collaboration with multiple professionals is a necessity for a new instrument. Child language experts, linguists, speech-language pathologists, developmental psychologists, psychometricians, pediatricians, teachers, focus groups of parents, and artists all bring different expertise and perspective to the problem. Our first endeavor was to assemble a team of experts in response to the need in China to design, test, and refine a new standardized language assessment, called DREAM-C (Diagnostic Receptive and Expressive Assessment of Mandarin–Comprehensive). The goal was to create an omnibus test that focused on children aged 2.5 to 8 years, with an emphasis on semantics and syntax.

Linguistic Differences

Languages differ, and the linguistic differences should change the content of a test. Translation of existing tests in English is all too common and must not be the standard (Bedore & Peña, 2008; Peña, 2007). It is important to gather as much information as possible about the normal path of language development and what might be a unique challenge in the language. It is also key to remain open-minded about what might be difficult, not judging from one's own adult intuitions, or data from acquisition of better-studied languages like English. Typically developing children have an extraordinary capacity for mastering intricate formal systems that can defeat adult learners (Naigles, 2002). On the other hand, children are cognitively and socially less adept.

The idea was not to model the DREAM-C on any existing test in other languages but to be sensitive to the new research on the nature and stages of Mandarin acquisition. As one example, classifiers are an important part of Mandarin, but few tests in the world have anything resembling tests of classifier use because such linguistic elements are rare in Western languages. One cannot ignore classifiers in the acquisition of Mandarin. Other phenomena, such as the tense deletion in Western languages considered to be a hallmark of language delay (Rice et al., 1998), were unusable in Mandarin. If tense exists at all, and many linguists says it is only *aspect* that is being expressed, it is only optionally expressed in typical adult speakers.

When a phenomenon had proved to be widespread across languages and useful for demarcation of stages in child language acquisition, the choice was made to include it in DREAM-C, even if there had been no work on it in Mandarin. As an example, there had been widespread testing of a deceptively simple, three-word, "wh-" question like "Who eats what?" across English and about 30 European languages (Schulz, 2015). The question reveals whether children know something about the "exhaustive" nature of "wh-" questions, in that one must answer by naming a set of individuals and not just name one; and second, that in an answer to such a question the sets must be paired (e.g., "Mary ate an apple, John ate a banana"). Nothing less will do. Examples of this were included even though no one had studied it in Mandarin. A different case comes from a new emphasis on the process of learning that has developed over the last decade or two in other languages (Dollaghan, 1987; Kalashnikova et al., 2018; Rice et al., 1990). These tasks ask can the child learn a new word or linguistic form from a limited example? That is, such tasks determine whether the child can learn fast from the example provided and make appropriate inferences. There was little work in Mandarin, with some contradictory results on verbs (Imai et al., 2008; Lee & Naigles, 2008), but the concept seemed important to include in the test (see Figure 12-1 for an example).

This item and subtest selection procedure involved consultation among linguists, psycholinguists, psychometricians, speech-language pathologists, pediatricians, and test experts from both China and the United States. Then began an extensive piloting of items to make sure that they worked as hoped, and that the foils—the alternative choices—for comprehension items contained all the ways that a child of any age might potentially answer an item. An example of a production item is included in Figure 12-2. The final structure of the DREAM-C assessment is included in Table 12-1.

The figure is from a subtest in the expressive part of the test, where a child is encouraged to use a certain type of sentence structure by hearing it modeled in a related context. The relative clause in Mandarin is marked by the particle DE (Chen & Shirai, 2015), and this is a task that requires the child to use a relative clause to distinguish between two referents.

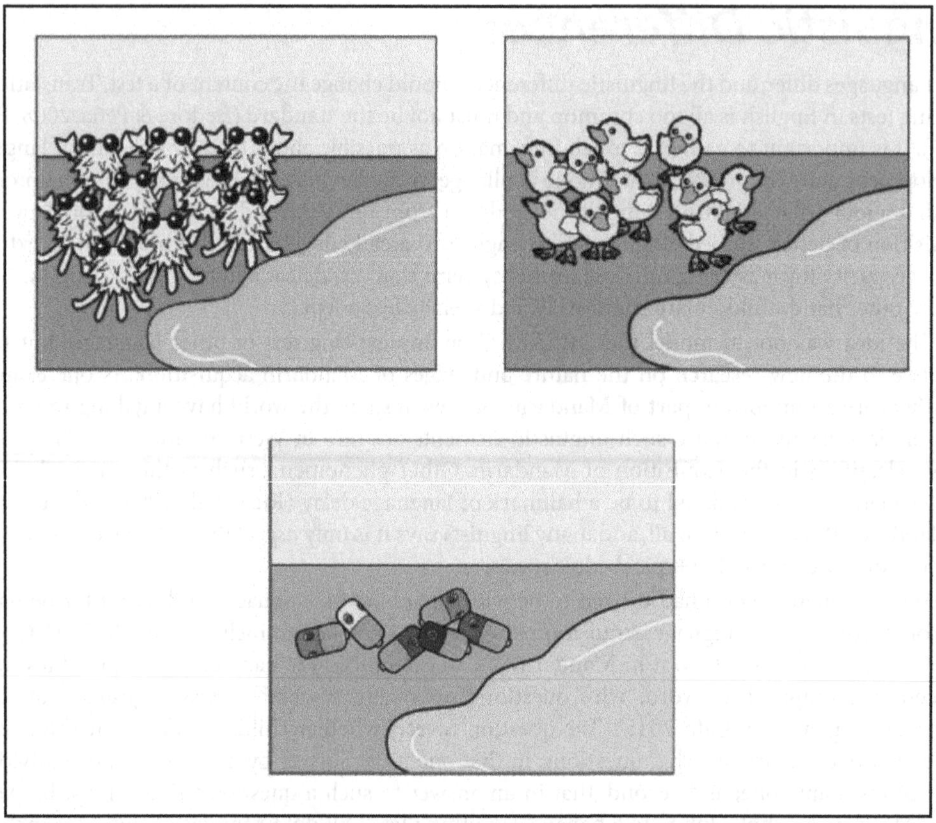

Figure 12-1. This figure provides an illustration of an item (1) in comprehension. The item involves a process-type problem, namely fast-mapping a novel word via cues from the sentence context, in this case, from the classifier that precedes it. (1) 看，河边有一群dafu。哪张图里的是dafu? Kan4, he2 bian1 you3 yi4 qun2 da1fu1. Na3 zhang1 tu2 li3 de shi4 da1fu1? "There is a flock of dafu by the river side. Which picture shows dafu?" (© 2014 Bethel Hearing and Speaking Training Center Inc. Reproduced with permission. All rights reserved.)

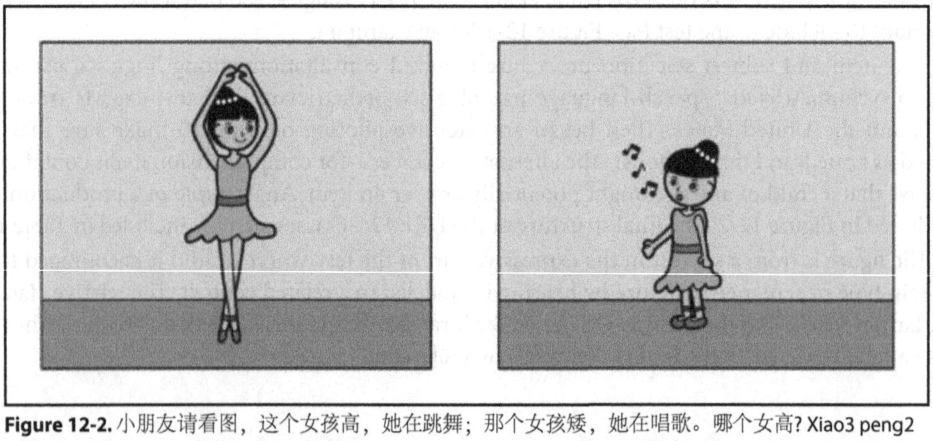

Figure 12-2. 小朋友请看图，这个女孩高，她在跳舞；那个女孩矮，她在唱歌。哪个女高? Xiao3 peng2 you3 qing3 kan4 tu2, zhe4 ge4 nü3 hai2 gao1, ta1 zai4 tiao4 wu3; na4 ge4 nü3 hai2 ai3, ta1 zai4 chang4 ge1. Na3 ge4 nü3 hai2 gao1? Elicitation: "Look at the picture: There is a girl. She is tall and she is dancing. There is another girl. She is short and she is singing." Question: "Which girl is tall?" An example of an event description item (from Ning et al., 2014). Diagnostic Receptive and Expressive Assessment of Mandarin (DREAM-C). (© 2014 Bethel Hearing and Speaking Training Center Inc. Reproduced with permission. All rights reserved.)

Table 12-1
Structure of the DREAM-C Assessment

CATEGORY	RECEPTIVE (N=165)					EXPRESSIVE (N=67)	
Subscale	*Vocabulary*	*Fast-Mapping*	*Closed Class*	*Logical Expressions*	*Sentence Contrasts*	*Event Description*	*Sentence Repetition*
Indices							
Receptive	X	X	X	X	X		
Expressive			X			X	X
Syntax					X	X	X
Semantic	X	X	X	X			
Total Language	X	X	X	X	X	X	X
Example	Point to where the cat is.	Which one is dafu? (See Figure 12-1)	Which picture shows an apple is in the bowl?	Which picture has a lot of apples?	Whose dog is eating the corn?	Elicit description of pictured event (e.g., Figure 12-2).	Repeat a sentence.

Designing for Children

Materials need to capture the eye of young children and contain culturally appropriate images of people and objects. Items also need to tap into vocabulary and grammar skills that are functional in children's everyday life and are in preparation for their social interactions and school learning. It is important to consider what chance responding would be, and to design "foils" for the target that are not just space fillers but represent choices a child might make if, say, their grammar or lexical knowledge is immature.

Four different indices were developed to characterize the child's performance. The tasks were either expressive or receptive and were also either semantic or syntactic in nature. These are not mutually exclusive categories, but different ways to look at the child's strengths or weaknesses. Some ways were devised to make the test adaptive, in the sense that children receive certain subsets of items matched for ability level so that in principle a child might receive some different items in retaking it.

Appropriate Sample for the Population

In test development, it is important that the sample population for the norms matches the population to which it is eventually to be generalized. Make sure the sample considers socioeconomic status, parental education, gender, and cultural/dialect variation. This is a very tall order, but effort is needed for fair assessment (de Villiers, 2017).

The sample for the assessment was chosen to match the census of China, the most recent being 2012, in terms of the distribution of parental education across the children. Parental education, especially maternal education, is generally considered the most likely predictor of the child's linguistic environment and rate of development. It is more awkward to make that assumption in China because of the widespread tendency for families to leave young children in the care of grandparents to allow both parents to work, and we collected data on the primary caregiver as well. It is also the case that there are widespread dialect variations in China, which necessitated testing in four main regions of the country and checking for differences in how test items behaved. Many children growing up in China speak a language other than Mandarin at first, such as Shanghainese, but by age 3 most children are now enrolled in preschools in which the language officially used is Mandarin. It is also important to mention that all the TV and cartoon programs are in Mandarin. Most of the time, even if grandparents are speaking the local dialect to the child, parents usually speak Mandarin to the child at home. By 2.5 years of age, Mandarin is L1 for most of the children in China living in the cities and suburbs, though for a very small portion of very young children Mandarin can be their L2.

A total of 969 Mandarin-speaking children between the ages of 2 years 6 months and 7 years 11 months were tested, with equal numbers of boys and girls. Half-year age groups were distinguished between 2 years 6 months and 5 years 11 months, with year-long age groups for 6- and 7-year-olds. Sampling included multiple cities and suburbs in both the northern and southern regions of China, and was stratified by multiple variables such as age, gender, urban versus suburban, region, and highest primary caregiver education level, according to the most recent census data (China Data Center, 2012).

Assessing the Assessment

In the light of initial results, a test must be further refined, limiting items to those that are most discriminating by age or ability and checking the reliability and validity of the test results against whatever exists in the way of clinical judgment, other tests, or a linguistically scored language sample. It is difficult in a new language to lay the groundwork, and tests will always be refined over time and practice; another property made easier by new technology. Revisions of materials, scoring, and norms can all be achieved much more quickly with an online test than with old-style paper publishing.

Once a large sample of children were tested, the adequacy of the assessment was evaluated in several standard ways. For example, one kind of test looks at the internal reliability of the test, measured by a metric called Cochran's Q. Rasch analysis involved asking whether the items behave in an orderly way, so that items can be sorted reliably into easy and difficult, and children into more or less successful at Mandarin. The internal reliability proved to be very high for DREAM-C.

The second metric of significance is the test's validity, or evidence that it predicts something real about the child's language performance. To achieve this, two procedures were developed to elicit more spontaneous language from the children. For children younger than 4.5 years who cannot usually sustain a narrative even when supported by pictures, we relied on a sample of speech recorded in a 15-minute play session. The materials were engineered to provide functional and natural opportunities to make requests, to ask questions, and to protest, for example, that a crayon was broken or missing in a coloring activity. Then a linguistically trained team evaluated the sample for vocabulary diversity, grammatical complexity on a scale, and the number and variety of different morphemes heard. These scales were developed based on previous literature in Mandarin, which is very limited, and data from mostly unpublished masters theses in linguistics in China, usually on fairly large samples of children. The children older than 4.5 years were shown three sets of wordless picture stories and asked to tell the experimenter about them. The narratives were recorded and analyzed in terms of several metrics of narrative complexity including time references, whether the child sufficiently distinguished characters, and references to mental states and not just behavior. In both sampling procedures, the result was a composite score that was then used to validate the DREAM-C categorizations. The DREAM-C correlated very well with each of these measures of spontaneous language production.

A third important metric is how well the assessment classifies children into those with language delays and those who were typically developing, and here we encounter a classic problem in making new tests in new countries: how do we know, independently of the test, who is language delayed? In established educational and clinical systems, it is considered very important that a test demonstrate high *specificity* and *sensitivity*. High sensitivity comes about when an assessment correctly identifies the children who have problems as at-risk. High specificity occurs when the test correctly excludes the typical children from the at-risk category. Most of the time, the a priori categorization depends on an existing gold standard, based on an established, respected test. But what happens when the test is the first one?

For DREAM-C, a further sample of 300 children were sampled to include a larger sample of children with potential language delays, using a major hospital in Shanghai. We relied on two indices for categorizing the children independently of the assessment. We relied on the judgment of a core group of pediatricians in China who received multiple trainings from the experienced developmental and behavioral pediatricians in the United States, who perform developmental examinations and ask parents questions based on guidelines about developmental milestones. At the same time, we also added another index other than experienced pediatricians' judgment from the spontaneous speech test to make sure the language issues are also indicated in the specifically designed functional language sample sessions. In addition to being referred for likely language problems by the pediatrician based solely on developmental tests and parent interview, the child also had to exhibit poor performance (z score <-1.25 SDs below the mean) on the language sample measures, whether that was the play session or the narrative. To count as typically developing, the child had to score above that level and not have an a priori judgment of disorder. With the two criteria combined, the sensitivity (95%) of DREAM-C proved to be very good, and therefore clinicians can have confidence that it identifies language-delayed children (Liu et al., 2017). Specificity was fair, but not high (82%), though in a case such as this with no alternative gold standard, relatively lower but good specificity still indicates that the test is adequate in not identifying children who do not have a language problem.

Multiple Assessments Are Needed

It is important to assess whether a single assessment is sufficient to meet the needs of a range of ages and circumstances. In a situation like the one in China, even the development of a good standardized language test is only a first step to meet the needs of the vast number of children who need to be served without adequate personnel. It is economically costly to screen children with a test that takes 45 minutes, yet appropriate diagnosis will take at least that long. What was needed is a shorter screener that could predict which children should be assessed more closely because they are at risk.

Screeners to Gauge Potential Risk

DREAM-S (Screener) was developed from the larger test, DREAM-C, to make that possible. To develop it, a new procedure was used called CART analysis (Lewis, 2000), which detects patterns of responding to items on the larger test, DREAM-C, that tend to lead to overall success or failure. This is not quite the same as finding the most discriminating items, because it allows for the possibility that different children might take different paths through the item sets to arrive at a similar outcome. CART analysis allowed the selection of a shorter test, DREAM-S, with good sensitivity and specificity against DREAM-C results. Ideally, a screener should detect almost all the children who will subsequently fail, even at the cost of over-including some typically developing children. Then the prediction was further tested by having a new group of children take DREAM-S followed by DREAM-C, with a pilot group of 33 LD (language disorder) and 22 TD (typically developing) children aged 2 years 6 months to 7 years 11 months. The predictions were borne out, with 82% of the children being correctly classified by the shorter test, which takes only 10 to 15 minutes. No short screener is perfect, but it can be a major help for detecting children who need more intensive assessment.

Assessments for the Youngest or Most Delayed

Following the successful launch of DREAM-C for children aged 2 years 6 months to 7 years 11 months, there was an almost immediate demonstration of need for an appropriate, evidence-based assessment of infants' and toddlers' early skills. This need was exacerbated by the increasing amount of research being conducted on the benefits of early intervention—the earlier, the better (Fricke et al., 2013; Calder et al., 2021). In addition, there appeared to be an added need for the assessment of children with severely delayed overall language and communication skills that fell below those skills assessed by an age-appropriate diagnostic tool, such as DREAM-C.

While some Mandarin-specific assessments for children under age 3 years exist, they focus primarily on vocabulary and did not include areas foundational to early communication and language development (Liu et al., 2023). In addition, due to a lack of language assessments, many clinical practitioners were using the communication subdomains of general developmental screeners as substitutes for language assessments, if they were using any instrument at all. We set out to determine the blueprint for our assessment.

What followed was an exhaustive review of the literature, research, and collaboration with expert linguists and speech-language pathologists who were highly experienced in the development of very young children from birth through 36 months. Clinically, we also worked closely with developmental behavioral pediatricians, developmental psychologists, and speech-language pathologists to select appropriate areas that might be discriminating of delay. From the evidence in both normal early language acquisition and areas clinically affecting language development (Liu et al., 2018), we confirmed that receptive language, expressive language, cognitive play, and social communication are the four foundational areas for our early communication and language assessment. After establishing the areas to be assessed, the mode of assessment was considered. Young children at this very early age range tend to be fairly difficult to assess in person. Research has demonstrated that for very young infants and toddlers, the use of parent report correlated well with assessments using a behavioral method and were in some cases better predictors of ability (Dale et al., 2003; Rescorla & Alley, 2001; Xue et al., 2015). For this reason, we chose to develop the assessment using the parent interview/report mode of assessment. The blueprint for DREAM-IT (Infant/Toddler) was thereby complete.

The development of the parent/caregiver questionnaire involved a review of existing language scales in languages other than Mandarin, considering that the availability of such scales was limited. This review took place in conjunction with input from experts in the fields of linguistics, speech-language pathology, and child development. A vast array of questions for parents/caregivers of children age 0 to 36 months related to the areas of receptive language, expressive language, cognitive play, and social communication was amassed, from which the best items could then be selected after testing. A set of standardized prompts to aid the parent/caregiver in answering each query was developed. Test administrators were trained to administer the parent questionnaire and to utilize the standardized prompts as needed to ensure that parent/caregiver clearly understood the questions. Parents/caregivers had to respond to statements using a simple Likert-type scale of "not yet," "sometimes," or "often" for many of the items asked. For example, "Does your child say single words?" Other queries asked for an approximate number of the child's responses. For example, "How many names of clothing items does your child understand?" These queries were included in a software program that was then loaded onto a tablet for ease of administration. Administrators indicated the parent/caregiver's response in real time and were able to access the standardized prompts as needed on the spot. The initial administration during the tryout was lengthy, as each administration took as long as 90 to 180 minutes. Two forms of the test were developed, spanning 2-year age ranges, 0 to 24 months and 12 to 36 months. In this way we could avoid asking "infancy"-type questions to parents of older children, and we could avoid asking mothers of young infants unsuitable questions about their children's grammar. However, the intermediate period of 12 to 24 months is a time of great variability, so we tested one group in this age range on one test and the other group on the second test, doubling the number of children participating in this age range.

The sample included the parents of 283 children ages 0 to 36 months. Data were collected in 3-month intervals (i.e., 0 to 2.99 months, 3 to 5.99 months ...). Every attempt was made to match the 2010 census data for China in terms of age, gender, and education level of the primary caregiver. We also attempted to gather respondents from both urban and suburban areas. The parents/caregivers were recruited to participate in the study from those coming in for well-baby checks to a clinic. No children with disorders such as autism spectrum disorder, intellectual disorder, specific language impairment, etc. were excluded from the study.

Following this first tryout administration of DREAM-IT, the data were analyzed using classic test theory by an experienced psychometrician. Items were reviewed by looking at item means within set, item total correlations, appropriate floor and ceilings, and items were removed that did not meet the prescribed parameters. This resulted in a significant total item number reduction, averaging 61% fewer items in each of the age bands. The second administration then became significantly shorter than the first administration.

The sampling plan for the second administration used the same stratification categories as the first administration and fewer items. The parents/caregivers of 193 of the previously tested children and 149 additional children ages 0 to 36 months were given the psychometrically refined and reduced number of test items using a similar protocol to the first. During this administration, items were scored using 0, 1, or 2 points. Data were analyzed and the final norms were developed using IRT (item response theory) analysis and resulting ability scores. In addition, the ability score information was used to develop growth charts to help identify how the child compares to their age peers. To further demonstrate validity of the assessment, both internal validity and external validity studies were completed.

As the pace of modern life in China is quite fast, and available resources are overloaded in clinics and hospitals, requests for a rapid means of assessing receptive and expressive language, cognitive play, and social communication skills for children 0 to 36 months were prevalent. The team decided to work to develop a rapid screener (10 minutes or less) that parents could take on their phones about their children's early communication levels. The resulting screening device, DREAM-IT-S, was developed utilizing the most discriminating items found in DREAM-IT. This process also involved the use of the cutting-edge psychometric procedure including CART analysis (Lewis, 2000). The resulting screener enables parents to know with a quick statement of "pass/has not passed" how their child is developing in relation to their peers. If a child receives a "has not passed" response, the child is considered at risk for language development and consequently should receive the full DREAM-IT. For children who have received a "pass" result, quartiles of performance within each of the four domains is also graphically presented to indicate possible uneven development of the four domains, which is also considered a risk factor for early language development.

DREAM-IT-S can also be used by community health care providers as a universal screener at certain age intervals when children come to receive immunizations. The screening reports also include three other functions to empower the frontline health care workers to provide basic parent education:

1. Reports also include early communication milestones expected in typical development for the child's age
2. Parent education articles on communication and language disorders and home activities that parents can read based on the child's general communication/language level as determined by the screening results
3. Locations of institutions where the DREAM-IT assessment can be administered

The Advantages of Technology

In modern times, technology is widespread and offers many advantages over paper and pencil administration. The DREAM assessment development projects benefited enormously from technology that provided automatic ways to present consistent materials, uniform narration, scoring, and reporting. Such investment is becoming less costly and will save time and money in the long run as well as providing greater accuracy and replicability.

To make the standardized use of the DREAM-C easier and to lessen the administrative load of practitioners who have limited experience using standardized, norm-referenced language assessments, special features were built into the assessment system. Administering assessments requires divided attention to multitask to ensure the correct administration of items, accurate observation of child's responses, tallying of correct and incorrect answers to arrive at the designated start and stop points in each subtest, all while managing the child's behavior. The development team wanted to support clinicians so they could allocate more of their focus on the child's behaviors and language performance rather than expending their efforts on the use of standard procedures. Therefore, DREAM-C was designed to automatically generate items for a child based on the child's age range and performance so that administrators need not locate the correct item to start and stop on in the stimuli book based on the child's age and consecutive number of items correctly answered. Unlike traditional paper and pencil assessments that require trained clinicians using stimuli materials (e.g., stimuli flipbook, manipulatives, toys), paper scoring record form, and a technical manual book that includes standard scores, DREAM-C, DREAM-S, DREAM-IT, and DREAM-IT-S are each administered via a single tablet or phone device. A comprehensive test report is automatically generated, including standard scores and the child's current language profile. These tests do not use the traditional start/stop rule. Instead, DREAM tests are semiadaptive. During the test administration, the DREAM-C and DREAM-IT program will present the most discriminating items for a particular age band and will also automatically adapt other presentation of items based on the best estimate of the child's ability from the child's response to previously administered items. The adaptive nature of the test maximizes the precision of the exam based on what is known about the examinee from the previous questions, so that different children of the same age receive appropriately different tests that yield equally accurate results. Compared to the traditional start/stop method, the semiadaptive method allows DREAM tests to attempt a wider variety of the linguistic skills expected for children within that age band with the items that are most close to their level.

The receptive part of the DREAM-C test includes the child viewing automated presentations of child-friendly, culturally appropriate pictures with prerecorded, standardized narratives. Artwork was drawn by a native Chinese artist to depict typical Chinese characters and culturally familiar environments and objects. All voice recordings were read by native Chinese vocal artists with children's broadcast journalism backgrounds. The most standard form of Mandarin pronunciation was spoken on all recordings per expert linguistic judgment. This design significantly reduced the dialectal influence from administrators from different parts of China.

After the child simultaneously listens to and views each receptive question prompt, the child touches a picture on the tablet to select their answer choice, and their selection is automatically recorded. Receptive item picture choices range from framed choices in sets of three to four or smaller objects and characters within a larger scene. Slightly opaque navigation and replay buttons at the corners of the screen allow the examiner to advance to the next screen or replay the audio with minimal distraction to the child. During the expressive portion of the test, the examiner touches icons, other pictures, and written word choices as the child is speaking their response. The response recording method and the scoring algorithm are designed to mimic a trained speech-language pathologist's clinical process. The online scoring is simple enough that examiners do not need special linguistic or speech-language pathology training. As with the receptive portion of the test, the child's responses are recorded live during the test administration, and the examiner does need to score, calculate, and/or convert scores afterwards. Midway through and at the end of the assessment administration, a list of the most commonly observed child testing behaviors, such as a child making multiple requests for repetitions or the child needing coaxing to participate, are displayed on a checklist so that the test administrators can quickly check off what they observed and type in any other specific observations. This pregenerated list of observations were designed to reduce the efforts of the test administrator to recall and record every relevant testing behavior encountered in the testing situation, and were based on the most common behaviors observed during the data collection process in the norming stage of the assessment development. After the test is electronically submitted, an assessment report is automatically generated. By using scoring algorithms to calculate, convert, and report standard and percentile scores in chart and table formats, the risk of human error and time spent calculating and reporting the scores is reduced. This is particularly important for the Chinese environment as the number of trained clinical practitioners to clients is very low and time constraints in the medical setting where assessments are administered are very high.

The self-generated report not only includes basic demographic information and relevant linguistic and medical history, but it also automatically calculates and generates the child's scaled scores in subdomains. Take DREAM-C as an example: scaled scores in five major linguistic areas (total language, receptive, expressive, semantics, and syntax skills) and corresponding confidence intervals and percentiles are automatically generated. In addition to the automatic score calculation and generation, the report also qualitatively describes particular areas of semantics and syntax that the child is beginning to master and specific linguistic areas that the child is having unusual difficulty with. Descriptions of linguistic areas are in mostly lay terms, but provide sufficient and useful guidance regarding the next steps in the child's language intervention process. These linguistic descriptions were designed based on extensive linguistic consultation and the review of the stages of Mandarin language development. A sample receptive language recommendation is, "These skills are usually the ones that the child's age peers either have mastered or are beginning to master. The level of the performance of the child on these skills is considerably behind their age peers."

1. Child does not seem to understand simple questions about "who," "what," and "which." Likewise, an example expressive language recommendation is (as stated above), "These skills are usually the ones that the child's age peers either have mastered or are beginning to master. The level of the performance of the child on these skills is mildly behind their age peers:"
2. Child is beginning to use a matching simple grammatical structure when describing a new event. This function to autogenerate a profile of language skills supports the clinical practitioner with the analysis and interpretation part of the assessment process and provides a starting point for intervention planning.

In a similar way, special features were built into the DREAM-IT (infant-toddler language) assessment and report. DREAM-IT is also delivered via a tablet with question presentation pre-selected according to child's age and according to parent's responses to an initial set of questions. Each question has standardized and clear examples to help users explain test items to parent. These examples were found to be the most easily understood and representative to Chinese caregivers during the data collection. Like DREAM-C, the system automatically records raw scores when each response is inputted, and upon submission of the assessment an automatic report is generated. Red, yellow, and green warning statuses along with percentiles on a growth curve chart and age equivalent scores are provided on the report. When a child has successive DREAM-IT assessments completed by a caregiver, the percentile of the newly administered test will be marked on the growth curve chart along with all previously tested percentiles to allow users to review child's progress over time in each domain. This type of graphical reporting is commonly used by Chinese pediatricians in other areas of development, such as in physical growth, so it is familiar and easily interpretable in the Chinese medical setting. To help guide intervention planning, the system also uses clusters of like-themed items with group cut-points to generate a profile of child's relative strengths and weaknesses in various areas compared to typically developing peers. The special DREAM-IT features allow clinical practitioners to understand a child's individualized communicative and language levels more easily as they develop the child's intervention plan. This is important, as some in the profession and general public have been misled by unregulated clinics into thinking that one generalized solution fits all language disorders.

The previous designs, including prerecorded standard test stimuli, the semiadaptive feature, automatic recording and calculating the test results through one simple electronic device, and automatically generated comprehensive test report (including standard scores and the child's current language profile) are all important for regions in which trained speech-language pathologists are limited.

Training and Guidance

For a test to be of value, the administrators and users need to be trained to give it and interpret it. The work is not finished when the tests are finally created, as then the training of parents, students, paraprofessionals, and medical experts must begin. In places where the training of speech-language pathology professionals and the knowledge of particular language and cultural variation are minimal, more training is essential to maximize the utility of the assessment in practice for diagnosis and intervention. Parents need training in ways that will help them interact and communicate more effectively. Zoom, webinars, and social media can all complement in-person training, where they are available.

The development team also recognized the need to give clinical practitioners who would use the assessments a foundational knowledge base in child speech-language development and disorders upon which to understand the context in which language assessments are used and to ensure the proper administration, interpretation, and use of assessment results, both in diagnostic and intervention practices. Therefore, for DREAM-C plus DREAM-S, a 4-day systematic intensive training was developed and conducted by the group's bilingual Bethel clinical training team with ASHA-certified speech-language pathologists and equivalent of ASHA-certified Canadian and British speech-language pathologists. The training was designed to help clinical practitioners gain an understanding of typical Mandarin language development, the characteristics of language disorders in various clinical populations, different forms of language assessments and their unique purposes in the overall evaluation process, the relevant stakeholders and stages of the assessment and intervention process, and therapy goal-planning principles, intervention strategies, and documentation. Within this context, participants are then specifically trained to administer DREAM-C and are given hands-on practicum opportunities to administer the assessment with children, explain assessment results to families, and use case studies to plan therapy. Only after successfully completing the practicum assessment and a certification exam are participants allowed to administer the DREAM-C and DREAM-S. When new institutions begin to use DREAM-C and/or DREAM-S, online supervision is also provided during initial test administrations and ongoing follow-up clinical support by the Bethel clinical training team. Online renewal trainings are also offered every 4 years to ensure that DREAM-C and DREAM-S clinical administrators are up-to-date on assessment information and procedures. Since the COVID-19 pandemic, the team clinicians have been offering part prerecorded and part live online DREAM-C trainings.

In a similar way, prospective clinical practitioners of DREAM-IT, the Infant Toddler assessment discussed following, are required to participate in a 3-day training that lays the foundation for understanding the process and milestones a young infant or toddler goes through when acquiring communication and language skills, how childhood language delays differ from other prevalent developmental disorders, the screening and assessment process for infants and young children, general therapeutic principles to use when working with young children and their families, and DREAM-IT specific test administration and related intervention planning. Just as in the DREAM-C training, participants engage in clinical practicum sessions that culminate in their assessment of a child using DREAM-IT with a caregiver, explanation of the DREAM-IT report with the family, and a debrief of their clinical case with others, under the guidance of the clinical trainers. When trained institutions are ready to begin using DREAM-IT, supervisory coaching is provided on initial assessments and ongoing follow-up support. Since 2016, when the first large-scale clinical assessment training was completed, until March of 2021, over 100 hospitals have participated in foundational assessment training sessions and over 1000 clinicians from these hospitals have received Bethel's certification.

To further support and enhance trainees who often have limited knowledge and experience in childhood language disorders, the clinical team has been developing and providing additional resources to help both professionals and families with children with language disorders.

For those children who are typically developing, at risk for delay, or in the monitoring stage due to mild language delays, a family training has also been developed to instruct both professionals and parents how to use basic communication strategies to facilitate the child's language development in naturally occurring situations in the child's daily life. Professionals from maternal child health centers, pediatric hospitals, and schools can attend the training and receive certification to replicate the training using the professionally developed and licensed materials and methods. Bethel's bilingual speech-language pathologists then supervise and coach institutions who are beginning to conduct trainings in their locales to ensure the quality of the trainings. These trainings have allowed a broad group of families across China to learn helpful knowledge and skills that will benefit their child's language develop.

User-friendly content, such as articles and video lessons, have been published to an official WeChat account since 2015 (Bethel Hearing & Speaking Training Center, 2015; https://s.ourbethel.cn/efadc2). WeChat is China's most used multi-purpose super-app that has billions of users. The WeChat platform also provides information to users on how to contact hospitals who can administer a DREAM assessment and clinics that can provide speech-language services, so that professional resources can be easily accessed. In 2020, we released an innovative app (Bethel HSTC, 2020)[1] that not only offers user-friendly content and links to resources, but also connects parents with their child's DREAM reports and specific, individualized intervention coaching videos made by Western-certified bilingual speech-language pathologists and articles based on the child's latest assessment report. The individualized intervention resources are accessed when a family sees a certified clinician who can guide the child's intervention plan and provide adequate counseling and coaching to caregivers through either 1:1 sessions or through a unique "Mom and Dad, Guide Me to Talk" (Bethel HSTC, 2018) family coaching program. The family coaching program is facilitated by a trained and certified family coaching provider who guides a group of about eight caregivers in both group and 1:1 intervention sessions using the individualized intervention resources on the parent app and the "Mom and Dad, Guide Me to Talk"[2] guidebook authored by bilingual clinicians. The "Mom and Dad, Guide Me to Talk" parent guide provides foundational knowledge on communication and language development; developmental stages in communication, play, and language; common parent strategies for facilitating productive communicative interactions; and suggested Chinese activities and books. The parent app's individualized intervention resources support both the professionals who deliver intervention and the families and children themselves. Through the additional intervention training and service programs and electronic media resources, those who are at-risk for language delays and those with language delays or disorders are provided with solutions for their needs.

[1]The Bethel Family Training for Early Communication & Language Development (Bethel Family Training Program, BFT) is the official name for the "Mom and Dad, Guide Me to Talk" family coaching program.

[2]美国培声听力语言中心/Bethel Hearing & Speaking Training Center, 2018. 《爸妈带我学说话·儿童语言发展家长指导手册/Mom and Dad, Guide Me to Talk: Parent Coaching Guidebook》人民出版社 /People's Publishing House.

Conclusion

The procedures followed by the team to develop a new standardized assessment where there were none, in a country with no established profession of speech-language practitioners, and without a tradition of recognition of language difficulties in children, might offer guidance and hope to those in other countries where similar circumstances prevail.

In summary, the team recognized that the effort must be collaborative across experts from different disciplines impacting on the child's language success. The problem of translation needs to be taken seriously, and the properties of the language considered carefully as it impacts what might be delayed. The assessment must be friendly to children, culturally appropriate to the population that is sampled, and utilize technology to its best advantage. It should be recognized that multiple assessments are needed for a wide age range, to tap different skills and concerns by age. The best scientific practice should be followed for testing, coding the results, and validation of the measures. However, even the best design will fail if parents and professionals are not on board with what it means, how they can best interpret the results, and help with the child's therapy when it is suggested.

An issue that is a continued concern is the degree of dialect variation, even multilingualism, among children growing up in China, despite the government mandate to have everyone learn Mandarin at age 3 and use it in schools. We were aware of this when the DREAM was developed, and the team has continued to pay attention to dialect influences, but more remains to be done. Other countries where there are multiple official languages may face even greater difficulty in assessment, as it is important to test bilingual children in each of their languages to assess the risk of language delay, and bilingualism exists on a continuum.

References

Bedore, L. M., & Peña, E. D. (2008). Assessment of bilingual children for identification of language impairment: Current findings and implications for practice. *International Journal of Bilingual Education and Bilingualism, 11*(1), 1-29.

Bethel Hearing & Speaking Training Center. (2015). *Official Our Bethel company account.* http://www.zwlhome.com/weixinPage/template/index.html#/template1?pageId=7594&defaultInit=1

Bethel Hearing & Speaking Training Center. (2020). *Bethel Parent App.* Bethel Hearing and Speaking Training Center.

Calder, S. D., Claessen, M., Ebbels, S., & Leitão, S. (2021). The efficacy of an explicit intervention approach to improve past tense marking for early school-age children with developmental language disorder. Journal of Speech, Language, and Hearing Research, 64(1), 91-104.

Chen, J., & Shirai, Y. (2015). The acquisition of relative clauses in spontaneous child speech in Mandarin Chinese. *Journal of Child Language, 42*(2), 394-422.

China Data Center. (2012). *China 2010 county population census data.* University of Michigan.

Dale, P. S., Price, T. S., Bishop, D. V., & Plomin, R. (2003). Outcomes of early language delay. *Journal of Speech-Language Hearing Research, 46*(3), 544-560.

de Villiers, J. G. (2017). Unbiased language assessment: Contributions of linguistic theory. *Annual Review of Linguistics, 3*, 309-330.

Dollaghan, C. A. (1987). Fast-mapping in normal and language-impaired children. *Journal of Speech and Hearing Disorders, 52*(3), 218-222.

Friberg, J. C. (2010). Considerations for test selection: How do validity and reliability impact diagnostic decisions? *Child Language Teaching and Therapy, 26*(1), 77-92.

Fricke, S., Bowyer-Crane, C., Haley, A. J., Hulme, C., & Snowling, M. J. (2013). Efficacy of language intervention in the early years. *Journal of Child Psychology and Psychiatry, 54*(3), 280-290.

Imai, M., Li, L., Haryu, E., Okada, H., Hirsh-Pasek, K., Golinkoff, R. M., & Shigematsu, J. (2008). Novel noun and verb learning in Chinese-, English-, and Japanese-speaking children. *Child Development, 79*(4), 979-1000.

Kalashnikova, M., Escudero, P., & Kidd, E. (2018). The development of fast-mapping and novel word retention strategies in monolingual and bilingual infants. *Developmental Science, 21*(6), e12674.

Lee, J. N., & Naigles, L. R. (2008). Mandarin learners use syntactic bootstrapping in verb acquisition. *Cognition, 106*(2), 1028-1037.

Lewis, R. (2000). *An introduction to Classification and Regression Tree (CART) analysis.* 2000 Annual Meeting of the Society for Academic Emergency Medicine, San Francisco, CA.

Liu, X. L., de Villiers, J., Ning, C., Rolfhus, E., Hutchings, T., Lee, W., Jiang, F., & Zhang, Y. W. (2017). Research to establish the validity, reliability, and clinical utility of a comprehensive language assessment of Mandarin. *Journal of Speech, Language, and Hearing Research, 60*(3), 592-606.

Liu, X. L., Lee, W., Rolfhus, E., Hutchings, T., Yao, L., Xie, J., Xu, Y., Peng, Y., & de Villiers, J. (2023). The development of a valid parent report instrument of early communication and language skills of infants and toddlers in mainland China. *International Journal of Language & Communication Disorders.* https://doi.org/10.1111/1460-6984.12874

Liu, X. L., Zahrt, D. M., & Simms, M. D. (2018). An interprofessional team approach to the differential diagnosis of children with language disorders. *Pediatric Clinics of North America: Pediatric Speech and Language: Perspectives on Interprofessional Practice, 65*(1), 73-90.

Naigles, L. R. (2002). Form is easy, meaning is hard: Resolving a paradox in early child language. *Cognition, 86*(2), 157-199.

Ning, C. Y., Liu, X. L., & de Villiers, J. G. (2014). *The diagnostic receptive and expressive assessment of Mandarin.* Bethel Hearing and Speaking Training Center.

Peña, E. D. (2007). Lost in translation: Methodological considerations in cross-cultural research. *Child Development, 78*(4), 1255-1264.

Rescorla, L., & Alley, A. (2001). Validation of the language development survey (LDS). *Journal of Speech, Language, and Hearing Research.*

Rice, M. L. (2013). Language growth and genetics of specific language impairment. *International Journal of Speech-Language Pathology, 15*(3), 223-233.

Rice, M. L., Buhr, J. C., & Nemeth, M. (1990). Fast mapping word-learning abilities of language-delayed preschoolers. *Journal of Speech and Hearing Disorders, 55*(1), 33-42.

Rice, M. L., Wexler, K., & Hershberger, S. (1998). Tense over time: The longitudinal course of tense acquisition in children with specific language impairment. *Journal of Speech, Language, and Hearing Research, 41*(6), 1412-1431.

Schulz, P. (2015). Comprehension of exhaustive wh- questions. In *Assessing Multilingual Children* (pp. 76-94). Multilingual Matters.

Xue, Y., E., Bandel, C. A., Vogel, & Boller (2015). *Measuring infant/toddler language development: Lessons learned about assessment and screening tools.* OPRE Brief 2015-52. Office of Planning, Research and Evaluation, Administration for Children and Families, U.S. Department of Health and Human Services.

Chapter 13

The Use of Sentence Repetition Tasks for Culturally and Linguistically Diverse Clients Across the Lifespan

Mellissa Bortz, PhD, CCC-SLP
and Christina Valenti, MA, CF-SLP, TSSLD

Definitions of Sentence Repetition Tasks

Sentence repetition tasks (SRTs), also known as elicited imitation tasks, are a "testing method that usually requires participants to listen to a series of stimulus sentences (or phrases, words, or sounds) and then repeat the sentences verbatim" (Yan et al., 2016, p. 2). The American Psychological Association defines sentence repetition as "a test in which the participant is required to repeat sentences of increasing difficulty and complexity, directly after the examiner reads them" (n.d.). Prutting and Connolly (1976) define these as "those imitations which occur when a child responds to an examiner's request to 'say what I say' and repeats a model sentence or phrase" (p. 415). Mumm et al. (1980) reports that because of sentence repetition during SRTs the child reduces the imitation to fit their own linguistic knowledge of a particular linguistic principle. Lust et al. (1998) define sentence repetition as the "overt, direct evidence of child's grammar construction for particular targeted aspects of grammar" (p. 63). The sentences that the child repeats utilize the rule that the child has for the particular structure "and not according to adult rules" (Lust et al., 1998, p. 63).

Bortz, M. (Ed.). *A Guide to Global Language Assessment: A Lifespan Approach* (pp. 263-272).
DOI: 10.4324/9781003524472-16

Benefits and Uses of Sentence Repetition Tasks

SRTs are a useful global language assessment for both developmental and acquired language disorders. They are used in both standardized language assessments such as the Test of Language Development Primary 5 (TOLD-P:5 and TOLD-I:5; Klem et al., 2014; Newcomer & Hammill, 2019) as well as stand-alone language assessments such as the Language Impairment in a Multilingual Society: Linguistic Patterns and the Road to Assessment (LITMUS) SRTs (LITMUS Sentence Repetition, n.d.). SRTs have been used to explore distinct aspects of syntactic, phonological, and morphosyntactic development (Polišenská et al., 2014, as cited in Kidd et al., 2007) as well as provide a holistic picture of how linguistic domains contribute to children's immediate sentence recall (Polišenská et al., 2014). SRTs can serve as a clinical marker for developmental language disorder (DLD), autism spectrum disorder (ASD), and aphasia in diverse populations. They allow for early identification in many languages. They also identify working memory components in impaired individuals compared to those who are typically developing and can serve as a measure of language proficiency. SRTs can distinguish typically developing children from children with DLD (Fleckstein et al., 2016; Gavarró, 2017). SRTs can be constructed in a large variation regarding sentence length (degree of complexity, and number of items), what is being evaluated (morphosyntax, memory capacity, or other cognitive functions), and how they are coded (identical repetition of stimulus sentences, correct repetition, or number of target words repeated correctly; Fleckstein et al., 2016). Sentence repetition is not a simple memorization task; grammatical reconstruction occurs when the sentences are repeated because the individual must first decode and interpret the sentence (Fleckstein et al., 2016). However, short-term memory capacities are included to some extent.

SRTs can be administered in a diverse array of settings for both first language (L1) and second language (L2) acquisition. It is important to note that SRTs make language assessment possible for communities that may not have materials and standardized tests readily available to them. They are especially beneficial to language communities with limited access to traditional language tests and materials such as Czech (Smolík & Vávrů, 2014). Furthermore, sentence repetition has been widely utilized to examine pediatric language disorders and neuropsychological activity (Yan et al., 2016). SRTs are a useful approach to assess grammatical skills in children and can serve as a diagnostic marker for various disorders. They are an effective and economical method for clinicians all around the world due to their adaptable nature (Polišenská et al., 2014; Smolík & Vávrů, 2014; van Compernolle & Zhang, 2014; Yan, 2019; Yan et al., 2016). There are numerous advantages to implementing SRTs in clinical, research, and pedagogical settings.

Measuring Progress

SRTs are useful considering the absence of standardized language tests for multilingual populations (Fleckstein et al., 2016). Sentence repetition as a test of L2 English morphology draws upon Vygotsky's zone of proximal development and dynamic assessment, in which human prompting links metalinguistic knowledge to performance abilities (van Compernolle & Zhang, 2014). In a prior study, prompts helped the learner transfer to tasks of increasing difficulty (van Compernolle & Zhang, 2014, p. 401). This sentence repetition test of grammatical competence provides information about a learner's zone of proximal development and helps "to provide a preliminary diagnosis of learner capacities" (van Compernolle & Zhang, 2014, p. 409).

CHILDREN

Sentence Repetition Tasks and Developmental Language Disorder

SRTs can target certain aspects of a given language that are known to be markers for DLD.[1] Lust et al. (1998) state that SRTs allow "researchers to assess children's knowledge of precise grammatical factors" (p. 59). They also allow for "testing of children's knowledge of specific hypothesized grammatical factors involving Universal Grammar" (p. 59). SRTs play an important role for children with DLD because they allow for early identification. SRTs can serve as a clinical marker for DLD in Czech (Smolík & Vávrů, 2014). The grammatical markers of DLD affect the parameters of each language differently, so it is important for each language to be identified distinctively (Smolík & Vávrů, 2014, p. 838). SRTs can be adapted for different languages, and can assess bilingual populations (Polišenská et al., 2014, p. 117, as cited in Chiat et al., 2013; Thordardottir & Brandeker, 2013).

Previous research showed significantly less accurate sentence imitations in a group of children with DLD than in a group of language-comparable children (Smolík & Vávrů, 2014). The pattern of imitation showed that a child's errors are caused by impaired syntactic foundation. The age sensitivity of SRTs highlights the clinical potential in identifying delay whereas "the consistency of patterns of performance ... indicates its potential for identifying atypical processes in recalling sentences across age" (Polišenská et al., 2014, p. 117). These tasks can therefore reliably diagnose DLD in clinical settings by identifying which grammatical categories are most challenging for children with language impairments across different ages, populations, and languages (Polišenská et al., 2014).

Theodorou et al. (2017) aimed to determine whether children with DLD can be identified by SRTs "in the context of diglossia in Cyprus, where no diagnostic tests designed for the particular situation are available." It was found that SRTs "can yield differences between groups of language-impaired versus nonimpaired participants in terms of morphosyntactic errors" (Theodorou et al., 2017, p. 2). There were significant differences for all four types of errors (i.e., omissions, substitutions, additions, and word order errors), which are clinical markers for DLD (Theodorou et al., 2017). Further, typically developing 9-year-old children did not reach the ceiling on the SRT, which is most likely because they have not yet fully acquired all morphosyntactic structures by 9 (Theodorou et al., 2017, p. 8). Significant differences between the younger and older groups (e.g., object relative clauses) show that developmental stages must be considered when selecting an appropriate SRT (Theodorou et al., 2017, p. 8).

"Sentence repetition has been found to be related to measures examining grammatical skills, namely, phonology, morphosyntax, and semantics" (Theodorou et al., 2017, p. 10). The findings of Theodorou et al. (2017) support the performance on SRTs as an indicator of a child's grammatical ability. The significant differences in performance of Cypriot Greek-speaking children with DLD and typical development confirms previous findings for other languages including English, Cantonese, Italian, and French (Theodorou et al., 2017). Although Theodorou et al. (2017) found SRTs to be a successful measure of DLD in bidialectal children in Cyprus, more research is suggested to generalize these findings to the linguistically diverse populations of the world.

Due to the malleable nature of SRTs, they can measure a variety of linguistic and cognitive abilities such as short-term memory and grammar (Gavarró, 2017). In a previous study, Gavarró (2017) aimed at core syntactic features that are affected in DLD including: canonical subject-verb-object sentences; sentences with a third person object; sentences with a clitic, long passive sentences; wh-questions; and sentences with finite and non-finite complement clauses (p. 5). Identical repetition

[1] Developmental Language Disorder is being used to refer to what was previously known as Specific Language Impairment, https://www.nidcd.nih.gov; CATALISE-2 Consortium.

was found in the majority of cases for typically developing children. However, in children with DLD there were higher instances of ungrammatical productions (Gavarró, 2017). Controlling for age, the typically developing children performed significantly better than the children with DLD on all sentence types during an SRT. SRTs are a reliable tool to discriminate typically developing children from children with DLD in both monolingual and bilingual populations.

Repetition abilities can therefore serve to distinguish typical versus atypical language development of children as well as account for a difference versus disorder. It is agreed that a child with DLD would have DLD in both of their languages (Fleckstein et al., 2016), so therefore the child must be tested in both languages. There is a lack of standardized tests normed for bilingual populations, which adds to the challenges for diagnosing DLD in multilingual contexts (Fleckstein et al., 2016; Gavarró, 2017). SRTs are therefore essential for children with DLD within multilingual contexts due to the lack of standardized language assessments, which leads to misdiagnosis. Speech-language pathologists must ensure that SRTs are used in combination with case history information "such as language exposure and language use, obtained from a parental questionnaire specifically tailored for bilingual contexts" (Fleckstein et al., 2016, p. 99).

Fleckstein et al. (2016) aimed to identify DLD in French bilingual children using the French LITMUS SRT. The French LITMUS SRT included five target structures known to pose difficulty to individuals with DLD: monoclausal sentences in the present and past tenses, wh-questions, as well as complement and relative clauses (Fleckstein et al., 2016). The SRT distinguished children with DLD from typically developing monolingual and bilingual children ages 5 to 8 (Fleckstein et al., 2016, p. 93). Since SRTs involve grammatical knowledge, there were significant differences between the four groups, such as singular versus plural verbs, in which children with DLD performed significantly worse (Fleckstein et al., 2016). French-speaking children with DLD experienced challenges with measures of composite past tense, plural verb agreement, object wh-questions, complement clauses, and relative clauses.

In children, SRTs are useful to detect and prevent language difficulties (Bishop, 2006; Rujas et al., 2021). Rujas et al. (2021) posit that performing these tasks with very young children increases the possibilities of early detection and prevention. They are useful for making differential diagnoses (Rujas et al., 2021). Seeff-Gabriel et al. (2010) used the Sentence Imitation Test 61 (SIT-61) to detect morphosyntactic challenges and reported that SRTs are good indicators of children's language skills. Polišenská et al. (2014) also describe the benefit of SRTs for morphosyntactic tasks.

Second Language Acquisition

In second language research, sentence repetition has been used to test "learners' knowledge of specific grammatical features, learners' interlanguage systems, and the memory system" (van Compernolle & Zhang, 2014, pp. 396-397). SRTs measure implicit linguistic competence and can minimize the potential for a test-taker to rely on rote memorization for L2 productions. As long as the participant has already acquired the grammatical features involved in the stimuli, repetition involves simple and adaptable task development (Yan et al., 2016). A meta-analysis from 1970 to 2014 by Yan et al. (2016) used sentence repetition to measure aspects of L2 proficiency in the fields of applied linguistics, L2 acquisition, and education. It has been found that higher proficiency speakers were more capable of repeating the sentences than lower proficiency speakers (Yan et al., 2016).

Language proficiency plays a role in a speaker's performance on SRTs (Yan, 2019). "Sentence length was the strongest predictor of task difficulty ... That is, as the sentence becomes longer, the level of cognitive pressure for elicited imitation tasks increases, requiring the speaker to be more automatic at chunking the sentences" (Yan, 2019, p. 470). SRTs are an effective measure of L2 proficiency across a variety of languages (Yan et al., 2016). Speech fluency is conditioned by the speaker's proficiency level and the task difficulty (Yan, 2019, p. 470). Longer sentences involved more pauses, which showed that speakers spend more effort to process information in longer sentences than shorter sentences (Yan, 2019, p. 475). For these reasons, sentence repetition "presents a clear advantage over open-ended speech tasks for measuring the processing of formulaic sequences" (Yan, 2019, p. 465).

Autism Spectrum Disorder

SRTs can be used to make differential diagnoses in ASD and attention-deficit/hyperactivity disorder (Redmond et al., 2011; Riches et al., 2010). SRTs were shown to be more challenging for individuals with ASD than for individuals with Down syndrome or typical development (Heimann et al., 2016). The responses on SRTs contribute to robust clinical knowledge of the repetition difficulties that children with ASD experience. Low performance of children with ASD on SRTs results from the lack of pragmatic skills such as theory of mind, joint attention to social stimuli, and "difficulties in mapping visual representations to motor output" (Heimann et al., 2016, p. 5). There was a higher success rate on SRTs for children with ASD when the tasks involved actions with a clear meaning or visual goal (Heimann et al., 2016, p. 3). Children with ASD are therefore more likely to imitate if a familiar object and interesting outcome are involved. The clinician has an advantage with the easily individualized nature of SRTs, which can help elicit responses of individuals with ASD.

Sentence Repetition Tasks as a Measure of Working Memory

SRTs reveal the relationship between language processing and phonological working memory on a complex metalinguistic level (Polišenská et al., 2014; Smolík & Vávrů, 2014). Given the close relationships between various components of working memory (Smolík & Vávrů, 2014, as cited in Alloway et al., 2004), limitations in other components of memory such as phonological short-term memory may contribute to performance on SRTs. Thus, "the differences in sentence imitation between typically developing children of different ages may be attributed to phonological short-term memory" (Smolík & Vávrů, 2014, p. 844). Measuring memory capacity "enables us to determine the extent to which [it] depends on linguistic knowledge," with implications for interpreting children's difficulties with repetition tasks, and the relationship between verbal short-term memory and pediatric language deficits (Polišenská et al., 2014, p. 109).

Challenges with sentence recall signify limitations in children's capacity for processing verbal phonological and morphosyntactic information (Polišenská et al., 2014). Poor performance on SRTs therefore indicates impairments in the linguistic domains that are crucial for immediate recall (Polišenská et al., 2014, p. 117). Furthermore, sentence length has been observed to condition the difficulty level of SRTs (Yan et al., 2016, p. 14). "In order to measure language comprehension (i.e., to minimize the effect of working memory), the length of sentence stimuli must exceed the learners' [short-term memory capacity]" (Yan et al., 2016, p. 14). There is evidence that sentence repetition requires the speaker to access implicit grammatical knowledge to comprehend the sentence before repeating" (Yan et al., 2016, p. 13).

Adults

SRTs have been widely used for differential diagnoses in adults, for example, the Anomalous Sentence Repetition Test (Weeks, 1988) is used to diagnose depression. SRTs have also been applied to progressive disorders, including aphasia, such as language production tasks in the Western Aphasia Battery (Eom & Sung, 2016). SRTs are also significant to diagnose the presence of different forms of dementia and primary progressive aphasia (Graham et al., 2019). Furthermore, the Bilingual Aphasia Test includes a seven-item SRT. These tasks could be sentences to the patient's mnemonic ability, particularly for patients with receptive difficulties (Paradis, 1987).

Collaboration in the Development of Cross-Linguistic Sentence Repetition Tasks

The European Union provides an important example of collaboration in developing multilingual SRTs for European languages. The purpose of the COST Action IS0804 LITMUS was to develop language assessments such as SRTs (Armon-Lotem & Grohmann, 2021) among multilingual societies and second-language learners (Bi/multilingualism and Specific Language Impairment, n.d.). According to LITMUS Sentence Repetition (n.d.), "sentence repetition tasks have been shown to be very sensitive and specific in identifying children with language impairment." The lack of multilingual assessments inspired the COST Action IS0804 (Bi/multilingualism and Specific Language Impairment, n.d.) to develop SRTs across several languages for multilingual children such as Catalan, French, German, Hebrew, Irish, Lebanese Arabic, Norwegian, Polish, Russian, Turkish, and Welsh (LITMUS Sentence Repetition, n.d.). Difficulties in multiple languages would result in language delay or impairment, whereas performance within normal limits in a child's L1 and difficulties in their L2 would represent limited proficiency in that language (LITMUS Sentence Repetition, n.d.).

Considerations for Developing Sentence Repetition Tasks

Rujas et al. (2021) states that when constructing SRTs in different languages it is important to remember that languages differ from each other in many linguistic features such as tone. For example, Vietnamese (Pham & Ebert, 2020) and most Bantu languages are tonal. "Additional work on languages outside English that calculates diagnostic accuracy metrics for these tasks is needed to evaluate their cross-linguistic potential" (Pham & Ebert, 2020, p. 1524). Readers should make use of the information provided about language families discussed in Chapters 1 and 3 to assist with the development of SRTs for multilingual clients.

Cross-Sectional Group Study Example: Assessment of the Passive in Setswana-Speaking Preschoolers

Aims and Hypothesis of the Study

The aim of this study was to investigate Setswana-speaking children's comprehension and production of the passive in terms of age, passive categories (reversible, negative/malefactive, nonreversible, psychological, and impersonal passives), and long passives that include a by-phrase and short passives. Specifically, the study aimed to describe the development of the passive of children aged 2 years 6 months to 5 years 5 months.

The hypothesis for this study is that Setswana-speaking children would develop the passive construction early in sentence repetition language acquisition. This is based on research that the passive has been found to develop by 3 years of age in Bantu languages such as Sesotho (Demuth, 1989; Demuth et al., 2009, 2010) and isiZulu (Suzman, 1985, 1987, 1991) and in Indo-European languages by 5 years (Armon-Lotem et al., 2016) and 8 years (Horgan, 1978).

Method

A total of 114 children divided into three age groups from 2 years 6 months to 5 years 5 months were the participants in this study. Picture-selection comprehension tasks elicited production, and SRTs were used to determine comprehension and production of the passive.

Setting

The participants were tested at three preschools in Pankop, Chief Maluke Trust in the Mpumalanga Province of South Africa. Pankop is a semirural/peri-urban area. Peri-urban areas form "belts of nonurban land" bordering cities. Usually, they are not fully urban nor rural but "form a mosaic of often incompatible and unplanned Socioeconomic Status [sic]" (periurban.org.au/index.htm). However, in South Africa peri-urban areas are beset by massive poverty (Cook, 2001). These are areas of absolute poverty—when a person lacks the basic needs required for a healthy life. Mpumalanga includes 7% of South Africa's population and has the fifth lowest total income of South Africa's nine provinces (Nag, 2018).

Requirements of Sentence Repetition Tasks

Slobin and Welsh (1967) in a sentence repetition seminal field manual for cross-cultural study of the acquisition of communicative competence recommend that elicited imitation tasks examine "major grammatical categories such as tense, mood and aspect." Lust et al. (1998) recommends the SRTs should "tax" the child's processing ability (e.g., by sentence repetition length). This assessment should be just enough so that children can and do attempt reconstruction without overtly involving sentence repetition grammar. Sentences, therefore, consisted of an average of 8 syllables for short passives and 11 syllables for long passives. Lust et al. (1998) recommended that sentences should be approximately 9 syllables long and not vary by more than 2 syllables. In this case study constructions were not longer than 11 syllables. It is interesting to note that pilot testing showed that both the standard form *kgarameditswa* "scratched" and the nonstandard, language mixed form *pushiwa* "push" needed to be provided to the children. Some children did understand the standard form, but the majority understood only the nonstandard form. Standardized forms of language are generally used in rural areas where sentence repetition is limited, as well as the chance of codeswitching and language mixing. In urban areas the opposite is true.

Results

The results showed variability among tasks. The results for comprehension tasks were at chance level. The elicited production task was unsuccessful as children found great difficulty with this task with 2 years 6 months to 3 years 6 months old children scoring 7% and the oldest group 14%. There was a significant difference on performance on SRTs between the youngest group (69%) compared to the middle (83%) and oldest age group (81%).

Discussion

The SRT was successful and confirmed the diagnostic value of such a measure. A possible reason for this is that rote learning is often used as a method of teaching in schools in South Africa (Makonye & Hlako, 2021, p. 70; Mda & Mothata, 2000; Prinsloo & Stein, 2004). Children are generally not familiar with learning using pictures as a task. This could be seen from the fact that there were few books or pictures in the classrooms. In addition, the SRTs proved to be very successful as they showed that the participants comprehended and produced the passive (Lust et al., 1998; Vinther, 2002).

The SRTs were also successful in that they showed significant developmental trends. They are therefore well suited to the way of learning of the participants and the broader South African population. To conclude, this study supports the fact that SRTs are powerful and useful tools for multilingual, culturally, and linguistically diverse clients.

Acknowledgments

It is with the utmost gratitude that I (C.V.) want to thank Dr. Mellissa Bortz for giving me the opportunity to contribute to this book as her graduate research assistant.

References

American Psychological Association. (n.d.). *APA dictionary of psychology.* https://dictionary.apa.org/

Armon-Lotem, S., & Grohmann, K. K. (2021). Language impairment in multilingual settings. *Language Impairment in Multilingual Settings,* 1-340.

Armon-Lotem, S., Haman, E., Jensen de López, K., Smoczynska, M., Yatsushiro, K., Szczerbinski, M., van Hout, A., Dabasinskiene, I., Gavarro, A., & Hobbs, E. (2016). A large-scale cross-linguistic investigation of the acquisition of passive. *Language Acquisition, 23*(1), 27-56.

Bi/multilingualism and Specific Language Impairment. (n.d.). *Home.* https://www.bi-sli.org/

Bishop, D. V. M. (2006). What causes specific language impairment in children? *Current Directions in Psychological Science, 15*(5), 217-221. https://doi.org/10.1111/j.1467-8721.2006.00439.x

Cook, V. (2001). Using the first language in the classroom. *The Canadian Modern Language Review, 57*(3), 402-423. https://doi.org/10.3138/cmlr.57.3.402

Demuth, K. (1989). Maturation and acquisition of the Sesotho passive. *Language, 65,* 56-80.

Demuth, K., Machobane, Malillo, & Moloi, F. (2009). Learning how to license null noun-class prefixes in Sesotho. *Language, 85*(4), 864-883. https://doi.org/10.1353/lan.0.0173

Demuth, K., Moloi, F., & Machobane, M. (2010). Three-year-olds' comprehension, production, and generalization of Sesotho passives. *Cognition, 115*(2), 238-251. https://doi.org/10.1016/j.cognition.2009.12.015

Eom, B., & Sung, J. E. (2016). The effects of sentence repetition-based working memory treatment on sentence comprehension abilities in individuals with aphasia. *American Journal of Speech-Language Pathology, 25*(4S). https://doi.org/10.1044/2016_ajslp-15-0151

Fleckstein, A., Prévost, P., Tuller, L., Sizaret, E., & Zebib, R. (2016). How to identify SLI in bilingual children: A study on sentence repetition in French. *Language Acquisition, 25*(1), 85-101. https://doi.org/10.1080/10489223.2016.1192635

Gavarró, A. (2017). Sentence repetition tasks for Catalan-speaking typically-developing children and children with specific language impairment. *Frontiers in Psychology, 8.* https://doi.org/10.3389/fpsyg.2017.01865

Graham, C. R., Borup, J., Pulham, E., & Larsen, R. (2019). K–12 blended teaching readiness: Model and instrument development. *Journal of Research on Technology in Education, 51*(3), 239-258. https://doi.org/10.1080/15391523.2019.1586601

Heimann, M., Nordqvist, E., Strid, K., Connant Almrot, J., & Tjus, T. (2016). Children with autism respond differently to spontaneous, elicited and deferred imitation. *Journal of Intellectual Disability Research, 60*(5), 491-501. https://doi.org/10.1111/jir.12272

Horgan, D. (1978). The development of the full passive. *Journal of Child Language, 5*(1), 65-80.

LITMUS Sentence Repetition. (n.d.). *Home: Litmus sentence repetition tasks.* https://www.litmus-srep.info/

Klem, M., Melby-Lervåg, M., Hagtvet, B., Lyster, S. A. H., Gustafsson, J. E., & Hulme, C. (2014). Sentence repetition is a measure of children's language skills rather than working memory limitations. *Developmental Science, 18*(1), 146-154. https://doi.org/10.1111/desc.12202

Lust, B., Flynn, S., & Foley, C. (1998). What children know about what they say: Elicited imitation as a research method for assessing children's syntax. In D. McDaniel, C. McKee, & H. Smith Cairns (Eds.), *Methods for assessing children's syntax* (pp. 55-76). MIT Press.

Makonye, J. P., & Hlako, V. W. (2021). *The 29th Annual Conference of the Southern African Association for Research in Mathematics, Science and Technology Education* (p. 70). University of the Witwatersrand, South Africa.

Mda, T. V., & Mothata, M. S. (2000). *Critical issues in south african education after 1994.* Juta.

Mumm, M., Secord, W., & Dykstra, K. (1980). *Merrill language screening test.* Psychological Corporation.

Nag, O. S. (2018). *The richest and poorest provinces of South Africa.* https://www.worldatlas.com/articles/the-richest-and-poorest-provinces-of-south-africa.html

Newcomer, P. L., & Hammill, D. D. (2019). *TOLD P 5: Test of language development. Primary.* Pro-Ed.

Paradis, M. (1987). Neurolinguistic perspectives on bilingualism. *The Assessment of Bilingual Aphasia,* 1-17.

Pham, G., & Ebert, K. D. (2020). Diagnostic accuracy of sentence repetition and nonword repetition for developmental language disorder in Vietnamese. *Journal of Speech, Language, and Hearing Research, 63*(5), 1521-1536. https://doi.org/10.1044/2020_jslhr-19-00366

Polišenská, K., Chiat, S., & Roy, P. (2014). Sentence repetition: What does the task measure? *International Journal of Language & Communication Disorders, 50*(1), 106-118. https://doi.org/10.1111/1460-6984.12126

Prinsloo, M., & Stein, P. (2004). What's inside the box? Children's early encounters with literacy in South African classrooms. *Perspectives in Education, 22,* 67-84.

Prutting, C. A. & Connolly, J. (1976). Imitation: A closer look. *Journal of Speech and Hearing Disorders, 41,* 412-442.

Redmond, S. M., Thompson, H. L., & Goldstein, S. (2011). Psycholinguistic profiling differentiates between specific language impairment from typical development and from attention-deficit/hyperactivity disorder. *Journal of Speech Language, and Hearing Research, 54,* 99-117.

Riches, N. G., Loucas, T., Baird, G., Charman, T., & Simonoff, E. (2010). Sentence repetition in adolescents with specific language impairments and autism: An investigation of complex syntax. *International Journal of Language & Communication Disorders, 45*(1), 47-60. https://doi.org/10.3109/13682820802647676

Rujas, I., Mariscal, S., Murillo, E., & Lázaro, M. (2021). Sentence repetition tasks to detect and prevent language difficulties: A scoping review. *Children, 8*(7), 578. https://doi.org/10.3390/children8070578

Seeff-Gabriel, B., Chiat, S., & Dodd, B. (2010). Sentence imitation as a tool in identifying expressive morphosyntactic difficulties in children with severe speech difficulties. *International Journal of Language & Communication Disorders, 45*(6), 691-702. https://doi.org/10.3109/13682820903509432

Slobin, D. I., & Welsh, C. A. (1967). *Elicited imitation as a research tool in developmental psycholinguistics.*

Smolík, F., & Vávrů, P. (2014). Sentence imitation as a marker of SLI in Czech: Disproportionate impairment of verbs and clitics. *Journal of Speech, Language, and Hearing Research, 57*(3), 837-849. https://doi.org/10.1044/2014_jslhr-l-12-0384

Suzman, S. M. (1985). Learning the passive in IsiZulu. *Papers and Reports on Child Language Development, 24,* 131-137.

Suzman, S. M. (1987). Passives and prototypes in IsiZulu children's speech. *Journal of African Studies, 7,* 241-254.

Suzman, S. M. (1991). *Language acquisition in IsiZulu* [Unpublished doctoral dissertation]. University of the Witwatersrand.

Theodorou, E., Kambanaros, M., & Grohmann, K. K. (2017). Sentence repetition as a tool for screening morphosyntactic abilities of bilectal children with SLI. *Frontiers in Psychology, 8.* https://doi.org/10.3389/fpsyg.2017.02104

Thordardottir, E., & Brandeker, M. (2013). The effect of bilingual exposure versus language impairment on nonword repetition and sentence imitation scores. *Journal of Communication Disorders, 46*(1), 1-16. https://doi.org/10.1016/j.jcomdis.2012.08.002

van Compernolle, R. A., & Zhang, H. (S. (2014). Dynamic assessment of elicited imitation: A case analysis of an advanced L2 English speaker. *Language Testing, 31*(4), 395-412. https://doi.org/10.1177/0265532213520303

Vinther, T. (2002). Elicited imitation:A brief overview. *International Journal of Applied Linguistics, 12*(1), 54-73. https://doi.org/10.1111/1473-4192.00024

Weeks, D. J. (1988). *The Anomalous Sentences Repetition test.* NFER-Nelson.

Yan, X. (2019). Unpacking the relationship between formulaic sequences and speech fluency on elicited imitation tasks: Proficiency level, sentence length, and fluency dimensions. *TESOL Quarterly, 54*(2), 460-487. https://doi.org/10.1002/tesq.556

Yan, X., Maeda, Y., Lv, J., & Ginther, A. (2016). Elicited imitation as a measure of second language proficiency: A narrative review and meta-analysis. *Language Testing, 33*(4), 497-528. https://doi.org/10.1177/0265532215594643

Part IV

ASSESSMENT OF LANGUAGE DISORDERS

Chapter 14

Augmentative and Alternative Communication

It Is About Having a Voice

Juan Bornman, PhD; Carla van Nieuwenhuizen; and Lebogang Sehako

Introduction

Successful communication is when one person shares something with another, that the communication partner did not know beforehand, but now does.

The word "communication" entered the English language between the 14th and 15th centuries and is derived from the Latin word "communicare," which means to impart, to share, or to make common (Kuyler et al., 2022). In other words, to create a shared meaning of something between two individuals. We use speech to express basic needs, wants, desires, thoughts, emotions, and knowledge. Hence, it provides a window to our inner self as it allows others to see who we are. Moreover, our speech also carries a personal signature—we are all able to identify a person by recalling the sound of their voice. While speaking, having a voice, and being understood are things that we often take for granted, we can all recall an example of the frustration we felt when we were temporary silenced (e.g., by laryngitis, or by the "mute" button on a device, or when immersed in a context where we do not speak [or understand] the language).

For some individuals this is not a temporary situation, as they have such significant communication disabilities that they cannot rely on their natural speech to meet their daily communication needs. These individuals need to be heard—and offered a platform to share their stories. Individuals like Carla van Nieuwenhuizen and Lebogang Sehako, two young South Africans who shared their stories in their own words (Tables 14-1 and 14-2).

Bortz, M. (Ed.). *A Guide to Global Language Assessment: A Lifespan Approach* (pp. 275-288).
DOI: 10.4324/9781003524472-18

Table 14-1
Carla van Nieuwenhuizen

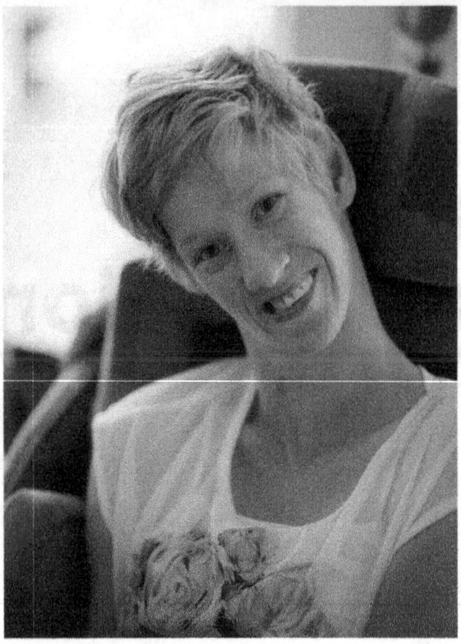

I am Carla, a 31-year-old from Krugersdorp. I have cerebral palsy. I got brain damage at 5 months old from a lack of oxygen to the brain. I was diagnosed with a genetic decease called Propionic Academia. It means my body is unable to use protein, so it builds up in my body as a poison. I completed my school years at the West Rand School. After leaving school I did a short course in beauty and makeup at the Blush Academy in Roodepoort. I have had a full-time job as social media manager at Blush Academy for the last 4 years. I am an augmentative and alternative communication (AAC) user since childhood and have done many courses at the CAAC at the University of Pretoria. I am a member of ISAAC and recently attended their World Congress proudly in August 2021.

I am a proud lobbyist for AAC and their users and do regular motivational speeches at churches, women's functions, and even schools. I am a great example of living a positive life with my disabilities. An example for anyone.

I use Grid 2 on my laptop with a clicker switch. I write all my speeches and poetry with my clicker.

Here is one of my poems, written in Afrikaans, with the English translation.

Soms

As ek my gedagtes loslaat
en die venster oopmaak
voel ek hoe jy binnewaai op die wind
en bly … tot die aand daal
en swyend bly sit langs my bed
wagtend tot my oë—moeg gekyk—
oorgee en dan sing tot ek slaap

—Carla van Nieuwenhuizen

Sometimes

When I set my thoughts free
and open the window
I feel how you enter blowing on the wind
and stay … till the evening comes
and silently sits by my bed
waiting till my eyes—tired from seeing—
surrenders and then sings until I sleep

—Carla van Nieuwenhuizen

Table 14-2
Lebogang Sehako

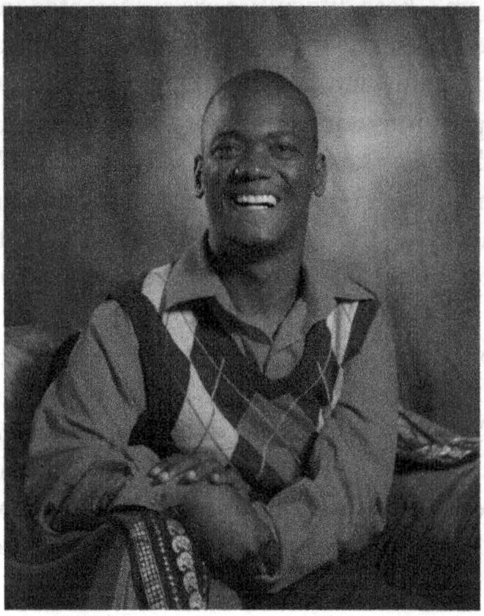

My name is Mr. Lebogang Sehako. I am a 41-year old person with cerebral palsy. I use a wheelchair and AAC device to communicate. The system that I use is Etriloquist, which is a program that I downloaded on my laptop. On this device I can type out any message and the device then "speaks" my message using text-to-speech software. I stay in a small rural town in the Northern Cape province in South Africa.

During my school-going years I attended three different special schools. I started my education as a 7-year-old at Re Tlameleng Special School in Kimberly, the capital city of the Northern Cape province. It is a public school and although it now focuses on learners with visual impairment, at the time when I attended it catered to all students with all types of disabilities. However, it only offered primary school education (thus up to Grade 7) and when I enrolled for Grade 8, I had to attend a new school. Elizabeth Conradie School for Learners with Special Needs is also in Kimberly, and is a public, urban school specifically for learners with physical disability, and ranges from preschool all the way to Grade 12. Unfortunately, I failed Grade 8 twice—which is not surprising given the fact that I had no communication device! I was then sent to Tlamelang special school, a commerce school for learners with special educational needs (in Gelukspan in the North West Province). Like the Elizabeth Conradie School, it is also a public school specifically for learners with physical disability, and ranges from preschool all the way to Grade 12.

In total, I attended school for 16 years and spent all of my schooling years living in the school hostel (boarding facility), as my home was too far away from the school to travel on a daily basis. During the time when I was attending school, South Africa did not have an inclusive education policy, but focused on special education. These "special schools" all had a specific focus (e.g., on hearing disability, visual disability, intellectual disability, or physical disability [which describes the schools I attended]). Unfortunately, I didn't pass my final Grade 12 exam, because I didn't have good resources at school. For example, I did not have access to either a communication device or to an electric wheelchair. However, I never gave up! I hope that when you read my story you will see what I mean.

Carla and Lebogang are not alone. Across the world, persons with disabilities have poorer health outcomes (Vergunst et al., 2017), lower education achievements (Carew et al., 2020), less employment possibilities (Morwane et al., 2021), and higher rates of poverty than peers without disabilities (Pinilla-Roncancio, 2015). This is partly because health services, education, employment, transport, information, and communication, are inaccessible to them. These difficulties are exacerbated in less-advantaged communities as confirmed in the extensive systematic review by Banks and colleagues (2017) that showed strong evidence for a link between disability and poverty in low-income settings.

Disability disproportionately affects vulnerable populations and is therefore both a cause and a consequence of poverty. However, not all people with disabilities are equally disadvantaged. Within the sphere of disability, individuals with complex communication needs are particularly vulnerable, as participation in all aspects of life is restricted. Furthermore, these individuals have a heightened risk of becoming the victim of crime, abuse, and neglect, because perpetrators see silent victims as perfect victims (White et al., 2021).

Beukelman and Mirenda (2013) estimated that approximately 1.3% of the American population cannot rely on speech alone to meet their daily communication needs, and the prevalence and complexity of communication disorders increase with age (Yorkston et al., 2010). If this percentage is applied to the global population (7.9 billion people in 2022 according to Worldometer), it would mean that globally there are approximately 10 million people who could be regarded as having complex communication needs. AAC offers great potential to enhance the communication and interaction of these individuals.

Defining Augmentative and Alternative Communication

Many definitions have been put forward to define what AAC is. According to the American Speech-Language-Hearing Association (ASHA; n.d), AAC is an area of clinical practice that supplements or compensates for temporary or permanent impairments, activity limitations and participation restrictions of persons with severe disorders of speech-language production and/or comprehension, including spoken and written modes of communication. Beukelman and Light (2020) expanded this definition in their seminal AAC textbook by alluding to the wide variety of systems that are available to meet the needs of all persons (including both children and adults) with complex communication needs. AAC systems are typically divided into unaided AAC (i.e., systems that do not require any equipment or technology external to the individual's body) and aided AAC, which requires some form of equipment or technology. Aided AAC includes low-technology options, (e.g., communication boards or picture exchange systems) and high-technology options (e.g., computer-based systems, typically with speech-output).

Unaided AAC ranges from intuitive nonlinguistic systems that can easily be understood by everybody to complex linguistic-based systems that require training. Examples of intuitive systems include simple vocalizations (including laughter and humming) and speech approximations; head nodding and head shaking (to indicate "yes/no"); pointing with the eyes or staring at an object; indicating with an outstretched arm or pointing with a finger (to request that you want/need something); taking somebody else's hand to request something (e.g., putting a person's hand on a container to request help opening the container); body posture and head, neck, and body movements; facial expressions (typically used to show emotion, such as smiling to show happiness, or frowning to show confusion); as well as natural gestures (gestures generally understood by people within a specific culture or society that require no additional training such as the gestures for come, stop, and phone; Bornman et al., 2023).

On the other hand, linguistic unaided AAC includes sign languages (e.g., American Sign Language [ASL] in the United States, or South African Sign Language [SASL] in South Africa); alphabet-based systems like finger spelling (one-handed and two-handed finger spelling are used, although the former is more common); as well as manually coded languages (e.g., Signed English).

When considering aided AAC, both the choice of symbol and display type should be considered. Symbols offer a visual representation of a word or an idea and typically develop along a complexity continuum that includes object symbols (e.g., real objects that are similar to the object that they represent, such as car keys to indicate "going for a drive" or a cup to indicate "drink"); partial objects (e.g., a leather strap to represent "horse-riding" or miniature objects such as doll utensils); photographs (e.g., photographs of friends at school or family members); hand-drawn pictures (i.e., these are especially effective if the person watches while you draw and explain: "look this is the dog's long ears and here is his fluffy tail ..."); line drawings (graphic symbols such as Picture Communication Symbols, SymbolStix, Bildstöd [a free symbol library], Widgit, Blissymbols, Makaton; or traditional orthography (written words that depend on literacy skills; Bornman et al., 2023).

Symbols are organized and displayed in many ways, depending on the specific system selected. In the past, such aided systems were classified as low technology (i.e., inexpensive, simple to make, easy to obtain, and requiring simple equipment) and high technology (i.e., sophisticated, usually programmable devices that typically use an integrated circuit). This definition would imply that low technology AAC would include communication books and boards, visual schedules, communication bracelets, pocket-sized communication passports, business card folders, flip-up photograph albums, etc. The list of creative display options is unlimited, and clinicians will be guided by the individual and their needs in designing the most appropriate communication display. In the early 1990s, Sarah Blackstone (1993) recommended that low technology should form a critical part of any person's communication system—a statement that is just as true today as it was 30 years ago.

With the rise of the fourth (and now fifth) industrial revolution, high technology—which would typically refer to devices with speech output (i.e., speech generating devices) and includes mobile technologies (tablets and phones) with a wide range of AAC applications and digital communication media (Beukelman & Light, 2020)—has grown exponentially. However, this once-clear distinction between low and high technology has become blurred (Bornman & Waller, 2023). For example, if a tablet is used to serve as a communication board without speech output, it could be considered "low tech," but adding speech output could turn the tablet into "high tech." When considering aided AAC, therapists should be cognizant of the different physical features of the system, such as the language of the system (e.g., non-English synthetic speech options are still limited, thereby impacting on multilingual AAC users), the input device that is needed (e.g., automatic speech recognition and brain computer interfaces, eye-gaze, keyboards, mice, switches, touch screens), the required access methods (e.g., direct or indirect access), the types of displays (e.g., fixed, dynamic or hybrid displays), voice (e.g., digitized [recorded] speech, text-to-speech and mixed mode or hybrid speech), and finally portability (Bornman & Waller, 2023).

The language option(s) of the system should also be considered. Multilingualism is a well-known international phenomenon, and it is estimated that more than half of the world's population is multilingual (i.e., uses two or more languages in everyday life; Grosjean, 2013). However, despite acknowledgment of the ubiquitous nature of multilingualism, many multilingual individuals who require AAC intervention still receive monolingual communication intervention, thereby reducing their communication opportunities, limiting their participation and interaction, and restricting their broader inclusion into society (Tönsing & Soto, 2020). Multiple reasons have been put forward, including but not limited to, the lack of available AAC systems that allow access to multiple languages (e.g., commercially available aided AAC systems in languages other than English are often limited [Soto & Yu, 2014], or if available, these systems are expensive); restricted preprogrammed non-English vocabulary sets and grammar support (Tönsing et al., 2019); family members who do not experience the AAC system as helpful, citing reasons such as unintelligible synthetic speech (McCord

& Soto, 2004); inappropriate graphic symbols, as these symbols might not be culturally sensitive or relevant to home activities (Pickl, 2011); limited knowledge and skill of speech-language therapists in both languages (Bornman & Louw, 2021); and misperceptions or myths around multilingual AAC (Tönsing & Soto, 2020). More recently, arguments around language ideology have been foregrounded as both the family and the interventionists' beliefs, feelings, and conceptions around language and multilingualism ultimately influence intervention goals and practices (Tönsing & Soto, 2020).

Despite a paucity of research related to AAC and multilingualism, there seems to be widespread agreement that AAC interventionists should be trained in multilingual practice and cultural awareness based on current evidence (Lindholm, 2020; Pickl, 2011; Soto & Yu, 2014; Tönsing & Soto, 2020). A recent Finnish study found diverse opinions amongst speech-language therapists regarding multilingual AAC intervention based on the heterogeneity of the AAC population and the wide range of available AAC systems and strategies (Lindholm, 2020).

Although the "golden standard" of providing multilingual AAC intervention does not (yet) exist, there is consensus amongst speech-language therapists that multilingual AAC users require an integrated linguistic repertoire that includes features from the different languages in the individual's life. Speech-language therapists should carefully consider how language resources and AAC are used in the individual's specific community and explore creative and novel solutions to allow the multilingual AAC user to engage in creating shared meaning. Translation of material is one method commonly used in aided low-technology AAC systems (e.g., displaying a written word [gloss] in two different languages: one above and one below the graphic symbol). However, limited practice guidelines exist regarding how translation can best be done (Bornman & Louw, 2021). AAC systems and strategies should provide multilingual users with the choice of language they would opt to use as L1, with the ability to code switch and code mix into a different language (L2), as code switching may not be a neutral act for multilingual individuals but an attempt to show respect, to promote belonging to and cohesion in a particular group, to align or distance oneself from a communication partner, or to achieve social closeness (King & Soto, 2022; Tönsing et al., 2019). More research on the topic of AAC and multilingualism is needed to ensure evidence-based practice ensuring equal services and support for multilingual AAC users.

Other attributes of the system could include their function such as single-function devices (e.g., attention-getting devices, voice recorders, and voice amplification), graphic-based AAC systems (e.g., visual scene displays [VSDs], dynamic screens, and semantic compaction), literacy-based AAC systems, and hybrid AAC systems. Systems can also make use of acceleration techniques such as layout optimization and language prediction. Apart from the positive impact of prediction on the speed of interaction, it may also assist those with limited literacy skills. Furthermore, prediction in languages other than English may also support multilingual AAC users (Herold et al., 2008). Despite these obvious benefits and possibilities afforded by AAC technology, one of the greatest threats is that an AAC device is sometimes seen as an appliance—like a washing machine or a coffee maker—something that one can operate and use without training.

Carla was asked to reflect on the question: "If you could design an ideal system for yourself, what would it look like?" This is what she had to say (verbatim):

> This is one of the most important questions ever. If I could design a system, it would be easier and lighter to carry than my laptop. It's quite heavy and definitely not easy to take with me where I go.
>
> The language is very important. Obviously English is a universal language, but I would love to speak in my native language, Afrikaans, too. The accent of the AAC programs cannot pronounce some words in Afrikaans and then my mother must help me find a spelling so that the word will be pronounced so that people can understand it. It's very funny sometimes to hear the American or British voice speak a word in Afrikaans. Especially our surnames.

> Cost is a major factor. The devices and programs are so expensive that parents cannot afford to buy it for their children who really need it. Being a disabled person, you already need so much additional things to assist you in living a normal life and if a device that can let you communicate costs so much that you cannot afford it, it makes life even harder. I had bought myself a new computer recently, but I had to get a bigger one because the program takes a lot of space. I wanted to upgrade to Grid 3 but neither my mother nor I could afford getting the upgraded program. So, I would definitely fight for cheaper, more accessible programs. I don't know how I would handle the upgrades and insurance. In our country WiFi is still not accessible by all. So automatic updates won't always be done.
>
> Relevancy to gender, age and culture are very important issues. Can you imagine if a 10-year-old girl talks with a 50-year-old male's voice? As if a disabled person doesn't look weird in any case, it will only look and sound weirder. We want to blend in not stand out.

In response to this same question, Lebogang also had definite ideas:

> If I can design an AAC system for me, it should look similar to my mobile phone so that I can carry my AAC system where I go. I want to be able to use it in all the different places where I go like, for example, the toilet/bathroom, sitting room, and my bedroom. I must not struggle to use it and I must not need another person to help me when I use that AAC system. It must not have too many apps like my phone. It should have only one communication app and the battery must be able to be charged with electricity and with the sun (solar power). It must have the two languages that I speak every day: Setswana and English. Every AAC user must be able afford to buy my designed AAC system.

When unpacking AAC, it is now clear where the term originates from. AAC is about:

- **Augmentative** (i.e., adds to or enhances). Everyone (natural speakers and persons who use AAC) augments their communication by using vocalizations, facial expressions, gestures, eye pointing, and body language.
- **Alternative** (i.e., substitutes or replaces). Some persons require alternatives to speech, which can include pointing to symbols using their eyes or hands, using a speech-generating device, signing, or writing/typing.
- **Communication** (i.e., creating shared meaning). This requires the sending and receiving of messages between at least two persons.

Augmentative and Alternative Communication as Voice

Although it is true that AAC is an area of clinical practice, a field of research, and that it includes both aided and unaided systems and strategies—it is more than that. Much more. Without access to speech, Carla and Lebogang, as well as the other 10 million people worldwide in need of AAC, are severely restricted in their communication and participation in all aspects of life: education, employment, family life, and citizenship. Therefore, when asking persons who use AAC how they would define AAC, they frequently describe it as their voice. For these individuals, AAC is not about systems and strategies, it is about having a voice, about communication, about connecting, about sharing, and about access to their human rights.

What does it mean to have a voice? Some dictionary definitions would refer to "human beings making sounds through the mouth like in talking or singing," some would refer to "giving expression" or "making sounds with resonance of the vocal cords." In speech-language therapy definitions, voice aspects such as quality, pitch, and loudness are considered (Boone et al., 2010). But voice is more than that. Having a voice is about agency. It is about not being reliant on others to hear you, to provide you with communication opportunities and allowing you to speak. Having a voice is about finding and having a voice that is your own, that is not controlled by anyone else. This allows all human beings to have a deep sense of purpose, self-worth, and quality of life. It opens up opportunities, and reminds us that just because a person cannot speak, it does not mean that they have nothing to say.

In 2005, the Centre for AAC at the University of Pretoria embarked on a weeklong youth empowerment project for persons who use AAC. This programme was named "Fofa," a Sesotho word that means "to soar" or "to fly." In Africa, youth with disabilities experience many external barriers that hamper the opportunities provided to them (e.g., policy barriers, practice barriers, as well as attitude and knowledge barriers) and also certain internal access barriers (e.g., related to their specific environments, their communication skills, and available resources; Beukelman & Light, 2020). These barriers are imposed by society and prevent individuals with complex communication needs from realizing their potential, rendering them unable to become valued participants in society. In the broader sphere of disability, individuals with complex communication needs have the least access to education and economic resources, which reinforces the vicious cycle between poverty and disability.

It is against this background that the Fofa project focused on the identification of youth with severe communication abilities who have the potential to become advocates for people with disabilities and become entrepreneurs within their own context. Lebogang was part of the first "Fofa fly-boys," and this is how he described his experience:

> In May 2005, the physiotherapist from the hospital where I attended therapy accompanied me to a consultation at the Centre for AAC at the University of Pretoria. I received some great tips for technology to help me access a computer and idea for high-tech AAC systems. I was then also invited to take part in the Youth Empowerment Program "Fofa" for young people using AAC, run by the Centre for AAC at the University of Pretoria from South Africa. The Sotho word "Fofa" means to fly, and it made me realize that I could fly as high as I was brave enough to dream!
>
> At the Fofa workshop in September 2005, when I was 24 years old, I received my first AAC device with support from the team from the Centre for AAC at the University of Pretoria. I will never forget how I felt when during that first Fofa week, on the Wednesday to be precise, the professor said, "This AAC device that is front of you is now yours. It can go to school with you. It can go home with you after the Fofa weekends." It was one of the happiest moments of my life! It meant no more struggles to try and use my mouth to speak. I was able to use my new AAC device to communicate with teachers and with the other learners in the classroom. The following week I also received my first electric wheelchair at PGC. Since receiving my AAC device and my electric wheelchair, I became a new person! I started to believe that disability is not inability but a matter of faith. There were also other things I started doing and this gave me more self-confidence, increased my determination to do things, and taught me patience. I thank my principal, Mr. Odendaal, very much who gave me permission to attend the Fofa week, because at that time I was writing preparatory exams. I was so happy when I returned to school after the Fofa week with my new AAC device. I continued attending the Fofa programme on a yearly basis from 2005 to 2010, and later also became a mentor in the project.

> During the years 2012 to 2015, I attended a disability project leadership training at Gelukspan Hospital, and the year 2016 I also attended a 3-week Carer-to-Carer Parent Facilitator course at Malamulele Centre Johannesburg. At this course I learned about different types of disability, especially cerebral palsy, as well as about disability severity levels, and how to train parents and community members about disability. This is very important because community awareness is the first crucial step in disability advocacy—and I regard myself as a community disability advocate!
>
> My work experience also took some interesting turns. Between 2010 until 2015, I volunteered as co-facilitator of the Disability Youth Empowerment Program at the Parents Guidance Centre in Gelukspan Hospital near Mahikeng. In the year 2011, I gathered together mothers who have children with disability to start a centre for children with disability in and around Kuruman in the broader John Taolo Gaetsewe District. Currently I am volunteering as a manager at Kuruman Children with Disability Centre and ward committees at Magojaneng community.
>
> Using AAC is a positive thing that happened in my life. I felt like a little baby who had started to walk and who wanted to walk inside the house without ever wanting to stop!

Carla also attended the Fofa project, and she recalls that this was the first time when she was assessed (as a young adult) for an AAC system. This is how she describes it:

> I was really assessed at the University of Pretoria by the Centre for AAC team. We were a group of disabled persons that spent the week at the University. We all had one person that assisted us. Our caregivers were also in attendance. That was great because my caregiver could also learn to assist me.
>
> We got different themes that we had to write about. Because of my involuntary movements, I got tired very quickly. So, in the beginning they tried different switches to find which one will work the best for me.
>
> I also used a communication board for when I was very tired. Just so that I could catch my breath. This helped a lot.
>
> I attended the "Fofa week" for 5 years and every time I learned something new. I became a mentor the third year and that was amazing. To show people how to use my device is the best feeling ever.

Deciding on an Augmentative and Alternative Communication System

AAC assessments generally differ for other forms as speech-language assessment—as not only are the skills of the individual assessed, but also the features of the proposed AAC (i.e., the functionality). Clinicians need to understand the different components of the AAC system to identify appropriate technology, which is often described as "feature matching" (Pitt & Brumberg, 2018). Feature matching is widely accepted as the established standard AAC assessment practice for choosing the AAC system (i.e., communication book, tablet), the symbol set/system as well as its layout, the access method (e.g., direct selection or scanning), as well as the intervention strategy that will best suit the specific person based on their current and future communication profile, their level of support, their preferences and needs and also their sensory, motor, cognitive, literacy, and socioemotional skills (Thistle & Wilkinson, 2015). When considering their specific communication skills, both receptive communication skills (such as the understanding of single-word vocabulary, syntax, and grammar) as well as subjective measurements (like ability to follow single- and multiple-step instructions, coherent language [narratives and conversation], and humor), and expressive communication skills should be included. Furthermore, communication intent or desire needs to be observed. When assessing expressive communication skills, communication functions should be assessed (e.g., greeting, protesting, requesting help or information, initiating interaction) as well as the multimodal communication means and modalities that are currently being used (e.g., ability to use natural speech and future prospects for increasing this, vocalizations, facial expressions, pointing, and gestures).

A "match" between the individual's capabilities and the features of the system does not automatically account for all the components needed to guarantee success. The high rate of technology abandonment (despite the obvious advantages thereof) is of high concern in the AAC field. Researchers attribute this to multifaceted reasons such as the lack of user-centered design when developing AAC devices, a poor match between user requirements and the features of the technology, and the changing needs of users and environments in practice (Bornman & Waller, 2023; van Niekerk et al., 2017).

Moreover, assessments tend to be dynamic in nature because at no one point does assessment end and intervention start—there is generally a fusion between the two as the person is provided with a potential system and is then assessed to determine how effective the specific device is and what further adaptations can be made.

Furthermore, it is generally accepted as best practice that AAC intervention involves an interprofessional team who works in a collaborative manner. The team members differ and vary according to the specific case (Binger et at., 2012), but generally include the following team members:

- *The person with the complex communication needs themself.* They are best suited to identify the current (and future) needs and goals for communication and should also assist with prioritizing intervention goals related to communication.
- *Close communication partner(s) (parents in the case of children, and a spouse or partner in the case of adults).* They know the person best and are also the only constant long-term team member. These individuals can also provide information about aspects that enhance the efficacy of assessment and intervention such as routines, about likes and dislikes, strengths and weaknesses, interests, etc.
- *Other family members or close friends (e.g., peers, siblings, paid carers).* They know what the typical activities and contexts are that the person is expected to communicate in. This will assist in developing functional age-appropriate assessment and intervention goals.
- *AAC clinician.* This person may have a variety of disciplinary backgrounds but should have an additional qualification or extensive clinical experience in the field of AAC. This team member will take the lead in conducting the feature matching and should thus be skilled in matching the technology features and the individual's skills and needs.
- *Teacher (in the case of children).* They know what is expected of the child in the classroom context in terms of communication that would facilitate learning and will also help to inform other children about the child's AAC system. In the case of adults who are working, this role might be taken up by a co-worker or a human resource practitioner.
- *(Educational) psychologist.* Psychologists can provide counseling to support the family and child—a role that is foregrounded when the person enters into a new life phase (e.g., transitioning into teenagerhood) and the grieving cycle might come to the forefront again.
- *Physiotherapist.* Physiotherapists are instrumental in providing advice on correct positioning, maintaining or achieving best possible posture, preventing contractures, etc.

- *Occupational therapist.* Occupational therapists promote and enhance independence and life skills, as well as adapting material and equipment for play and learning and increasing participation in activities of daily living.
- *Speech-language therapist.* Speech-language therapists focus on enhancing and facilitating communication and language learning. They can also assist with implementing and expanding the AAC system and address literacy skills. In cases where needed, they are also equipped to skillfully address any feeding problems.
- *Audiologist.* Audiologists assess hearing skills and provide intervention if needed (e.g., hearing aids, cochlear implants, or referral to ear-nose-throat surgeon [ENT]).
- *Social worker.* Social workers support families, for example, by providing help with accessing disability grant and other social grants. In some cases, they also run community training programs aimed at raising awareness around specific disability challenges.
- *Rehabilitation engineer/software specialist.* These individuals have specialized knowledge about the different AAC devices and possible adaptations and can also assist in the personalization of systems.
- *AAC manufacturer/vendor.* Vendors may provide information about the most current and recent devices and systems that are available, about new devices that will soon be launched, and can also arrange for a person to receive a device for a loan period.
- *Medical practitioner.* There may be a whole range of medical practitioners who are involved with the person at a given time. Their practitioners are not necessarily constant members of the team but may provide expert opinions or guidance to the interprofessional team.
- *Pediatric neurologist.* They may assist with the diagnosis and medical treatment (e.g., anti-epileptic drugs).
- *Ophthalmologist.* They may assist with the diagnosis of visual impairments, including cortical visual impairment. They might also be able to make valuable suggestions related to visual intervention by providing guidance of the visual acuity and the visual field, which has implications for the type and size of symbols selected as well as the visual layout of the system.
- *ENT.* They can assist with the diagnosis and treatment of auditory impairments, as many individuals may have hearing difficulties and/or chronic middle ear infections.
- *Orthopedic surgeon.* They can aid in the case of joint deformities and if a person requires surgery.
- *Genetic nurse/genetic counselor.* They have knowledge in cases where the cause of the disability is genetic and the family requires advice with respect to family planning.
- *Nurse.* They can act as advocates and counselors and provide basic medical routines and help to monitor medication (e.g., anti-epileptic drugs).

Interprofessional collaboration, which is widely regarded as best practice in assessment and intervention, entails that multiple practitioners (as listed earlier) from different disciplines work together with the person requiring assessment and intervention, with their families, and with members of the general community to deliver the highest possible quality of care to these individuals (Hlongwa & Rispel, 2021). Carla was asked that if she should design an ideal assessment and intervention team for herself, what this team would look like. This is what she thinks:

> Obviously the team must consist of persons that know about technology. I would also put a speech-language therapist and an occupational therapist on the team. I don't only have a speech problem. My whole body becomes more spastic when I try to do something. So, the occupational therapist will assist in helping me with posture, neck, hand control, etc.
>
> With my disability I will include my parents and caregiver too. They know me the best and will know what I need. Or at least what is needed to let me communicate the best.

My mother and her friend came up with wonderful plans to make my clicker switch more user friendly. At my Centre they also changed my communication board with words and sentences that I regularly use, to make it easier for me to communicate.

I would like the team to listen to my suggestions and not just assume that they know what I need because they have encountered a person with a similar disability. We all differ and so do our needs. Our environments and needs are not the same.

In a follow-up question, Carla was asked if she could train a speech-language therapist to do an assessment for a person who uses AAC, what she would tell them:

I think that not only a speech-language therapist should be involved but also an occupational therapist. Because of my disability I need help with posture, easy controls, etc.

To train the therapists I would ask them to go in open minded. Again, not all people with certain disabilities are the same. So don't let preset mindsets get in the way of evaluating the person in front of you. Interact with the person. Don't make any judgment before you have seen the disabled person in a few scenarios. And please be patient with that person. Don't tell them to relax because that is not possible. We all tense up in any situation. So just give me a chance to express myself.

The therapist should think of ways to communicate other than the AAC device. Like, for instance, in a shopping mall. How will I communicate without my laptop? Remember I might not have a tablet or some smaller device to take with me. So other options must also be available.

My caregiver's daughter is studying speech therapy at Medunsa [a medical university in South Africa where speech-language therapists are trained]. She is currently busy with her practical year at the hospital. She has assisted me a couple of times as a caregiver. And one thing she has shared with me is that what they learn at university is not always applicable in my situations. Therapists tend to cling to book education. I can teach them the practical side. They must just give me a chance.

The family is very important in this process. No one knows that person better than the people who share their lives every day. My mother came up with very neat plans to make my life easier. So, it's important to have their input. They might think of something that might work that the therapist doesn't think of. Sometimes the silliest thing is the easiest way to cross a huge hurdle. So, when a device is set up, ask the family if it will work in the home setting. Ask them for their experience. They should share their needs for communication and be part of getting a solution.

In response to this same question, this is what Lebogang expressed:

One day, when I get the opportunity to train a speech-language therapist, I will tell them they must be patient, loving, and take good care of the AAC user. They must bring about change in the life of the AAC user and should not bring challenges in our life.

Conclusion

The silence as a result of speechlessness is never golden. It is crucial for all humans to engage and establish connections with each other, exploring various avenues of communication, not limiting ourselves to just one. Communication is a basic human need as it provides a window into who we are and what knowledge we have. It shapes how others perceive us (M. Romski, personal communication). Communication is a basic human right—it is power.

The late Stephen Hawking (2018), black hole theorist and possibly the most iconic and inspirational AAC user, shared his thoughts on communication with this profound quote:

> For millions of years, mankind lived just like the animals. Then something happened which unleashed the power of our imagination. We learned to talk and we learned to listen. Speech has allowed the communication of ideas, enabling human beings to work together to build the impossible. Mankind's greatest achievements have come about by talking, and its greatest failures by not talking. It doesn't have to be like this. Our greatest hopes could become reality in the future. With the technology at our disposal, the possibilities are unbounded. All we need to do is make sure we keep talking.

References

American Speech-Language Hearing Association. (n.d.). *Practice portal's augmentative and alternative communication.*https://www.asha.org/practice-portal/professional-issues/augmentative-and-alternative-communication

Banks, L. M., Kuper, H., & Polack, S. (2017). Poverty and disability in low- and middle-income countries: A systematic review. *PLOS ONE, 12*(12), e0189996. https://doi.org/10.1371/journal.pone.0189996

Beukelman, D. R., & Light, J. C. (2020). *Augmentative and alternative communication: Supporting children and adults with complex communication needs* (5th ed.). Paul Brookes.

Beukelman, D. R., & Mirenda, P. (2013). *Augmentative and alternative communication: Supporting children and adults with complex communication needs* (4th ed.). Paul Brookes.

Binger, C., Ball, L., Dietz, A., Kent-Walsh, J., Lund, S., McKelvey, M., & Quach, W. (2012). Personnel roles in the AAC assessment process. *Augmentative and Alternative Communication, 28*, 278-288.

Blackstone, S. (1993). Low-tech communication displays: Are we considering anything? *Augmentative Communication News, 6*(1), 1-7.

Boone, D. R., McFarlane, S. C., Von Berg, S. L., & Zraick, R. I. (2010). *The voice and voice therapy.* Allyn & Bacon.

Bornman, J., Gouws, H., Moolman, E., Robberts, A., & Tönsing, K.M. (2023). Using augmentative and alternative communication strategies in schools in Namibia. In U. Lüdtke, E. Kija, & M. K. Karia (Eds.*), Handbook of communication disabilities and language development in sub-Saharan Africa* (pp. 643-671). Springer.

Bornman, J., & Louw, B. (2021). A model for cross-cultural translation and adaptation of speech-language pathology assessment measures: Application to the Focus on the Outcomes of Communication Under Six (FOCUS). *International Journal of Speech-Language Pathology, 23*(4), 382-393. https://doi.org/10.1080/17549507.2020.1831065

Bornman, J., & Waller, A. (2023). Background, features, and principles of AAC technology. In D. Fuller & L. L. Lloyd (Eds.), *Principles and practices in augmentative and alternative communication* (pp. 192-215). SLACK Incorporated.

Carew, M., Deluca, M., Groce, N., Fwaga, S., & Kett, M. (2020). The impact of an inclusive education intervention on learning outcomes for girls with disabilities within a resource-poor setting. *African Journal of Disability, 9*, 1-8. https://dx.doi.org/10.4102/ajod.v9i0.555

Grosjean, F. (2013). Bilingualism: A short introduction. In F. Grosjean & P. Li (Eds.), *The psycholinguistics of bilingualism* (pp. 5-25). Wiley-Blackwell.

Hawking, S. (2018, March 14). In my mind I am free: Notable quotes from Stephen Hawking. *Associated Press.* https://apnews.com/general-news-international-news-cc460330580f439796b5c6015a5ca8e0

Herold, M., Alant, E., & Bornman, J. (2008). Typing speed, spelling accuracy, and the use of word-prediction. *South African Journal of Education, 28*, 117-134.

Hlongwa, P., & Rispel, L. C. (2021). Interprofessional collaboration among health professionals in cleft lip and palate treatment and care in the public health sector of South Africa. *Human Resources for Health, 19*(1), 1-9. https://doi/org/10.1186.s12960-021-00566-3

King, M. R., & Soto, G. (2022). Code-switching using aided AAC: Toward an integrated theoretical framework. *Augmentative and Alternative Communication, 38*(1), 67-76. https://doi/org/10.1080/07434618.2022.2051603

Kuyler, A., Johnson, E., & Bornman, J. (2022). Unaided communication behaviours displayed by adults with severe cerebrovascular accidents and little to no functional speech: A scoping review. *International Journal of Language and Communication Disorders, 57*(2), 403-421. https://doi.org/10.1111/1460-6984.12691

Lindholm, J. (2020). Multilingualism and AAC: A study of Finnish SLPs' opinions and practices of multilingual AAC. Unpublished master's dissertation in speech-language pathology, Åbo Akademi University, Turku, Finland.

McCord, M. S., & Soto, G. (2004). Perceptions of AAC: An ethnographic investigation of Mexican-American families. *Augmentative and Alternative Communication, 20*(4), 209-227. https://doi.org/10.1080/07434610400005648

Morwane, R. E., Dada, S., & Bornman, J. (2021). Barriers to and facilitators of employment of persons with disabilities in low- and middle-income countries: A scoping review. *African Journal of Disability, 10*. https://doi.org/10.4102/ajod.v10i0.833

Pickl, G. (2011). Communication intervention in children with severe disabilities and multilingual backgrounds: Perceptions of pedagogues and parents. *Augmentative and Alternative Communication, 27*(4), 229-244. https://doi.org/10.3109/07434618.2011.630021

Pinilla-Roncancio, M. (2015). Disability and poverty: Two related conditions. A review of the literature. *Revista de la Facultad de Medicina, 63*(Suppl. 1), 113-123. https://doi.org/10.15446/revfacmed.v63n3sup.50132

Pitt, K. M., & Brumberg, J. S. (2018). Guidelines for feature matching assessment of brain-computer interfaces for augmentative and alternative communication. *American Journal of Speech-Language Pathology, 27*(3), 950-964. https://doi.org/10.1044/2018_AJSLP-17-0135

Soto, G., & Yu, B. (2014). Considerations for the provision of services to bilingual children who use augmentative and alternative communication. *Augmentative and Alternative Communication, 30*(2), 83-92. https://doi.org/10.3109/07434618.2013.878751

Thistle, J. J., & Wilkinson, K. M. (2015). Building evidence-based practice in AAC display design for young children: Current practices and future directions. *Augmentative and Alternative Communication, 31*(2), 124-136.

Tönsing, K. M., & Soto, G. (2020). Multilingualism and augmentative and alternative communication: Examining language ideology and resulting practices. *Augmentative and Alternative Communication, 36*(3), 190-201. https://doi/org/10.1080/07434618.2020.1811761

Tönsing, K. M., van Niekerk, K., Schlünz, G., & Wilken, I. (2019). Multilingualism and augmentative and alternative communication in South Africa: Exploring the views of persons with complex communication needs. *African Journal of Disability, 24*(8), 507-518. https://doi/org/10.4102/ajod.v8i0.507

van Niekerk, K., Dada, S., Tönsing, K. M., & Boshoff, K. (2017). Factors perceived by rehabilitation professionals to influence the provision of assistive technology to children: A systematic review. *Physical and Occupational Therapy in Pediatrics, 38*(2), 168-189.

Vergunst, R., Swartz, L., Hem, K. G., Eide, A. H., Mannan, H., MacLachlan, M., Mji, G., Braathen, S. H., & Schneider, M. (2017). Access to health care for persons with disabilities in rural South Africa. *BMC Health Services Research, 17*, 741. https://doi.org/10.1186/s12913-017-2674-5

White, R., Johnson, E., & Bornman, J. (2021). Giving voice to the voices of legal practitioners with disabilities. *Disability and Society, 38*(8), 1451-1475. https://doi.org/10.1080/09687599.2021.1997719

Yorkston, K. M., Bourgeois, M. S., & Baylor, C. R. (2010). Communication and aging. *Physical Medicine and Rehabilitation Clinics of North America, 21*(2), 309-319.

Chapter 15

Addressing Multicultural and Multilingual Aspects in the Assessment of Individuals With Autism Spectrum Disorder

Kakia Petinou, PhD, SLP; Maria Christopoulou, EdD; and Kyriakos Antoniou, PhD

Introduction

The purpose of the current chapter is to present recent advances in the area of multilingual and multicultural issues in the management of individuals diagnosed with autism spectrum disorder (ASD). In addition, the chapter is set to recommend clinical protocols relevant to the challenges associated with the assessment and intervention practices for individuals with ASD who come from diverse linguistic and cultural backgrounds. Notably, the discussion of such topics is necessitated by the significant influx of refugees across Europe and across the globe (Grech, 2019; Guiberson & Atkins, 2010). A particular focus is given on the themes related to multilingualism and multiculturalism facets of the disorder. In the introduction, the authors describe the behavioral and communicative symptomatology associated with ASD, provide information related to the prevalence of the disorder across the globe, and underscore the need to develop awareness related to the linguistic and cultural diversity of populations given the influx of immigrant population in Europe and across the world. In the second part of the chapter, the authors present the theoretical underpinnings of bilingualism and multilingualism vis-à-vis populations with developmental language challenges including ASD. The multilingual/bilingual advantage is discussed along with research findings that either support or refute myths and realities behind the use of one versus two languages by individuals with ASD. For purposes of clarity the term *multilingualism* will be used thought the chapter, including reference to the term *bilingualism*. The third part of the chapter focuses on the implementation of assessment

Bortz, M. (Ed.). *A Guide to Global Language Assessment: A Lifespan Approach* (pp. 289-303).
DOI: 10.4324/9781003524472-19

protocols and diagnostic tools in the context of clinical management of ASD. The challenges of such endeavors are discussed. The overall goal of the chapter is to encourage health practitioners and especially speech-language therapists to capitalize on available global information related to the management of ASD. Recent reports suggest that important evidence-based findings and information related to ASD management (including the topic of multilingualism) appear to be an "Achilles tendon" as most of the time such outcomes do not reach the mainstream clinicians who, after all, find themselves in the "front line" during their interaction with individuals and their families (Gillon et al., 2017; Law et al., 2019).

Characteristics, Terminology, Prevalence

ASD is an umbrella term referring to a range of conditions secondary to complex neurobiological underpinnings. As such, the condition results in aberrant brain circuitry that surfaces during infancy (Baron-Cohen, 1991, 1995; Petinou & Minaidou, 2017; Tager-Flusberg, 2016; Westby, 2014). The pathogenesis of ASD is triggered by complex mechanisms traced in utero and in synergy with environmental and genetic factors (Wolff & Piven, 2013). The disorder affects children and families regardless of language background, religion, and/or socioeconomic status across the globe (American Psychiatric Association [APA], 2013; Gillon et al., 2017; Health Resources & Services Administration, 2019; Richard, 1997; World Health Organization [WHO], 2019; World Health Organization Resolution on ASD, 2019). The prevalence of ASD reported by WHO (2019) is estimated to be 1:160 individuals, although this represents an average figure. ASD prevalence is higher in males as compared to females with a ratio of 4:1. Although global occurrence of ASD is difficult to estimate, the consensus converges toward a notable increase according to recent reports by the Centers for Disease Control and Prevention (CDC; 2020) indicating that in the United States alone during 2016 around 1 in 54 children presented with a diagnosis of ASD. Moreover, prevalence has also been estimated to be 222 per 10,000 children worldwide (Elflein, 2020). Nevertheless, there is scarcity of ASD figures from underrepresented and remote populations, a topic that warrants further investigation as it remains underexplored. ASD does not appear to be more prevalent in a specific geographic area within particular ethnic groups (Gillon et al., 2017). Such observations underscore the need to increase examinations and screening for underrepresented and underserved populations who might present with communication, social, and behavioral profiles consistent with ASD. Notably, the WHO resolution on ASD, according to the 67th World Health Assembly (WHO, 2012), presents a plan in relation to a series of comprehensive and coordinated efforts for the management of ASD. This serious effort has been endorsed by more than 60 countries across the globe. Such actions form the springboard for the advancement of suitable and collective clinical tools and checklists (e.g., questionnaires) in an effort to develop homogeneous clinical assessment tools, albeit the heterogeneity of ASD symptomatology. This alone forms a paramount challenge for all professionals who are involved in the current task force (for further details, see Part III). This is an encouraging endeavor, in the sense that the resolution seeks to collaborate with member states and stakeholders to strengthen national support and services to individuals with ASD.

Communication Skills, Challenges and Characteristics of Children With Autism Spectrum Disorder

Individuals with ASD form a heterogeneous group. Symptoms of onset are diverse and long-term outcomes vary from individual to individual. Although early symptomology and clinical characteristics of ASD are evident early in life (e.g., poor eye-gaze and lack of joint attention skills; Baron-Cohen, 1991; Lombardo et al., 2015; Pierce et al., 2016), the actual diagnosis comes much later. ASD impacts on the typical course of language development, affects social-emotional behaviors, hinders adaptive capacity and sensory modulation, affects typical play skills, and poses challenges for achieving life-long literacy and academic abilities. Specifically, challenges presented by individuals with ASD include social-pragmatic deficits such as low affect and poor eye contact, aberrant behaviors such as repetitive gestures, obsessive preferences and insistence on "sameness," difficulty in transition from one activity to the another, fixated obsession to details, poor sensory integration skills, circumscribed interest, and irregular sensory responsivity to name a few. In as much, communication skills in verbal children with ASD include echolalia; phonological errors; restricted semantic and syntactic skills, challenges, and lack of coherence in narrative ability; and deficits in using language for social and pragmatic purposes. Furthermore, since many individuals with ASD are nonverbal, communication goals are targeted via alternative and augmentative channels (for a review see Hus et al., 2021; Westby, 2014; Westerveld et al., 2021). Notwithstanding, in cases where individuals do use verbal language, the output is characterized by prosodic errors, phonological challenges, and speech patterns consistent with apraxia of speech (Health Resources & Services Administration, 2019; Hus et al., 2021; Paul, 1997; World Health Organization Resolution on ASD, 2019). On parallel lines, comorbid conditions are associated with cognitive, intellectual, and learning limitations including academic and literacy difficulties (APA, 2013; Levy et al., 2009).

Challenges in the Management of Individuals With Autism Spectrum Disorder From Multilingual and Multicultural Backgrounds

The management of individuals with ASD regarding diagnosis and service support is a complex issue. Many factors play a significant role in determining best clinical practices across the world. Despite challenges in the aforementioned context, there are also solutions and suggestions in alleviating difficulties as a result of lack of specially trained personnel and scarcity of available diagnostic batteries and tools appropriate for individuals who come from diverse language and cultural backgrounds. In a recent special issue report, Levy, Grech, Moonsamy, and Garcia de Goulart (2019) advocate for the special needs of such populations and underscore the importance of improving professionals' awareness of the needs of these populations. In addition, a number of internationally held projects provide suggestions and solutions that can be implemented when assessing multilingual individuals, including those with ASD. Approximately 12 million children in the United States speak more than one language (Bialystok, 2017). Children with ASD form no exception, in the sense that about one out of four children with ASD come from multilingual home environments (Wang et al., 2018). Such figures alone necessitate increased awareness of these factors among health professionals in an effort to provide these populations and their families with appropriate services. Despite a keen research interest and data output in the area of multilingual and multicultural aspects related to communication disorders, such information rarely reaches the mainstream clinicians (Law et al., 2019). In a recent paper, Grech (2019) discusses the particular challenges faced by speech-language pathologists who are working with multilingual and multicultural populations, with a special focus on immigrants. Constraints such as the lack of suitable assessment tools and language-specific diagnostic batteries might lead to misdiagnosis. Furthermore, scarcity of translators hinders adequate communication between clinician-patient and clinician-caregiver. In this context, clinicians who are faced with the challenging aspect of assessing and diagnosing children with complex communication needs, including ASD, need to adapt to the linguistic diversity observed by people who do present with adequate language proficiency in the resident country. American Speech-Language-Hearing Association (2008) highlights a number of beliefs and attitudes of speech-language pathologists working with diverse populations. These include a sense of "insecurity" and "reduced competence" in managing culturally and linguistically diverse populations, including individuals with ASD. Such shortcomings may stem from a lack of adequate training that clinicians receive during academic or clinical fellowship years, as well as may be due to a language barrier between clinician and patient. In the following sections the authors discuss the impact of bilingualism/multilingualism on language skills within the ASD context and provide suggestions on the management of these populations based on current research findings. Furthermore, the issue of cultural diversity is discussed, along with its impact and challenges when assessing individuals with ASD and addressing the person's family environment.

Theoretical and Empirical Aspects of Autism Spectrum Disorder—Bilingualism-Multilingualism-Multicultural

There is a widespread impression in Western societies that monolingualism is the norm, but in fact most people are bilinguals; that is, they grow up and function with more than one language or dialect (Grosjean & Li, 2013). It is estimated, for example, that about two-thirds of children in the world are raised in bilingual settings (Crystal, 1998). Bilingualism is expected to further rise due to globalization, increased population mobility, migration, the use of English as a *lingua franca*, and the adoption of bilingual policies in countries around the globe. European policy, for instance, considers language learning as a priority and aims for Europeans to master two additional languages and seeks to protect and promote minority languages (European Council, 2002).

Recently, research on how bilingualism affects language and nonverbal cognition in children has seen a steep increase, reflecting an awareness that findings with monolinguals might not apply to a substantial portion of the child population and that language and cognitive development possibly proceed differently in bilinguals (Barac et al., 2014). This growing body of work has revealed two groups of findings. First, some studies have linked bilingualism to a slower rate of language development (specifically, for some complex grammatical phenomena) and to lower language performance (e.g., slower lexical access, smaller vocabulary size), when each of bilinguals' languages is considered separately (Bialystok & Feng, 2009). This has been attributed to an "input deficit" rather than a developmental or cognitive problem, in that bilinguals have less experience with each of their languages compared to monolinguals because their language use is divided between two or more languages. Second, some research has reported bilingual advantages in aspects of nonverbal cognition, such as executive control (Antoniou et al., 2016; Bialystok, 2017) and theory of mind (Schroeder, 2018). Executive control (EC) refers to a set of cognitive processes that are thought to underlie flexible, goal-directed behavior (Miyake et al., 2000). There is no broad consensus on the structure of EC, but researchers most often assume three executive functions: *switching* (the ability to switch between tasks), *updating or working memory* (roughly, the ability to maintain and manipulate information in mind), and *inhibition* (the ability to inhibit irrelevant information). In addition, Theory of Mind (ToM) is a cognitive system that is responsible for attributing mental states (e.g., beliefs, intentions) to oneself and to others and for using them to understand other people's linguistic and nonverbal behavior (Baron-Cohen et al., 1985).

Against this background, researchers have also started to investigate how bilingualism interacts with common neurodevelopmental disorders such as ASD. Understanding cognitive development in bilingual children with ASD is an urgent societal priority in a predominantly bilingual world, especially given the increased prevalence of ASD (Elflein, 2020).

As mentioned earlier in the chapter, it has been claimed that individuals with ASD present consistent difficulties in pragmatic language use (e.g., Andrés-Roqueta & Katsos, 2017); that is, the use and interpretation of language in context (Taguchi et al., 2009). Moreover, ASD is often associated with various other cognitive impairments that are not considered core symptoms for diagnosis, including deficits in EC and ToM (Demetriou et al., 2018). EC impairments have been suggested to underlie the inflexible, stereotypical behavior and some of the social and communicative difficulties of children with ASD (Hill, 2004). Addressing this question is also even more urgent given the widely held, but not evidence-based, beliefs that children with ASD cannot develop and function bilingually and that learning an additional language might have further negative effects on the development of children who are already facing severe difficulties (Howard et al., 2020). As a result of these misconceptions, professionals working with children with ASD often advise parents to raise them monolingual (in the majority language) and children with ASD (and other developmental disorders) have limited access to bilingual education programs (e.g., they are less likely to enroll in such programs or in optional foreign language classes at school; Bird et al., 2016). This practice, however, deprives the child of the right to become bilingual, to effectively communicate in important contexts of everyday life (e.g., with family members who are not native speakers of the majority language), participate in an increasingly bilingual reality, and to benefit from a range of advantages associated to bilingualism, for instance, enhancing the opportunities for employment, travel, cross-cultural communication, and socialization in an increasingly mobile and globalized world. It further ignores some research (though controversial) suggesting that bilingualism confers cognitive benefits specifically in EC and ToM (e.g., Bialystok, 2017; Schroeder, 2018).

Research that has examined language and cognitive functioning in bilingual children with ASD has generally led to the conclusion that multilingualism does not impair development over and above the effects of disorder (e.g., Lund et al., 2017; Ulijaverić et al., 2016). To the contrary, there is some evidence (though still scarce and inconclusive) of bilingual advantages, particularly in nonverbal domains such as EC and ToM.

Studies that have compared ASD bilingual and monolingual children on the achievement of early language milestones and on aspects of core language development (vocabulary and grammar) have mostly focused on young, preschool-aged children and tested children in the majority language (usually English), which was not necessarily the bilinguals' L1 (Wang et al., 2018). These studies found mixed results, with some reporting no group differences and others reporting inconsistent effects that favored either monolingual or bilingual children. Ulijaverić et al. (2016), for example, reported that all studies in their review observed no group differences in various aspects of language (including presence of babbling and vocalization, age of first words and phrases, receptive total vocabulary, expressive vocabulary, and general receptive and expressive language), except one that found a bilingual advantage in a measure of expressive vocabulary. Based on their findings, they conclude that there is little evidence to support the widely held belief that bilingualism has negative effects on the linguistic development of bilingual children with ASD (or other developmental disorders). More recent reviews reach the same conclusion, reporting that, despite small and varied differences (some of which indicate a bilingual disadvantage and others a bilingual advantage), overall bilingual and monolingual children with ASD exhibit comparative language development (Lund et al., 2017; Wang et al., 2018). There is also some evidence that children with more experience in the language of testing (e.g., children who started learning their two languages from birth versus children who started learning the additional language a bit later) achieve better language outcomes (e.g., Gonzalez-Barrero & Nadig, 2019; Hambly & Fombonne, 2014). It is also important to note that many studies compared bilingual and monolingual children with ASD (rather than bilingual children with and without ASD) where a slower rate of development or lower performance in some aspects of language is actually expected to occur based on the research with typically developing bilingual and monolingual children. This fact further reinforces the conclusion that there is no reason to avoid raising a child with ASD with two languages because of fear that a bilingual experience is detrimental for language development.

Research that examined communicative or pragmatic aspects of language use is more limited but has generally revealed no differences between bilingual and monolingual children with ASD. Reetzke, Zou, Sheng, and Katsos (2015) compared bilingually exposed and monolingual Chinese-speaking children on the Children's Communication Checklist (CCC-2; Bishop, 2006), a parental rating scale that assesses aspects of structural language (speech, syntax, semantics, and coherence) and pragmatics (inappropriate initiation, scripted language, use of context, nonverbal communication). Their results showed no effect of the group in any of the CCC-2 scales and no effects of onset age of second language exposure or balanced exposure to two languages. Ohashi et al. (2012) examined functional communication (measured with Vineland Adaptive Behavior Scale-2, v-scale; Sparrow et al., 2005) and severity of ASD-related communication impairments (as measured by the Autism Diagnostic Observation Schedule) in bilingual-exposed and monolingual-exposed 2- to 3-year-old children. Moreover, Iarocci, Hutchison, and O'Toole (2017) compared the functional communication skills (measured with the functional communication scale of the Behavior Assessment System-2 for children and adolescents, Parent Rating Scales) of bilingual children with and without ASD, but in a wider age range (6 to 16 years). Both studies reported no group effects, suggesting that bilingualism in ASD is not associated with a delay in aspects of communication either as compared to ASD monolinguals or relative to typically developing bilinguals. With regards to ASD, Dosi and Sotiriadis (2020) concluded in their study that the "advantage" of bilingual children in cognitive and pragmatic abilities has a positive effect on ASD difficulties due to the equal support of the two languages. Finally, a recent study (Peristeri et al., 2020) investigated narrative production (among other skills) in bilingual and monolingual 7- to 12-year-old children with and without ASD (using the Edmonton Narrative Norms Instrument; Schneider et al., 2005). Results of this research revealed differences on various measures of storytelling; particularly, bilingual children achieved overall higher scores for story structure complexity, the use of mental-state terms, and subordinate and adverbial clauses, while monolingual children produced more complement clauses. For children with ASD specifically, again, most differences favored bilingual children (in adverbial clauses, story structure complexity, use of fewer ambiguous terms), while other effects favored monolinguals (complement clauses). Thus, overall, the few studies on communicative and pragmatic language use suggest that bilingual children with ASD are similar to monolinguals, with one study reporting a bilingual advantage in aspects of narrative production.

In recent years, a few studies have also investigated the effect of multilingualism on domains of nonverbal cognitive functioning, such as EC and ToM, in children with ASD. This research has provided some indications for positive effects of bilingualism, even though the evidence base is currently small and the findings have been so far mixed. A handful of studies that employed direct tests of EC reported a bilingual performance advantage in switching (Gonzalez-Barrero & Nadig, 2019; Peristeri et al., 2020) and working memory tasks (Andreou et al., 2020; Peristeri et al., 2020). However, other findings indicate no bilingual-monolingual differences in tests tapping into the same cognitive processes (Li et al., 2017; Peristeri et al., 2020). For inhibition, one study found a bilingual advantage (Li et al., 2017), but this benefit was evident in only one of three inhibition tests, and even for this task it was restricted to one of its two versions administered. Similarly, using parent-reported measures, one study found fewer EC problems for dual-language learners (Ratto et al., 2020), but again, other research reported no bilingual effects for similar outcomes (Gonzalez-Barrero & Nadig, 2019; Iarocci et al., 2017). These mixed results might be attributed to a range of methodological factors (e.g., the use of small sample sizes, the use of tasks that do not show convergent validity, the different characteristics of bilingual samples; for a discussion of these factors as related to neurotypical individuals, see Bialystok, 2017; Paap et al., 2015). However, overall the limited literature has been inconclusive as to the existence of a bilingual advantage in EC and its specific cognitive locus. Finally, to our knowledge, only two studies to date (with possibly overlapping samples) have investigated the effect of bilingualism on ToM in school-aged children with ASD (Andreou et al., 2020; Peristeri et al., 2020). Both studies reported that bilingualism boosts ToM skills, even though in Andreou et al. (2020) the advantage was detected in only one of two ToM tasks; specifically, the one that posed low verbal demands. Thus, in general, research on the cognitive effects of bilingualism in ASD has provided some evidence for positive effects on EC and ToM. However, given the limited research thus far (and the mixed findings especially for EC), it is premature to conclude that bilingualism confers any definite benefits on executive functions or ToM. It is nevertheless clear that bilingualism does not have any further detrimental effects on children with ASD's cognitive development.

Assessment in Autism Spectrum Disorder From a Multilingual and Multicultural Perspective

The promotion of awareness related to multilingual and multicultural aspects in ASD can contribute to the development of specialized assessment and accurate and sensitive diagnostic tools and protocols, with an additional focus on differential diagnosis (Hambly & Fombonne, 2014; Jordaan, 2008; McLeod & Verdon, 2017). On parallel lines, an equally significant focus should be on the establishment of interdisciplinary teams involved with each clinical case (e.g., speech-language pathologists, occupational therapists, special educators, social workers, psychiatrists, family counselors, teachers). Further to the aforementioned, members of the interdisciplinary team need to become aware of the individual's linguistic and cultural idiosyncrasies. Best practices for assessing multilingual children require multiple measures across time over a number of variables including vocabulary, phonological skills, grammatical competency, daily living skills, cognitive-linguistic status, pragmatic ability, etc. In a recently published thematic volume titled *The Many Facets of ASD in Children, Youth and Young Adults,* Hus, Segal, and Petinou (2021) address the diverse challenges of ASD, discuss the challenges of diversity across cultures, and share cross-linguistic research findings on topics including phonological intervention, autobiographical memory, reading skills, feeding and swallowing, prosodic processing, semantic processing, and narrative skills. This body of research along with relevant resources has been the product of an ongoing keen work of specialized professional teams and associations (i.e., ad hoc committees of the International Association of Communication Disorders and Sciences [IALP]) underscore the challenges faced by speech-language pathologists who are called to manage and service populations from diverse immigrant backgrounds and multilingual language status. Along these lines, published data associated with refugees and ethnic minority groups indicate that team collaborations and shared knowledge and sources adds to better service provisions (Levy et al., 2019). A number of international projects include the Crosslinguistic-Phonology Project (for details see Stemberger & Bernhardt, 2017), Literacy in South Africa (Moonsamy, 2019), and Collaboration with Families and Educators in increasing awareness on ASD in China (see Huang et al., 2013). Such endeavors provide information and resources for evaluating children who come from diverse language backgrounds and cultures.

Some General Comments on the Assessment Tools and Resources for Autism Spectrum Disorder From Diverse Backgrounds

Clinical management warrants early identification as the cornerstone for long-term prognostic outcomes. This framework will ultimately set intervention goals for the alleviation of aberrant symptomatology, always from the perspective of a multidisciplinary approach. Further to this, speech and language assessment processes should take into consideration linguistically and culturally appropriate communicative interactions that support the participation of children in everyday and special activities, including the family context dynamics (Gillon et al., 2017). Although research findings regarding the assessment of bilingual and multilingual children with ASD from diverse ethnic backgrounds await further exploration, available findings indicate more accurate diagnostic outcomes when services are provided in both the child's languages (Lang et al., 2011; Seung et al., 2006; Summers et al., 2017; Zhou et al., 2018). Research today indicates that exposure of a child in both languages offers a head start when it comes to adaptive functioning, social, and pragmatic communication, but most importantly allows the child to maintain important interaction with caregivers (in case the parents do not adequately speak the mainstream language; Frith, 2008; Prior & Roberts, 2012; Wang et al., 2018). Cross-cultural differences have been found in caregivers when they reported symptoms of ASD. Notably though, findings suggested that although manifestation of socialization and communication behaviors may be "more universal," identification of aberrant clinical markers associated with ASD may be more "culturally subjective," resulting in delayed identification (Matson et al., 2017). Language acquisition results from the active participation of the child. Language learning is not a passive process; on the contrary, language development is a dynamic process with all elements interacting in various ways as a function of chronological age (Petinou et al., 2021). Similarly, faster learning occurs when a child with linguistic challenges is actively involved in an event. In general, the more actively the child is involved, the better and more accurate the generalization to other linguistic and communicative contexts—suggesting that intervention should consist of participatory activities aimed at using a variety of language characters (Bencini & Valian, 2008). Interventions aim to advance the human rights of a child. Interventions for children with ASD are most often designed and used with the aim to help children develop new skills and/or reduce behaviors that are perceived to act as barriers to their learning and participation in home and community activities. Individuals with ASD vary widely in their profiles of strengths, support needs, and behavioral characteristics.

Specific Assessment Tools and Suggestions in the Context of Bilingual Multicultural Autism Spectrum Disorder

The abilities of children with ASD vary with heterogeneity usually constituting the rule than the exception. A paramount skill to assess, if possible, is the child's current cognitive and linguistic capacity. While some individuals with ASD present with typical cognitive skills, unfortunately, the majority exhibit restricted cognitive and speech output ability, which needs to be addressed during the diagnostic sessions (Paul, 1997; Paul & Roth, 2011; Richard, 1997). When examining cognitive skills of multilingual children with suspected ASD, research recommends the use of nonverbal tests such as the Raven's Coloured Progressive Matrices (Raven et al., 2004) or the Test of Nonverbal Intelligence (TONI; Brown et al., 2010) for children ages 6 years and above or the Primary Test of Nonverbal Intelligence (PTONI; Ehrler & McGhee, 2008). However, the implementation of such tools comes with caveats in the sense that some testing items might be less sensitive to cultural and/or linguistic biases. Caution is warranted when interpreting the results.

For linguistic assessment, resources do exist but there is a mixed picture regarding the implementation, ethnographic bias, evidence-based support, adaptation versus translation, validation, sensitivity, and specificity issues (Gillon et al., 2017; McLeod et al., 2012; Thandeka, 2019). Despite the concerns regarding the appropriateness of a certain tool, choices do exist, and resources are ample (for phonology see McLeod & Goldstein, 2012). Nowadays, there is a rich mix of cross-linguistic diagnostic clinical tools clinicians can use when called upon to examine a child with ASD who speaks a language other than English. When considered together, such tools in the form of checklists, parental questionnaires, and locally standardized tests (e.g., adaptation of available tests and their standardization on the bases of local norms) can provide the streamline for systematic use in many clinical settings (McLeod et al., 2012). Without this being an exhaustive list, such tools are presented in the section to follow as a function of specific language subsystem.

Expressive and Receptive Vocabulary

A widely used tool that has been standardized and adapted cross-linguistically includes the MacArthur-Bates CDI Words and Gestures (adapted in more than 30 languages; Fenson et al., 1994). This parentally reported list can be one of the first tools to measure expressive, receptive vocabulary, gestures, and the emergence of phrase combinations. The speech-language pathologist through the collateral help from a translator (in case caregivers do not speak the mainstream language) can assist the caregiver to complete this task (Sussman, 1999).

Phonological Skills

Numerous resources are available when it comes to addressing and assessing speech sound output and overall phonological skills. Clinicians need to be aware that during the assessment they might need to work with an interpreter and become familiar with the cultural and linguistic idiosyncrasies of the client, patient, or child. A significant resource to capitalize on comes from the keen effort and research output of the International Expert Panel on Multilingual Children's Speech (McLeod & Verdon, 2017). Suggestions include the examination of the child's early vocal motor schemes and phonetic inventory profiles (if existent; McLeod et al., 2012; McLeod & Goldstein, 2012) as well as the implementation of the international version of the "Intelligibility in Context Scale," which assesses the child's intelligibility in different communication contexts, including the home environment (McLeod et al., 2012; Petinou, 2021).

Narrative Skills

A significant resource database for assessing narrative skills in children across the world, including children with ASD, come for the "Global Tales" project within the auspices of the Child Language Committee (CLC) of the IALP. Seminal research output suggests that a standard probe of personal narrative question (available in several languages) can be used when examining 9- and 10-year-olds' skills on microstructure and macrostructure of language use (Westerveld et al., 2022). In addition, the Multilingual Assessment Instrument for Narratives (MAIN) can be implemented when analyzing language output in neurotypical and language impaired children ages 3 to 10 (Gagarina et al., 2012).

Clinical Markers/Observation Scales and Questionnaires

The most widely used instrument for the diagnosis and assessment of developmental levels and communication skills in ASD is the Autism Diagnostic Observation Schedule (ADOS-2, revised version; Gotham et al., 2007) with its use mainly limited to English-speaking populations. Its translation and adaptation in other languages are still at the initial stages. Nevertheless, its use can be adapted in other languages and cultures (Soto et al., 2015) without, of course, some caveats especially in areas related to cultural appropriateness and unique idiosyncrasies of the given language. Cultural and linguistic modifications are always needed when using tools with limited psychometric standardization data as per a certain language/cultural adaptation process. Soto et al. (2015) provides a list of diagnostic ASD screening tools in 10 languages in South Africa. A series of questionnaires address skills across different developmental age windows through parentally reported information in an effort to screen for early signs of ASD. Such tools include the Modified-Checklist for Autism in Toddlers (M-CHAT-R; Robins et al., 2001) and the Checklist for Autism in Toddlers (CHAT; Baron-Cohen et al., 2000) designed to target early and timely diagnosis as well as toddlers who might be at risk for ASD around the ages of 18 to 24 months. Carefully designed methodology for cross-cultural and cross-language adaptation of such tools remains a challenge to all researchers and clinicians. Notwithstanding, such tools can still be promising in examining children of all backgrounds. Further to the aforementioned is the Autism Spectrum Screening Questionnaire (ASSQ; Ehlers et al., 1999) for school-aged children ages 9 and above. Reportedly, ASSQ was found to adhere to validity and reliability, with good specificity and sensitivity indexes in clinical settings. Since then, the ASSQ has become one of the most widely used instruments for ASD assessment across the globe in different countries including Sweden, Norway, China, Denmark, Korea, and Estonia. Some of the items focus on "social interaction," six with "communication issues," five with "limited and repetitive behavior," and five with "motor clumsiness" and other related symptoms, such as "motor and vocal tics." Such instruments are currently going under a series of validity studies especially in understudied dialects including Cypriot Greek (Theodorou et al., 2022). Preliminary results remain promising in terms of specificity and sensitivity aspects which will allow the existence of an additional tool in assessing school-aged children who might be exhibiting ASD characteristics.

Conclusion

WHO (2019) underscores the importance of implementing integrated services in accordance with the person's individual needs and preferences. People with ASD do not differ from the rest of the population when it comes to health problems. Nevertheless, their special needs and co-occurring conditions necessitate awareness from politicians and ad hoc committees who can support the societal needs and the level of support in the effort to increase quality of life, access to services, family support, and availability to resources of best service provision according to the *Declaration of Human Rights* (United Nations, 1948). ASD is a lifelong condition requiring continuous management and support toward the afflicted individual and their family circle. When adding the factors of cultural diversity and multilingualism, ASD outcomes become less clear due to the fact that such issues are understudied. Moreover, resourcing diagnostic materials is even less accessible and nonexistent in many languages. Over the past 10 years, numerous research and clinical teams, organizations, and task forces related to ASD had research-based findings which translate to clinical context and inform evidence-based practice. Thus, health care professionals, educators, and stakeholders can capitalize on such findings and information in an effort to improve and support the lifelong challenges of individuals with ASD in the best possible way.

In this chapter, we presented recent advances regarding the characteristics and management of individuals with ASD, especially as they relate to multilingualism and multiculturalism. Multilingualism and multiculturalism are now the norm rather than exception in most countries around the globe, and their interaction with developmental disorders, and particularly ASD, presents clinicians and speech-language therapists with unique challenges. The chapter began by discussing the increased prevalence and symptomatology of ASD. Recent figures suggest that ASD may affect up to 2% or more of children worldwide. ASD is characterized by considerable heterogeneity, but affected individuals typically present social and pragmatic communicative deficits and often cognitive and language difficulties, which altogether might pose significant challenges to their everyday functioning as well as their literacy and academic attainment. Next, we presented the findings of recent research on the language, communicative, and cognitive development of multilingual children with ASD. This research shows that, contrary to common belief, children with ASD can develop bilingually and that growing up with more than one language does not add to the language, communicative, or cognitive difficulties that children with the disorder face in the course of development. To the contrary, there is some evidence (though still mixed and inconclusive) that bilingualism may have a positive effect on children with ASD's cognitive skills. In the final section, we focused on issues related to the assessment, diagnosis, and treatment of individuals with ASD in a clinical setting, especially as they relate to the linguistic and cultural idiosyncrasies of multilingual children. The authors underscore the need for an evidence-based clinical service (assessment, diagnosis, and intervention) provision to children with ASD, factoring in linguistic and cultural diversity as in the case of multilingual children. All the aforementioned issues underscore the pressing need for developing adequate policies and protocols for addressing multilingual and multicultural populations. According to Grech, "... diversity should be perceived as an opportunity for increased democracy, while equity should be considered a positive opportunity for a country's growth ..." (2019, p. 144).

Acknowledgments

The writing of this chapter has been supported by an award from the Cyprus Research and Innovation Foundation (CULTURE/AWARD-YR/0421B/0005) to the first and last authors.

References

American Psychiatric Association. (2013). *Diagnostic and statistical manual of mental disorders (DSM-5)*. American Psychiatric Pub. https://doi.org/10.1176/appi.books.9780890425596

American Speech-Language-Hearing Association. (2008). *Roles and responsibilities of speech-language pathologists in early intervention: Guidelines*. American Speech-Language-Hearing Association.

Andreou, M., Tsimpli, I. M., Durrleman, S., & Peristeri, E. (2020). Theory of mind, executive functions, and syntax in bilingual children with autism spectrum disorder. *Languages, 5*, 67.

Andrés-Roqueta, C., & Katsos, N. (2017). The contribution of grammar, vocabulary and theory of mind in pragmatic language competence in children with autistic spectrum disorders. *Frontiers in Psychology, 8*, 996.

Antoniou, K., Grohmann, K. K., Kambanaros, M., & Katsos, N. (2016). The effect of childhood bidialectalism and multilingualism on executive control. *Cognition, 149*, 18-30.

Barac, R., Bialystok, E., Castro, D. C., & Sanchez, M. (2014). The cognitive development of young bilingual children: A critical review. *Early Childhood Research Quarterly, 29*, 699-714.

Baron-Cohen, S. (1991). The development of a theory of mind in autism: Deviance and delay?. *Psychiatric Clinics, 14*(1), 33-51.

Baron-Cohen, S. (1995). *Mindblindness: An essay on autism and theory of mind*. MIT Press.

Baron-Cohen, S., Leslie, A. M., & Frith, U. (1985). Does the autistic child have a "theory of mind"? *Cognition, 21*(1), 37-46.

Baron-Cohen, S., Wheelwright, S., Cox, A., Baird, G., Charman, T., Swettenham, J., & Doehring, P. (2000). Early identification of autism by the Checklist for Autism in Toddlers (CHAT). *Journal of the Royal Society of Medicine, 93*(10), 521-525.

Bencini, G. M., & Valian, V. V. (2008). Abstract sentence representations in 3-year-olds: Evidence from language production and comprehension. *Journal of Memory and Language, 59*(1), 97-113.

Bialystok, E. (2017). The bilingual adaptation: How minds accommodate experience. *Psychological Bulletin, 143*, 233-262.

Bialystok, E., & Feng, X. (2009). Language proficiency and executive control in proactive interference: Evidence from monolingual and bilingual children and adults. *Brain and Language, 109*, 93-100.

Bishop, D. V. (2006). *CCC-2: Children's Communication Checklist-2*. Pearson.

Bird, E. K. R., Trudeau, N., & Sutton, A. (2016). Pulling it all together: The road to lasting bilingualism for children with developmental disabilities. *Journal of Communication Disorders, 63*, 63-78.

Brown, L., Sherbenou, R., & Johnsen, S. *Test of Nonverbal Intelligence-4*. (2010). Pearson Publications.

Centers for Disease Control and Prevention. *Launching on ASD*. https://www.cdc.gov/ncbddd/autism/index.html

Centers for Disease Control and Prevention. (2020). *Culture & health literacy: Tools for cross-cultural communication and language access can help organizations address health literacy and improve communication effectiveness*. https://www.cdc.gov/healthliteracy/culture.html.

Crystal, D. (1998). *Language play*. Penguin Books.

Demetriou, E. A., Lampit, A., Quintana, D. S., Naismith, S. L., Song, Y. J. C., Pye, J. E., Hickie, I., & Guastella, A. J. (2018). Autism spectrum disorders: A meta-analysis of executive function. *Molecular Psychiatry, 23*(5), 1198-1204.

Dosi, I., & Sotiriadis, S. (2020). Interventions for early language development in monolingual and bilingual children with autism spectrum disorders: Two case studies. *International Journal of Research, 9*(7), 1-11.

DuBay, M., Watson, L. R., Méndez, L. I., & Rojevic, C. (2021). Psychometric comparison of the English and Spanish Western-Hemisphere versions of the Modified Checklist for Autism in Toddlers-Revised. *Journal of Developmental and Behavioral Pediatrics*, 42(9), 717-725. doi:10.1097/DBP.0000000000000968

Ehlers, S., Gillberg, C., & Wing, L. (1999). A screening questionnaire for Asperger syndrome and other high-functioning autism spectrum disorders in school age children. *Journal of Autism and Developmental Disorders, 49*(2), 129-141.

Ehrler, D. J., & McGhee, R. L. (2008). *Primary-test of non-verbal intelligence* (PTONI). Pro-Ed.

Elflein, J. (2020). *Prevalence of autism spectrum disorder among children in select countries worldwide as of 2020*. Statista. https://www.statista.com/statistics/676354/autismrate-among-children-select-countries-worldwide/

European Council. (2002). *Barcelona European Council. Presidency Conclusions*. https://ec.europa.eu/commission/presscorner/detail/en/DOC_02_7

Fenson, L., Dale, P. S., Reznick, J. S., Bates, E., Thal, D. J., & Pethick, S. J. (1994). Variability in early communicative development. *Monographs of the Society for Research in Child Development, 59*, 1-173.

Frith, U. (2008). Weak central coherence. *Autism. A very short introduction.* Oxford University Press.

Gagarina, N., Klop, D., Kunnari, S., Tantele, K., Välimaa, T., & Balčiūnienė. (2012). Part I. MAIN: Multilingual Assessment Instrument for Narratives. *ZAS Papers in Linguistics, 56*, 1-139.

Gillon, G., Hyter, Y., Dreux F., Ferman S., Hus, Y., Petinou, K., Segal, O., Tumarova, T., Vogindroukas, I., Westby, C., & Westerveld, M. (2017). International survey of speech-language pathologists' practices in working with children with autism spectrum disorder (ASD). *Folia Phoniatrica et Logopedica, 69*, 8-19.

Gonzalez-Barrero, A. M., & Nadig, A. (2019). Brief report: Vocabulary and grammatical skills of bilingual children with autism spectrum disorders at school age. *Journal of Autism and Developmental Disorders, 49*, 3888-3897.

Gonzalez-Barrero, A. M., & Nadig, A. S. (2019). Can bilingualism mitigate set-shifting difficulties in children with autism spectrum disorders? *Child Development, 90*, 1043-1060.

Gotham, K., Risi, S., Pickles, A., et al. (2007). The Autism Diagnostic Observation Schedule: Revised algorithms for improved diagnostic validity. *Journal of Autism and Developmental Disorders, 37*, 613. https://doi.org/10.1007/s10803-006-0280-1

Grech, H. (2019). Impact of forced migration on communication and social adaptation. *Folia Phoniatrica et Logopaedica, 71*(4), 137-145.

Grosjean, F., & Li, P. (2013). *The psycholinguistics of bilingualism.* Wiley-Blackwell.

Guiberson, M., & Atkins, J. (2010). Speech-language pathologists' preparation, practices, and perspectives on serving culturally and linguistically diverse children. *Communication Disorders Quarterly, 33*(3), 169-180.

Hambly, C., & Fombonne, E. (2014). Factors influencing bilingual expressive vocabulary size in children with autism spectrum disorders. *Research in Autism Spectrum Disorders, 8*, 1079-1089.

Health Resources & Services Administration. (2019). *Health literacy.* https://www.hrsa.gov/about/organization/bureaus/ohe/health-literacy/index.html

Hill, C. E. (2004). *Helping skills: Facilitating exploration, insight, and action* (2nd ed.). American Psychological Association.

Howard, K., Gibson, J., & Katsos, N. (2020). Parental perceptions and decisions regarding maintaining bilingualism in autism. *Journal of Autism and Developmental Disorders, 51*, 179-192.

Huang A. X., Jia, M., & Wheeler, J. J. (2013). Children with autism in the People's Republic of China: Diagnosis, legal issues, and educational services. *Journal of Autism and Developmental Disorders, 43*(9), 1991-2001.

Hus, Y., Petinou, K., & Segal, O. (2021). The many facets of ASD in children, youth and adults. *Folia Phoniatrica et Logopedica, 73*(3), 161-163. doi:10.1159/000516048

Iarocci, G., Hutchison, S. M., & O'Toole, G. (2017). Second language exposure, functional communication, and executive function in children with and without autism spectrum disorder (ASD). *Journal of Autism and Developmental Disorders, 47*, 1818-1829.

Jordaan H. (2008). Clinical intervention for bilingual children: An international survey. *Folia Phoniatr Logop, 60*(2), 97-105. https://doi.org/10.1159/000114652

Lang, R., Rispoli, M., Sigafoos, J., Lancioni, G., Andrews, A., & Ortega, L. (2011). Effects of language of instruction on response accuracy and challenging behavior in a child with autism. *Journal of Behavioral Education, 20*(4), 252-259.

Law, J., McKean, C., Murphy, C. A., & Thordardottir, E. (Eds.). (2019). *Managing children with developmental language disorder: Theory and practice across Europe and beyond.* Routledge.

Levy, S., Grech, H., Moonsamy, S., & de Goulard. (2019). Special issue topic: Communication disorders associated with immigrants, refugees and ethnic minorities. *Folia Phoniatrica Et Logopaedica, 71*(2-3).

Levy, S. E., Mandell, D. S., & Schultz, R. T. (2009). Figure: Children reported to our study who first developed symptoms of Guillain-Barré syndrome or Fisher's syndrome. *Lancet, 374*, 2115-2201.

Li, H., Oi, M., Gondo, K., & Matsui, T. (2017). How does being bilingual influence children with autism in the aspect of executive functions and social and communication competence? *Journal of Brain Science, 47*, 21-49.

Lombardo, M. V., Pierce, K., Eyler, L. T., Barnes, C. C., Ahrens-Barbeau, C., Solso, S., & Courchesne, E. (2015). Different functional neural substrates for good and poor language outcome in autism. *Neuron, 86*, 567-577.

Lund, E. M., Kohlmeier, T. L., & Durán, L. K. (2017). Comparative language development in bilingual and monolingual children with autism spectrum disorder: A systematic review. *Journal of Early Intervention, 39*, 106-124.

Matson, J. L., Matheis, M., Burns, C. O., Esposito, G., Venuti, P., Pisula, E., Misiak, A., Kalyva, E., Tsakiris, V., Kamio, Y., Ishitobi, M., & Goldin, R. L. (2017). Examining cross-cultural differences in autism spectrum disorder: A multinational comparison from Greece, Italy, Japan, Poland, and the United States. *European Psychiatry, 42*, 70-76.

McLeod, S., & Goldstein, B. (2012). *Multilingual aspects of speech sound disorders in children*. Multilingual Matters.

McLeod, S., Harrison, L. J., & McCormack, J. (2012). The intelligibility in Context Scale: Validity and reliability of a subjective rating measure. *J Speech Lang Hear Res*. 55(2), 648-656. doi: 10.1044/1092-4388(2011/10-0130). Epub 2012 Jan 3. PMID: 22215036.

McLeod, S., & Verdon, S. (2017). Tutorial: Speech assessment for multilingual children who do not speak the same language(s) as the speech-language pathologist. *American Journal of Speech and Language Pathology, 26*(3), 691-1055. https://doi.org/10.1044/2017_AJSLP-15-0161

Miyake, A., Friedman, N. P., Emerson, M. J., Witzki, A. H., Howerter, A., & Wager, T. D. (2000). The unity and diversity of executive functions and their contributions to complex "frontal lobe" tasks: A latent variable analysis. *Cognitive Psychology, 41*(1), 49-100.

Moonsamy, S., & Carolus, S. (2019). Emergent literacy for children from marginalized populations. *Folia Phoniatrica et Logopedica, 71*, 57-59. https://doi.org/10.1159/000499421

Ohashi, J. K., Mirenda, P., Marinova-Todd, S., Hambly, C., Fombonne, E., Szatmari, P., & The Pathways in ASD Study Team. (2012). Comparing early language development in monolingual- and bilingual-exposed young children with autism spectrum disorders. *Research in Autism Spectrum Disorders, 6*, 890-897.

Paap, K. R., Johnson, H. A., & Sawi, O. (2015). Bilingual advantages in executive functioning either do not exist or are restricted to very specific and undetermined circumstances. *Cortex, 69*, 265-278.

Pappas, N. W., McLeod, S., McAllister, L., & McKinnon, D. H. (2008). Parental involvement in speech intervention: A national survey. *Clinical Linguistics & Phonetics, 22*(4-5), 335-344.

Paul, R. (1997). Communication and its development in autism spectrum disorders. In F. Volkmar (Ed.), *Autism and pervasive developmental disorders* (2nd ed., pp. 129-155). Cambridge University Press.

Paul, D., & Roth, F. P. (2011). Guiding principles and clinical applications for speech-language pathology practice in early intervention. *Language, Speech, and Hearing Services in Schools, 42*(3), 320-330. doi:10.1044/0161-1461(2010/09-0079)

Petinou, K. (2021). Promoting speech intelligibility in toddlers with Autism Spectrum Disorders, Special issue: "The many faces of ASD". *Folia Phoniatrica & Logopaedica, 73*(3), 174-184. https://doi.org/10.1159/000511346

Petinou, K., & Minaidou, D. (2017). Neurobiological bases of autism spectrum disorders and implications for early intervention: A brief overview. *Folia Phoniatrica et Logopaedica, 69*(1-2), 38-42.

Petinou, K., Taxitari, L., Phinikettos, I., & Theodorou, E. (2021). Interconnectedness and variability in toddlers. *Journal of Psycholinguistic Research*. https://doi.org/10.1077/s10936-020-09747-y

Peristeri, E., Baldimtsi, E., Andreou, M., & Tsimpli, I. M. (2020). The impact of bilingualism on the narrative ability and the executive functions of children with autism spectrum disorders. *Journal of Communication Disorders, 85*, 105999.

Pierce, K., Marinero, S., Hazin, R., McKenna, B., Barnes, C. C., & Malige, A. (2016). Eye-tracking reveals abnormal visual preference for geometric images as an early biomarker of an ASD subtype associated with increased symptom severity. *Biological Psychiatry, 79*(8), 657.

Prior, M., & Roberts, J. (2012). *Early intervention for children with autism spectrum disorders: Guidelines for good practice*. http://www. Dss.gov.au/our-responsibilities/disability-and-carers/program-services/for-people-with-disability/early-intervention-for-children-with-autism-spectrum-disorders-guidelines-for-good-practice-2012

Ratto, A. B., Potvin, D., Pallathra, A. A., Saldana, L., & Kenworthy, L. (2020). Parents report fewer executive functioning problems and repetitive behaviors in young dual-language speakers with autism. *Child Neuropsychology, 26*, 917-933.

Raven, J., Raven, J. C., & Court, J. H. (2004). *Manual for Raven's Progressive Matrices and Vocabulary Scales. Section 3: The Standard Progressive Matrices, including the Parallel and Plus versions*. Harcourt Assessment.

Reetzke, R., Zou, X., Sheng, L., & Katsos, N. (2015). Communicative development in bilingually exposed Chinese children with autism spectrum disorders. *Journal of Speech, Language and Hearing Research, 58*(3), 813-825.

Richard, G. J. (1997). *The source for autism*. LinguiSystems, Inc.

Robins, D. L., Fein, D., Barton, M. L., & Green, J. A. (2001). The Modified Checklist for Autism in Toddlers: An initial study investigating the early detection of autism and pervasive developmental disorders. *Journal of Autism and Developmental Disorders, 31*(2), 131-144.

Schneider, P., Dubé, R. V., & Hayward, D. (2005). *The Edmonton Narrative Norms Instrument.* http://www.rehabmed.ualberta.ca/spa/enni

Schroeder, S. R. (2018). Do bilinguals have an advantage in theory of mind? A meta-analysis. *Frontiers in Communication, 3*, 36.

Seung, H., Siddiqi, S., & Elder, J. H. (2006). Intervention outcomes of a bilingual child with autism. *Journal of Medical Speech-Language Pathology, 14*(1), 53-64.

Soto, S., Linas, K., Jacobstein, D., & Biel, M. (2015). A review of cultural adaptations of screening tools for autism spectrum disorders. *Autism, 19*(6), 646-661. https://doi.org/10.1177/1362361314541012

Sparrow, S. S., Cicchetti, D. V., & Balla, D. A. (2005). *Vineland Adaptive Behavior Scales* (2nd ed.). AGS Publishing.

Stemberger, J. P., & Bernhardt, B. M. (2017). Investigating typical and protracted phonological development across languages. In E. Babatsouli, D. Ingram, & N. Müller (Eds.), *Crosslinguistic encounters in language acquisition: Typical and atypical development* (pp. 71-108). Multilingual Matters.

Sussman, F. (1999). *More than words: Helping parents promote communication and social skills in children with autism spectrum disorder.* The Hanen Centre.

Summers, J., Shahrami, A., Cali, S., D'Mello, C., Kako, M., Palikucin-Reljin, A. & Lunsky, Y. (2017). Self-injury in autism spectrum disorder and intellectual disability: Exploring the role of reactivity to pain and sensory input. *Brain Sciences, 7*(11), 140.

Tager-Flusberg, H. (2016). Risk factors associated with language in autism spectrum disorder: Clues to underlying mechanisms. *Journal of Speech, Language, and Hearing Research, 59*(1), 143-154.

Taguchi, T., Magid, M., & Papi, M. (2009). The L2 Motivational Self System among Japanese, Chinese and Iranian Learners of English: A comparative study. In Z. Dornyei & E. Ushioda (Eds.), *Motivation, language identity and the L2 Self* (pp. 66-97). Multilingual Matters.

Thandeka, M. (2019). The cat on a hot tin roof? Critical considerations in multilingual language assessments. *South African Journal of Communication Disorders, 66*(1), 610.

Theodorou, E., Kitromilidou, M., Kyriakidou, S., Kaminaridou, E., Petinou, K., & Makris, C. (2022 submitted). A national survey evaluating routine behaviors and skills of primary school children in Cyprus: The use of the Autism Spectrum Screening Questionnaire (ASSQ). *PLoS ONE.*

Uljarević, M., Katsos, N., Hudry, K., & Gibson, J. L. (2016). Multilingualism and neurodevelopmental disorders: An overview of recent research and discussion of clinical implications. *Journal of Child Psychology and Psychiatry, 57*(11), 1205-1217.

United Nations. (1948). *Declaration of Human Rights.* General Assembly resolution 217A.

Wang, M., Jegathesan, T., Young, E., Huber, J., & Minhas, R. (2018). Raising children with autism spectrum disorders in monolingual vs bilingual homes: A scoping review. *Journal of Developmental & Behavioral Pediatrics, 39*, 434-446.

Westby, C. E. (2014). Social neuroscience and theory of mind. *Folia Phoniatrica et Logopaedica, 66*(1-2), 7-17.

Westerveld, M., Nelson, N., Khaloob., K., Kuvak., J., Theodorou, E., Petinou, K., et al. (2022). Global TALES feasibility study: Personal narratives in 10-year-old children around the world. *PLoS ONE.* PONE-D- 22-10735R1 31.

Westerveld, M., Paynter, J., & Adams, D. (2021). Brief report: Associations between autism characteristics, written and spoken communication skills, and social interaction skills in preschool-age children on the autism spectrum. *Journal of Autism and Developmental Disorders*, 1-6.

Wolff, J. J., & Piven, J. (2013). On the emergence of autism: Neuroimaging findings from birth to preschool. *Neuropsychiatry, 3*(2), 209.

World Health Organization. (2019). *International Classification of Diseases* (10th ed.). https://www.who.int/classifications/classification-of-diseases

World Health Organization. (2012). World Health Assembly resolution WHA67.8: Comprehensive and coordinated efforts for the Mayada et al. "Global prevalence of autism and other pervasive developmental disorders". *Autism Research,* 5(3), 160-179.

World Health Organization. (2019). *ASD fact sheet newsroom.* https://www.who.int/news-room/fact-sheets/detail/autism-spectrum-disorders

Zhou, B., Xu, Q., Li, H., Zhang, Y., Wang, Y., Rogers, S. J., & Xu, X. (2018). Effects of parent-implemented Early Start Denver Model intervention on Chinese toddlers with autism spectrum disorder: A non-randomized controlled trial. *Autism Research, 11*(4), 654-666.

Part V

ADULT LANGUAGE ASSESSMENT

Chapter 16

Assessment in Aphasia
Global Perspectives

Mira Goral, PhD, CCC-SLP
and Elizabeth E. Galletta, PhD, CCC-SLP

Introduction

In this chapter we review assessment practices for language and communication impairments associated with aphasia (an acquired language disorder) in multilingual people. We briefly define *aphasia* and *multilingualism*, and then review assessment tools in aphasia generally and those available for multiple languages. In the third section of the chapter, we suggest guidelines for good assessment practices with people who are multilingual, considering tools, procedures, and interpretation of performance.

Aphasia

Aphasia is a language disorder secondary to an acquired brain injury, most commonly due to stroke. In addition to stroke, other acquired brain injuries, such as traumatic brain injury, tumor, and neurologic disease, can also cause aphasia. In this chapter we focus primarily on post-stroke aphasia; the abbreviation PWA (people with aphasia) is used throughout this chapter.

Aphasia has historically been described as a result of focal brain damage to regions in the language-dominant hemisphere (left in most people), including cortical and subcortical areas, and/or damage to the white matter tracks connecting these regions (e.g., Fridriksson et al., 2018). More

Bortz, M. (Ed.). *A Guide to Global Language Assessment: A Lifespan Approach* (pp. 307-321).
DOI: 10.4324/9781003524472-21

recently, the importance of the white matter pathways has been a focus of discussions regarding aphasia etiology and prognosis (e.g., Fridriksson et al., 2018; Meier et al., 2020). In aphasia, oral language impairment can include oral expressive and/or auditory comprehension deficits. Both oral expressive and oral receptive language impairment may be evidenced in any of the linguistic domains of phonology, semantics, morphology, or syntax (with pragmatic skills often preserved). In addition, language impairment in the visual language domain may be evidenced in reading (*alexia*) and/or writing (*agraphia*); manual language (sign language) and gesture can also be affected.

Along with this impairment-focused aphasia definition, aphasia is defined from an activities and participation perspective. The A-FROM model, short for Living with Aphasia, Framework for Outcome Measurement (Kagan et al., 2008), promotes a framework for outcome measurement in aphasia and defines aphasia based on its linguistic limitations (e.g., severity of word-finding difficulty) as well as its effect on life participation (e.g., making a phone call). The A-FROM is based on the *International Classification of Functioning, Disability and Health*, a model updated by the World Health Organization (WHO; 2001) that defines a health condition at the level of impairment, as well as its effect on activities and participation. The A-FROM includes four domains: impairment, actual participation in life situations, environmental barriers or aids to communication, and characteristics of the PWA including feelings, emotions, and self-identity.

Although it is generally agreed that aphasia is not an intellectual deficit (e.g., aphasia.org), aphasia is sometimes referred to as a cognitive-linguistic disorder that can be defined based on the cognitive processes that underlie language use (Hillis & Newhart, 2008). Nonlinguistic executive function skills, often impaired post-stroke, can affect language and communication and therefore impact PWA, which is a basis for the cognitive-linguistic perspective on the definition of aphasia.

Multilingualism

More than half the world's population uses more than one language regularly and can be considered multilingual (e.g., Grosjean, 2013). This means that monolingualism, or the use of only one language, is almost the exception not the rule. The definitions of who bilingual and multilingual people are vary, as are the types of multilingualism. There are several areas, each on a continuum, by which multilingual people can be defined (we use the term *multilingual* to refer to both "bilingual"—those who use two languages—and those who use more than two languages), including age of acquisition, language proficiency, language typology, and language use.

- *Age of Acquisition:* Some multilingual people acquire all their languages from an early age (i.e., simultaneous or early multilinguals), others start with one language and later learn the other languages (sequential or late multilinguals). Multilingual people may learn their languages informally, by *immersion*, or *formally, as a foreign language.*
- *Language Proficiency:* Some individuals have equally high proficiency in two or more languages (balanced multilinguals), but many multilingual people have one language that is more dominant—of higher proficiency and/or more frequent use—than other languages (dominant multilinguals).
- *Language Typology:* Multilingual people use languages that are similar in their grammatical structures, pragmatics, and vocabulary, or have languages that are different in typology.
- *Language Use:* A person who uses more than one language in their daily life can be considered multilingual. Some people use their different languages in differing contexts (e.g., one language at home, another at work, another with certain family members), and some use multiple languages in the same context and often within the same conversations (e.g., a multilingual family in a multilingual society). Some people use only some modalities of a language (e.g., can only read and write; can speak and comprehend, but not read and write). People who use and are

exposed to more than one language may belong to multilingual communities or may be immersed in only one of these languages in their environment.

These variables are not independent of one another (e.g., typically high proficiency is associated with early age of acquisition and/or frequent language use) and are not static—multilinguals' language proficiency and use patterns change over time. People anywhere along these continua can be considered multilingual individuals.

The extent of cross-linguistic influences among the languages of multilingual people depends on the type of multilingualism and of the languages in question. Languages differ in their sound systems (e.g., English has an interdental fricative, such as in the word "there," French does not have this fricative), in their syntactic and morphosyntactic rules (e.g., word order, noun-verb agreement), in their semantic systems (e.g., the word "uncle" in English refers to both the brother of the mother and the brother of the father; in Arabic two different words are used: one for the brother of the mother and another for the brother of the father), and in pragmatic conventions (e.g., English does not distinguish polite versus casual registers for verb conjugation, Korean does). Cross-linguistic influences include transfer errors during language learning (e.g., a Spanish-speaking beginner learner of English produces the phrase "I have hunger" in English, transferring the structure of the expression in Spanish "tengo hambre"), lexical transfer or atypical use of lexical items (e.g., an English speaker uses the word "demonstration" in Spanish instead of "manifestation," thinking it means the same as street "demonstration"), or assuming a noun's gender based on the form in one language (e.g., an Italian speaker producing the Spanish word for *fork* as "la tenedor" in line with "la forchetta" in Italian, instead of using the correct Spanish determiner "el tenedor"), and transferring a pronunciation from one language to another (e.g., producing the cognate "student" in English as "estudent" in Spanish).

In addition, a hallmark feature of cross-linguistic influence is language mixing. Multilingual people who speak with other multilingual people often mix words and phrases from more than one language in an utterance and in a conversation. Language mixing has been studied extensively among multilingual people. Researchers have distinguished between code switching, referring to the change from one language to another between utterances, and code mixing, referring to the insertion of elements from more than one language within an utterance (e.g., Muysken, 2000). Psycholinguistic factors (such as the momentary inability to retrieve a word in one language) and sociolinguistic factors (such as choosing to include or exclude another speaker) have been implicated as reasons for language mixing (e.g., Walters, 2005). Language learners may mix due to a lack of proficiency in the target language whereas proficient users may mix as part of their language use patterns with no indication of difficulty. Different communities of speakers manifest greater or lesser incidence of language mixing and of types of mixing. Assessment of language and communication in multilingual people best considers these cross-linguistic phenomena.

Assessment of Aphasia in Monolingual and Multilingual People

Assessment in Aphasia

Aphasia assessment includes standardized and nonstandardized appraisal of all modalities of language: oral expressive, oral receptive, reading, writing, and manual/gesture.

Standardized Assessment

Several assessment batteries for aphasia have been published with information about standardized administration and scoring and with normative data. Two widely used standardized assessments in English in the United States are the Boston Diagnostic Aphasia Examination-3 (BDAE-3) and the Western Aphasia Battery-Revised (WAB-R), each assessing degree of impairment in oral expressive, oral receptive, reading, and writing skills. Similar batteries are commonly used in other countries, for example, in England clinicians use the Comprehensive Aphasia Test (CAT) and in Germany it is the Aachen Aphasia Test (AAT). In addition, tests designed to assess specific linguistic aspects, such as reading (e.g., the Reading Comprehension Battery for Aphasia [RCBA]), naming (e.g., the Boston Naming Test [BNT]), and verb production and comprehension (e.g., the Northwestern Assessment of Verbs and Sentences [NAVS]) are used.

To assess functional communication, clinicians use tools that consider the use of language and communication in the real world. The Communicative Abilities of Daily Living (CADL-3) is an individually administered assessment of communication ability and includes a variety of contexts. The American Speech-Language-Hearing Association Functional Assessment of Communication Skills for Adults (ASHA-FACS) is a rating where the clinician rates the PWA in four contexts: social communication, communication of basic needs, reading/writing/number concepts, and daily planning. Other patient-reported outcomes include the Aphasia Communication Outcome Measure (ACOM), where the patient self-reports communicative functioning; the Communicative Effectiveness Index (CETI), where the patient self-reports information related to their communication skills in a variety of contexts; as well as the aphasia-friendly Visual Analog Mood Scales. For a list of commonly used standardized aphasia instruments, see Table 16-1.

Nonstandardized Assessment

Nonstandardized impairment-focused assessments include the assessment of expressive and receptive language at the single word, sentence, and discourse levels. Single-word expressive language tasks typically include informal naming using visual confrontation naming and responsive naming, for example. Here, the clinician can show pictures of common objects such as a picture of a tool or of food items typical of the local environment and ask the individual to name the item depicted in the picture. Sentence-level expressive tasks include instructions to describe a picture or respond to a question with a one-sentence response (e.g., "What did you do before coming here today?"). Nonstandardized discourse tasks include elicited conversational discourse, pictured scene description, and procedural discourse tasks. For example, the examiner can elicit connected language by asking the individual with aphasia to talk about a recent event or to describe a common procedure, such as preparing a typical meal. Interviews and counseling may be considered as a part of nonstandardized methods of functional communication assessment.

Assessment in Multilingual Contexts

Standardized Assessment

Standardized tests for aphasia that have been developed in English as well as in other languages typically include norms from PWA who are monolingual users of the respective language. Several batteries and tests developed originally in English (or another language) have been adapted to additional languages, with a particular attention to language- and culture-specific aspects (Ballard et al., 2019; Ivanova & Hallowell, 2013). These include aphasia batteries such as the BDAE-3, which was adapted to several languages, including Greek and (an earlier BDAE version) Spanish, among other

Table 16-1
Assessment Instruments in Various Languages

BATTERY	LANGUAGE	REFERENCE
Boston Diagnostic Aphasia Examination (BDAE-3)	English	Goodglass et al. (2000)
	Greek	Tsapkini et al. (2010)
	Spanish	Rosselli et al. (1990)
Western Aphasia Battery (WAB-R)	English	Kertesz (2006)
	Korean	Kim & Na (2004)
	Bengali	Keshree et al. (2013)
Comprehensive Aphasia Test (CAT)	English	Swinburn et al. (2004)
	Norwegian	Fyndanis et al. (2017)
	Croatian	Kuvač Kraljević et al. (2020)
Aachen Aphasia Test (AAT)	German	Huber et al. (1983)
	Italian	Luzzatt et al.(1996)
	Dutch	Graetz et al. (1992)
	Portuguese	Lauterbach et al. (2008)
Communicative Abilities of Daily Living (CADL-3)	English	Holland et al. (2018)
American Speech-Language-Hearing Association Functional Assessment of Communication Skills for Adults (ASHA-FACS)	English	Frattali (1995)
Aphasia Communication Outcome Measure (ACOM)	English	Hula et al. (2015)
Communicative Effectiveness Index (CETI)	English	Lomas et al. (1989)
	Finnish	Rautakoski et al. (2008)
Visual Analog Mood Scales	English	Haley et al. (2015)
Psycholinguistic Assessments of Language Processing in Aphasia (PALPA)	English	Kay et al. (1992)
	Dutch	Bastiaanse et al. (1995)
	Spanish	Valle & Cuetos (1995)
	Hebrew	Gil & Edelstein (2001)
Reading Comprehension Battery for Aphasia (RCBA)	English	Lapointe & Horner (1998)
Boston Naming Test (BNT)	English	Kaplan et al. (2001)
	Spanish	Kaplan et al. (1986)
	Maltese	Grima & Franklin (2016)
	Greek	Patricacou et al. (2007)
Northwestern Assessment of Verbs and Sentences (NAVS)	English	Thompson (2012)
	Italian	Barbieri et al. (2019)

languages. The WAB original edition (Kertesz, 1982) was adapted to Korean and to Bengali, among other languages; the Psycholinguistic Assessments of Language Processing in Aphasia (PALPA) is available in multiple languages including English, Dutch, Spanish, and Hebrew.

The CAT, another aphasia battery based on the psycholinguistic approach, was developed in British English and has been adapted into multiple other languages (e.g., Norwegian, Dutch, Croatian) in a way that retains its psycholinguistic features (e.g., word frequency, word length). Other tests have been adapted into other languages, for example, the German AAT has versions in Italian, Dutch, and Portuguese, among other languages.

In addition, several of the aphasia tests designed to assess specific language abilities (e.g., reading, naming) have been adapted to various languages. For example, the RCBA, the BNT, and the NAVS have been adapted to languages such as Spanish and Italian. Of the functional communication assessment tools, the CETI has been adapted to multiple languages (e.g., Finnish; See Table 16-1.)

Despite the careful adaptation of several batteries and tests to multiple languages, it is often challenging to make such tests culturally appropriate to a variety of contexts (e.g., illiterate communities, Indigenous groups, highly multilingual people; see Penn & Armstrong, 2017). Moreover, when changes are made to accommodate linguistic and culturally specific characteristics of the target population, there is little evidence whether the different language versions of the same test are comparable in levels of difficulty, and there are no published norms from multilingual people with aphasia. Best practices for using standardized tests with multilingual patients are addressed below.

Nonstandardized Assessment

To circumvent some of the challenges associated with adapting standardized aphasia tests, nonstandardized forms of assessment for multilingual PWA are often used. These include a set of probes that are used to examine language production and comprehension abilities (but do not have normative data associated with them), specific tasks that were designed for the purpose of assessing efficacy of experimental treatment methods, and the elicitation of connected language production. Nonstandardized assessment requires little adaptation to the context of multilingualism, although language mixing is one factor that needs to be managed. Tests that are designed to determine treatment efficacy are typically experimental and are developed by researchers in the language in which the treatment is administered and for the population in question. One challenge here is to develop measures that can assess treatment benefits in the treated language as well as in the other, untreated languages of the multilingual patient.

Typically, the elicitation of semispontaneous connected language production is based on minimal prompts, such as giving a person a topic and asking them to talk about it (e.g., "Tell me about your stroke") or showing the person a picture or a picture sequence and asking them to tell the story depicted in the pictures (e.g., Lerman et al., 2019). These materials and prompts can be easily adapted to multiple languages, although attention should be paid to cultural considerations, including the use of culturally appropriate pictures (e.g., Norvik & Goral, 2021). The challenge here is the implementation of a careful, systematic analysis of the language produced. We turn next to some recommendations for best practices when assessing multilingual individuals with aphasia with standardized and nonstandardized assessments.

Guide to Clinicians and Clinical Researchers

In this section, we offer suggestions for assessment with multilingual people with aphasia. We review aspects of available materials, of conducting the testing session, working with interpreters, and making sense of the performance observed. See Table 16-2 for a summary checklist.

Materials

In the prior section on assessment, we listed several aphasia tests that are available in a variety of languages. A great deal of thought has often guided the adaptation of those tests to additional languages. Nevertheless, any normative data available for such tests are mainly from monolingual individuals. Therefore, even if the test is available in the relevant languages of a person with aphasia, the normative data are typically not applicable. Many clinicians opt for using the standardized tests available in the different languages, but are careful in interpreting the results. For example, examining performance qualitatively (e.g., which language tasks appeared difficult for the person) rather than quantitatively (e.g., calculating a severity score) may be best. Moreover, if the pre-stroke proficiency in a particular language was not high, severity measures such as the WAB-R will not simply reflect the aphasia severity but rather the post-stroke ability, combining pre-stroke lack of proficiency and stroke-related impairments (e.g., Lerman et al., 2020). Therefore, considering WAB-R in any language of multilingual PWA should be done cautiously as it may not reflect aphasia severity alone.

The Bilingual Aphasia Test (BAT; Paradis & Libben, 1987) is one aphasia test that was designed specifically with bilingualism in mind. It aims to offer comparable versions across multiple languages and to provide normative data from bilingual individuals (although normative data for speakers of more than two languages are unavailable). The BAT is now available (for free) in over 70 languages (https://www.mcgill.ca/linguistics/research/bat). Each version was constructed with highly specific guidelines, with a collaboration between Paradis and native speakers of the target new language. It can be used as a comprehensive assessment in multiple languages, with the caveats that some of its versions have been criticized for how the adaptation of specific items was done, and for the limited assessment of structures that do not exist in English, such as inflectional morphology.

One avenue for resolving the adaptation problem is to develop assessment tools that allow for language-specific features to be tested in each language, rather than attempting to translate and adapt an original version created in one language into additional languages (Bortz, 2023). This is an innovative approach, but its execution is proving challenging and is yet to be implemented. Finally, using nonstandardized measures, such as elicited language production, can be used in multiple languages; this will allow for natural language mixing, as discussed next.

Examiners and Language Mode

When providing assessment for multilingual people with aphasia, the concept of language mode needs to be considered. According to Grosjean (2001), multilingual individuals dynamically move along a continuum of greater or lesser activation of their languages. For example, when communicating in a monolingual sociolinguistic context with a person who knows only one of their languages, multilingual individuals will be in a relatively monolingual mode, whereas in a communication context with fellow speakers of the same languages, multilingual individuals will likely be closer to the completely multilingual end of the continuum, and all their languages will be active. A robust body

Table 16-2 Guide for Clinicians
GUIDE TO MULTILINGUAL ASSESSMENT: QUESTIONS TO CONSIDER
Materials
Is there an existing test in the language(s) of the PWA?
Is there a BAT version for the languages of the PWA?
How would qualitative information add to the quantitative scores?
Examiners
What languages are shared between the examiner and the PWA?
What is the examiner's experience working with interpreters?
Should each language be assessed by a different examiner?
Working With Interpreters
Should each language be assessed by a different examiner?
What should be discussed to ensure the examiner accurately conveys the PWA's actual responses?
What should be discussed in the debriefing with the interpreter?
Making Sense of Results
Who should code the PWA's responses?
How should responses that include language mixing be scored?
How should the language(s) used for therapy be determined?

of laboratory experiments provides evidence that all the languages of multilingual individuals are always active, such that words from all languages can be candidates for retrieval at any moment (Kroll et al., 2008). Such evidence suggests that no multilingual person is ever at the monolingual extreme of the language mode continuum. Nevertheless, factors such as the linguistic context, the interlocutors, and degree of language impairment in the case of aphasia, can all influence the extent to which one language will be more or less active than the others.

Monolingual Versus Multilingual Sessions and Examiners

For language assessment sessions with multilingual PWA, two main decisions need to be made prior to the assessment. These involve whether to assess one language at a time or multiple languages together, and if the former, whether or not the examiner should be a monolingual speaker or a multilingual person who shares the languages with the person with aphasia. For example, when assessing an isiZulu-Sesotho bilingual individual, assessment can be done in isiZulu only on day one and then in Sesotho only on day two, or in each language in two contiguous sessions on the same day. Moreover, a bilingual isiZulu-Sesotho examiner can administer the assessment in each language, or two different examiners—one a speaker of isiZulu and another of Sesotho—could administer the assessment in each language, respectively. Often, this latter decision is made based on practical considerations; in many communities, few if any clinicians share the full language repertoire of the person with aphasia, although the employment of interpreters can be a solution to this problem.

In the clinical setting, the patient may be best served by choosing one language for the initial assessment and then choosing the other language(s) for further assessment to best determine the pattern of linguistic strengths within each language. Moreover, if the person is evaluated in a country with one majority language, it may be possible to find a monolingual speaker of the majority language, but not for the other language(s) as the person who would evaluate the other (minority) language(s) will likely at the very least be a bilingual who knows the majority language, rather than a monolingual speaker of the minority language(s). This creates an asymmetric evaluation condition for the two languages. Perhaps the best practice then, is to have, to the extent possible, an examiner (a clinician or an interpreter) who shares the same multiple languages evaluate a multilingual speaker with aphasia.

If the decision is made to utilize a multilingual examiner, the next question then is the degree to which the evaluation should attempt to create a monolingual mode. That is, should the examiner only use the target language for the duration of the assessment of that language, or should the multilingual examiner foster a multilingual mode (e.g., by using more than one language in the testing interaction). A monolingual testing mode will allow for a more thorough investigation of the ability in each language, whereas a multilingual testing mode will allow for a better assessment of the overall communicative ability of the person with aphasia. And, often, a multilingual examination will likely foster language mixing, whereas a monolingual mode can minimize the opportunity for language mixing. The decision is thus between assessing communication in a relatively natural context versus a more structured evaluation of the abilities in each language separately. Allowing all languages as part of the assessment sessions is consistent with a translanguaging view of multilingualism (e.g., Garcia & Alvis, 2019). That is, accepting that multilingual individuals do not have separate "named" languages that might be mixed, rather, they use their one repertoire of their languages to communicate.

If the decision was made to assess each language separately (an approach that is inconsistent with translanguaging), additional decisions follow. One can assess the multiple languages in separate sessions administered sequentially on the same day or on different days. If multiple sessions (e.g., multiple baseline design) are administered, the order of the languages can be counter-balanced to avoid order and fatigue effects. Order should be considered, for example, because if multiple languages are assessed with comparable similar materials, "priming" from one language to another could occur. Using different sets of stimuli across multiple baselines is a potential solution for such priming effects (Borodkin et al., 2020).

Working With Interpreters

In the clinical setting there are competing priorities for the completion of best practice under the increased constraints of a limited timeframe. When the monolingual clinician does not speak the primary language(s) spoken by the person with aphasia, an interpreter is often used for the language assessment. Interpreters may be part of the session in-person, over the telephone, or via video-conferencing. When using telepractice with patients seen virtually, interpreters are increasingly not in-person with the patient but may be in-person with the evaluator. Since the clinical setting is an environment where patients are scheduled back-to-back, with assessment times generally ranging from 45 to 60 minutes, typically only one language is assessed at the initial clinical evaluation. With both the clinician and the interpreter in the assessment session, keeping a monolingual mode 100% of the time is basically impossible (as the clinician and the interpreter are likely to communicate in their shared language even if the interpreter communicates with the patient only in their shared language).

When a decision to assess one language at the initial session is made, there needs to be a method for selecting the language of assessment, because in most cases there is time for only one language to be assessed. One method to determine which language to assess at the initial evaluation is to ask during scheduling which language is spoken in the home environment. However, for some individuals multiple languages may be used at home, and given the dynamic nature of multilingualism, prior history of premorbid and current use of each language should be assessed to determine the best language for the initial assessment. Nevertheless, to the extent possible, all languages of the individual should be assessed. In the clinical setting, one language may be assessed at the initial evaluation with additional languages assessed during subsequent diagnostic therapy sessions.

Working with interpreters can be challenging. Several speech-language organizations provide best-practice guidelines for working with interpreters (e.g., the American Speech-Language-Hearing Association in the United States; Speech Pathology Australia in Australia; The Royal College of Speech and Language Therapists in the UK). These include numerous recommendations for conduct prior to the assessment, during the assessment, and after the assessment, where it is recommended that the evaluator spends time speaking with the interpreter to educate the interpreter (e.g., https://www.asha.org/practice-portal/professional-issues/collaborating-with-interpreters/). Depending on the work environment, the clinician may or may not be able to implement some of these recommendations. For example, it is generally recommended that family members do not serve as the interpreters (see Hyter & Salas-Provance, 2022, Chapter 8), but in many instances, if professional interpreters are not available, clinicians resort to using whoever may be available, including family members.

It is important to consider at the minimum a conversation with the interpreter regarding the assessment practices and the need to interpret specifically what the patient said rather than what the interpreter thinks the patient meant. Despite efforts to educate interpreters about the goal of assessment in aphasia and the impartial role of the examiner, successfully conveying these ideas is often challenging (e.g., Roger & Code, 2011). In the in-person setting, the evaluator and interpreter are seated across from the patient, where the interpreter should sit next to the evaluator in the ipsilateral space of the patient's lesion. In the virtual setting, the interpreter's location on the screen is difficult to manage, yet if possible, the interpreter should be in the ipsilateral space virtually, as well (Figure 16-1). In all assessments, the clinician will direct the evaluation. The clinician should conference with the interpreter regarding all aspects of the test administration, including the use of cueing. For example, semantic cueing from the clinician (e.g., "it is a fruit") can more easily be translated than phonemic cues (e.g., "it starts with /b/), and so the management of these cues needs to be considered prior to the assessment. Phonemic cues, such as in the administration of the BNT, can only be provided by an interpreter who understands the assessment process, since the evaluator does not know the form of the targets in the language of assessment and would therefore not know the appropriate phonemic cues.

Interpreting the Results

Similar to the pre-evaluation conference with the interpreter, the clinician speaks to the interpreter after the evaluation. These may be short exchanges, yet this information may be crucial to be able to provide an accurate representation of language and communication strengths and challenges in the language assessed. Here the therapist can ask the interpreter for clarification of responses, if needed; this may help the clinician score a section using the interpreter's knowledge of the language assessed. As mentioned previously, when using versions of standardized tests, scores can be obtained for each language but normative data can be largely ignored.

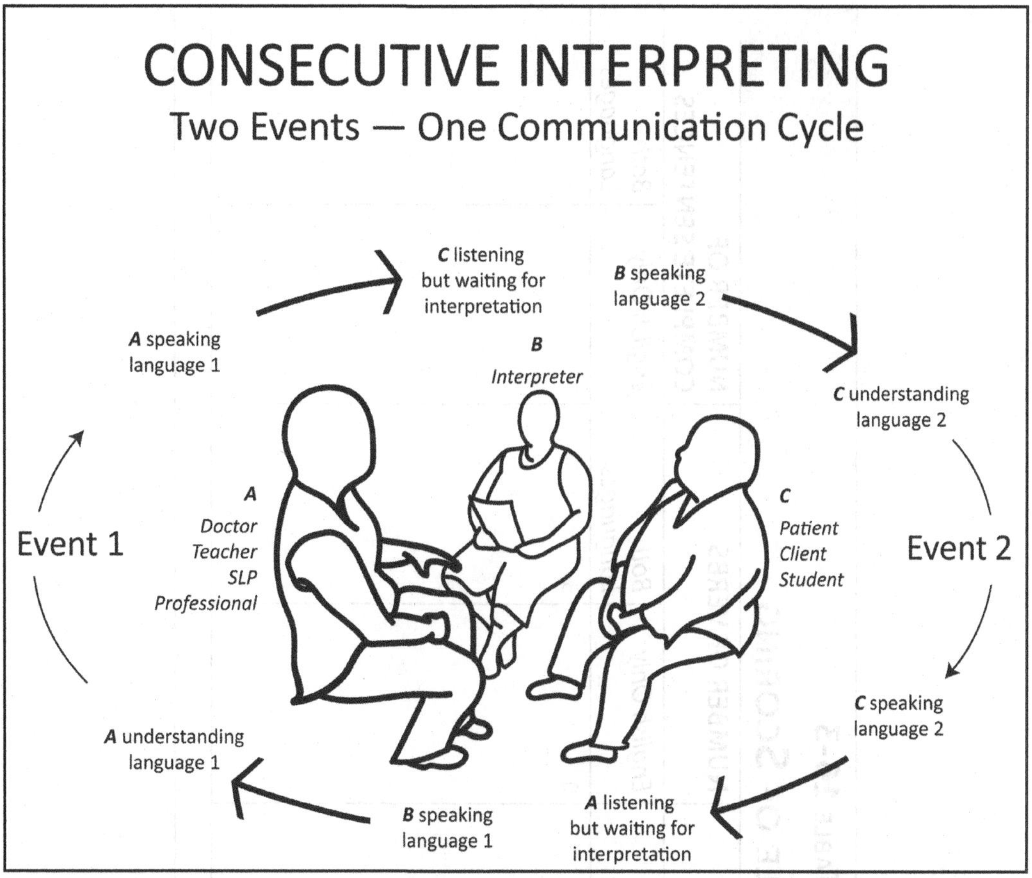

Figure 16-1. Consecutive interpreting. (From *Culturally Responsive Practices in Speech, Language, and Hearing Sciences, Second Edition* [pp. 1-448] by Hyter, Y. D., & Salas-Provance, M. Copyright © 2023. Plural Publishing, Inc. All rights reserved. Used with permission.)

Whether working with an interpreter or not, one challenge for scoring the assessment results with multilingual PWA is the presence of language mixing. When each language is tested separately, accurate responses in the target language may be counted more easily if the goal is to determine the person's abilities in each language. Alternatively, accurate responses in whichever language the person used may be counted as correct responses, for a more global picture of their language and communication abilities (Table 16-3). It may be useful to generate multiple scores: one for each language, and one regardless of language targeted (translanguage). This approach has been used in studies with multilingual children, for example, when counting "conceptual naming" rather than the vocabulary scores in each language (e.g., Peña et al., 2016). We note that sometimes determining the language in which the person answered is straightforward; in some instances, however, when a cognate word is produced with an accent, it is difficult to determine whether the response was produced in the target or the nontarget language. Within a translanguaging approach to assessment, responses regardless of language would be counted toward an overall communication success (Otheguy et al., 2015). Language mixing will likely depend on the context of the testing and the examiners, as mentioned previously (e.g., Grosjean, 2001). For example, the speech-language therapist may instruct the patient to use only one language or any of their languages throughout the evaluation session.

Table 16-3
Example of Scoring

NARRATIVE EXCERPT	TARGET LANGUAGE	NUMBER OF WORDS		NUMBER OF VERBS		NUMBER OF COMPLETE SENTENCES	
		English Only	*Both Languages*	*English Only*	*Both Languages*	*English Only*	*Both Languages*
And nine-eleven. **Ve ishti** call me. Eh eh eh **matos nasa ve** house **ve nasa 19ee in** house **19ee in** house. **Ve televizia ba bikor. Televizia ba bikor sheli eh ve matos nasa 20ee in** house **20ee in** house.	English	10	35	0	3	0	3

*Bold grey font=Hebrew words; black font=English words.

Language mixing may be particularly common during elicited connected language production tasks. Several variables that have been reported in the literature can be used to assess fluency, efficiency, and the content and the form of the language produced. For example, the Quantitative Production Analysis (QPA; Berndt et al., 2000) offers guidelines to examine use of lexical, grammatical, and morphological components, another measure often used is the Correct Information Unit analyses (CIU; Nicholas & Brookshire, 1993). For CIUs, a decision can be made to count only content units in the target language or in any language. For best practice, multilingual speakers of the languages of the person assessed would perform such analyses, to avoid any misinterpretation of cross-linguistic influences in the output produced.

Conclusion

In this chapter, we reviewed existing assessment tools for aphasia, including options available for a variety of languages. We highlighted procedure-related aspects that need to be considered when assessing multilingual people with aphasia, acknowledging challenges associated with choosing the languages examined, working with interpreters, and understanding the results. We brought up possible solutions for the lack of normative data for assessment of multilingual individuals and the possibility of evaluating one language at a time or embracing a translanguaging approach to assessing aphasia in multilinguals.

References

Ballard, E., Charters, H., & Taumoefolau, M. (2019). A guide to designing a naming test for an under-researched bilingual population: Adapting the Boston Naming Test to Tongan. *Clinical Linguistics & Phonetics, 33*, 376-392.

Barbieri, E., Brambilla, I., Thompson, C., & Luzzatti, C. (2019). Verb and sentence processing patterns in healthy Italian participants: Insight from the Northwestern Assessment of Verbs and Sentences (NAVS). *Journal of Communication Disorders, 79*, 58-75.

Bastiaanse, R., Bosje, M., & Visch-Brink, E. (1995). *PALPA: De Nederlandse Versie.* Lawrence Erlbaum Associates.

Berndt, R., Wayland, S., Rochon, E., Saffran, E., & Schwartz, M. (2000). *Quantitative production analysis: A training manual for the analysis of aphasic sentence production.* Psychology Press.

Borodkin, K., Goral, M., & Kempler, D. (2020). Measuring performance stability in persons with aphasia: identical versus comparable testing forms. *Aphasiology, 34*, 376-390.

Bortz, M.A. (2023). Tasks for assessing language in Africa: The passive construction. *Handbook of Communication Disabilities and Language Development in Sub-Saharan Africa.* Springer Publications.

Frattali, C. (1995). *Functional Assessment of Communication Skills for Adults (ASHA FACS).* American Speech Language Hearing Association.

Fridriksson, J., den Ouden, D., Hillis, A. E., Hickok, G., Rorden, C., Basilakos, A., Yourganov, G., & Bonilha, L. (2018). Anatomy of aphasia revisited. *Brain, 141*(3), 848-862. https://doi.org/10.1093/brain/awx363

Fyndanis, V., Lind, M., Varlokosta, S., Kambanaros, M., Soroli, E., Ceder, K., Grohmann, K. K., Rofes, A., Simonsen, H. G., Bjekic, J., Gavarro, A., Kuvac Kraljevic, J., Martinez-Ferreiro, S., Munarriz, A., Pourquie, M., Vuksanovic, J., Zakarias, L., & Howard, D. (2017). Cross-linguistic adaptations of the Comprehensive Aphasia Test: Challenges and solutions. *Clinical Linguistics and Phonetics, 31* (7-9), 697-710.

Garcia, O., & Alvis, J. (2019). The decoloniality of language and translanguaging: Latinx knowledge-production. *Journal of Postcolonial Linguistics, 1*, 26-40.

Gil, M., & Edelstein, C. (2001). *Hebrew Version of the PALPA.* Loewenstein Hospital Rehabilitation Centre.

Goodglass, H., Kaplan, E., & Barresi, B. (2000). *The Boston Diagnostic Aphasia Examination.* Lippincott.

Graetz, P., De Bleser, R., & Willmes, K. (1992). *Akense Afasie Test.* Nederlandstalige Versie (Swets and Zeitlinger).

Grima, R., & Franklin, S. (2016) A Maltese adaptation of the Boston Naming Test: A shortened version. *Clinical Linguistics & Phonetics, 30*(11), 871-887.

Grosjean, F. (2001). The bilingual's language modes. In J. Nicol (Ed.), *One mind, two languages: Bilingual language processing* (pp. 1-22). Blackwell.

Grosjean, F. (2013). Bilingualism: A short introduction. In F. Grosjean & P. Li (Eds.), *The psycholinguistics of Bilingualism* (pp. 5-26). Wiley-Blackwell.

Haley, K., Womack, J. L., Harmon, T., & Williams, S. W. (2015). Visual analog rating of mood by people with aphasia. *Topics in Stroke Rehabilitation, 22*(4), 239-245.

Hillis, A., & Newhart, M. (2008). Cognitive neuropsychological approaches to treatment of language disorders: Introduction. In: R. Chapey (Ed.), *Language intervention strategies in aphasia and related neurogenic communication disorders.* Wolters Kluwer.

Holland, A. L., Fromm, D., & Woznial, L. (2018). *Communicative Abilities in Daily Living-3.* Pro-Ed.

Huber, W., Poeck, K., Weniger, D., & Willmes, K. (1983). *Aachener Aphasie test (AAT), Protokollheft und handanweisung.* Göttingen, Germany, Hogrefe.

Hula, W. D., Doyle, P. J., Stone, C. A., Hula, S. N. A., Kellough, S., Wambaugh, J. L., Ross, K. B., Schumacher, J. G., & St. Jacque, A. (2015). The Aphasia Communication Outcome Measure (ACOM): Dimensionality, item bank calibration, and initial validation. *Journal of Speech, Language, and Hearing Research, 58*, 906-919.

Hyter, Y., & Salas-Provance, M. (2022). *Culturally responsive practices in speech, language, and hearing sciences* (2nd ed.). Plural Publishing.

Ivanova, M. V., & Hallowell, B. (2013). A tutorial on aphasia test development in any language: Key substantive and psychometric considerations. *Aphasiology, 27*(8), 891-920.

Kagan, A., Simmons-Mackie, N., Rowland, A., Huijbregts, M., Shumway, E., McEwen, S., Threats, T., & Sharp, S. (2008). Counting what counts: A framework for capturing real life outcomes of aphasia intervention. *Aphasiology, 22*(3), 258-280.

Kaplan, E., Goodglass, H., & Weintraub, S. (2001). *Boston Naming Test* (2nd ed.). Pro-Ed.

Kaplan, E., Goodglass, H., & Weintraub, S. (1986). *Test de Vocabulario de Boston.* Panamericana.

Kay, J., Lesser, R., & Coltheart, M. (1992). *PALPA: Psycholinguistic Assessments of Language Processing in Aphasia.* Erlbaum.

Kertesz, A. (1982). *Western Aphasia Battery.* Grune & Stratton.

Kertesz, A. (2006). *Western Aphasia Battery-Revised test manual.* The Psychological Corporation.

Keshree, N. K., Kumar, S., Basu, S., Chakrabarty, M., & Kishore, T. (2013). Adaptation of the Western Aphasia Battery in Bangla. *Psychology of Language and Communication, 17*(2),189-201. https://doi.org/10.2478/plc-2013-0012

Kim, H. & Na, D. L. (2004). Normative data on the Korean version of the Western Aphasia Battery. *Journal of Clinical Experimental Neuropsychology, 26*(8), 1011-1020. https://doi.org/10.1080/13803390490515397

Kroll, J. F., Bobb, S. C., Misra, M., & Guo, T. (2008). Language selection in bilingual speech: Evidence for inhibitory processes. *Acta Psychologica 128*, 416-430. http://dx.doi.org/10.1016/j.actpsy.2008.02.001

Kuvač Kraljević, J., Matić, A., & Lice, K. (2020). Putting the CAT-HR out: Key properties and specificities. *Aphasiology, 34*(7), 820-839. https://doi.org/10.1080/02687038.2019.1650160

Lapointe, L. L., & Horner, J. (1998). *Reading Comprehension Battery for Aphasia-2.* Pro-Ed.

Lauterbach, M., Martins, I. P., Garcia, P., Cabeça, J., Ferreira, A. C., & Willmes, K. (2008). Cross linguistic aphasia testing: the Portuguese version of the Aachen Aphasia Test (AAT). *Journal of the International Neuropsychological Society: JINS, 14*(6), 1046-1056.

Lerman, A., Edmonds, L., & Goral, M. (2019). Cross-language generalisation in bilingual aphasia: What are we missing when we do not analyse discourse? *Aphasiology, 33*(9), 1154-1162.

Lerman, A., Goral, M. & Obler, L. K. (2020). The complex relationship between pre-stroke and post-stroke language abilities in multilingual individuals with aphasia. *Aphasiology, 34*(11), 1319-1340. https://doi.org/10.1080/02687038.2019.1673303

Lomas, J., Pickard, L., Bester, S., Elbard, H., Finlayson, A., & Zoghaib, C. (1989). The Communicative Effectiveness Index. Development and psychometric evaluation of a functional communicative measure for adult aphasia. *Journal of Speech and Hearing Disorders, 54*(1), 113-124. https://doi.org/10.1044/jshd.5401.113

Luzzatti, C., Willmes, K., & De Bleser, R. (1996). *Aachener Aphasie Test: versione Italiana.* Organizzazioni Speciali.

Meier, E., Breining, B., Sheppard, S., Goldberg, E., Tippet, D., Tsapkini, K., Faria, A., & Hillis, A. (2020). White matter hyperintensities contribute to language deficits in Primary Progressive Aphasia. *Cognitive and Behavioral Neurology, 33*, 179-191.

Muysken, P. (2000). *Bilingual speech: A typology of code-mixing.* Cambridge University Press.

Nicholas, L. E., & Brookshire, R. H. (1993). A system for quantifying the informativeness and efficiency of the connected speech of adults with aphasia. *Journal of Speech and Hearing Research, 36,* 338-350.

Norvik, M., & Goral, M. (2021). Assessment challenges in acquired aphasia in multilingual individuals. In R. Blackwood & U. Røyneland (Eds.), *Multilingualism across the lifespan* (1st ed., pp.189-208). Routledge. https://doi.org/10.4324/9781003125815

Otheguy, R., García, O., & Reid, W. (2015). Clarifying translanguaging and deconstructing named languages: A perspective from linguistics. *Applied Linguistics Review 6*(3), 281-307.

Paradis, M., & Libben, G. (1987). *The assessment of bilingual aphasia.* Lawrence Erlbaum Associates.

Patricacou, A., Psallida, E., Pring, T., & Dipper, L. (2007) The Boston Naming Test in Greek: Normative data and the effects of age and education on naming. *Aphasiology, 21*(12), 1157-1170.

Peña, E. D., Bedore, L. M., & Kester, E. S. (2016). Assessment of language impairment in bilingual children using semantic tasks: Two languages classify better than one. *International Journal of Language & Communication Disorders, 51*(2), 192-202.

Penn, C., & Armstrong, E. (2017). Intercultural aphasia: New models of understanding for indigenous populations. *Aphasiology, 31*(5), 563-594.

Rautakoski, P., Korpijaakko Huuhka, A.-M., & Klippi, A. (2008). People with severe and moderate aphasia and their partners as estimators of communicative skills: A client-centred evaluation. *Aphasiology, 22*(12), 1269-1293. https://doi.org/10.1080/02687030802374788

Roger, P., & Code, C. (2011). Lost in translation? Issues of content validity in interpreter-mediated aphasia assessments. *International Journal of Speech Language Pathology, 13*(1), 61-73.

Rosselli, M., Ardila, A., Florez, A., & Castro, C. (1990). Normative data on the Boston Diagnostic Aphasia Examination in a Spanish-speaking population. *Journal of Clinical and Experimental Neuropsychology, 12*(2), 313-322. https://doi.org/10.1080/01688639008400977

Swinburn, K., Porter, G., & Howard, D. (2004). *Comprehensive Aphasia Test.* Routledge/Psychology Press.

Thompson, C. K. (2012). *Northwestern Assessment of Verbs and Sentences (NAVS).* Northwestern University.

Tsapkini, K., Vlahou, C. H., & Potagas, C. (2010). Adaptation and validation of standardized aphasia tests in different languages: Lessons from the Boston Diagnostic Aphasia Examination—Short Form in Greek. *Behavioural Neurology, 22*(3-4), 111-119. https://doi.org/10.3233/ben-2009-0256

Valle, F., & Cuetos, F. (1995). *EPLA: Evaluacion del procesamiento linguistic en la afasia.* Lawrence Erlbaum Associates.

Walters, J. (2005). *Bilingualism: The sociopragmatic-psycholinguistic interface.* Erlbaum.

World Health Organization. (2001). *International classification of functioning, disability and health.* Author.

Chapter 17

Neuropsychological Assessment in Dementia for Global Populations

Avanthi Paplikar, PhD, SLP; Aparna Venugopal, MSc, SLP; and Suvarna Alladi, DM Neurology

Introduction

Dementia is a common public health problem (Prince et al., 2015). Globally, 50 million people are living with dementia (World Health Organization [WHO], 2018) and approximately 60% of them are from a majority world. According to World Alzheimer Report, East Asia is the region with the most people living with dementia (9.8 million), followed by Western Europe (7.4 million), South Asia (5.1 million), and North America (4.8 million). The prevalence of dementia is expected to increase to 63% in 2030 and 68% in 2050 in the majority world (Prince et al., 2015) due to the highest growing older adult population (Ferri et al., 2005). One of the most common challenges in diagnosing dementia is low awareness in many majority-world societies. The majority of the patients being diagnosed in health care settings are in severe or advanced stages of cognitive impairment due to fewer specialised services for dementia diagnosis and management (Alladi & Hachinski, 2018). There is an added scarcity in experienced personnel and resources to provide diagnosis and care services to patients with cognitive disorders. Currently, due to low awareness and lack of skilled professionals in health care settings, more than 50% of those individuals with cognitive impairment are not being diagnosed globally (Prince et al., 2015). Hence, there is a need to improve diagnostic rates for dementia to institute management strategies and reduce burden of disease.

Bortz, M. (Ed.). *A Guide to Global Language Assessment: A Lifespan Approach* (pp. 323-354).
DOI: 10.4324/9781003524472-22

According to criteria from the *Diagnostic and Statistical Manual of Mental Disorders, Fifth Edition* (DSM-5), neurocognitive disorders should have significant impairment in cognitive performance based on standardized multi-domain neuropsychological testing and loss of independence in daily living (American Psychiatric Association [APA], 2013). Information obtained from neuropsychological assessment is important for (Alladi & Hachinski, 2018; Harvey, 2022): diagnostic formulation for detection of Alzheimer's disease and other related dementias (ADRD), systematic profiling of cognitive domains, differential diagnosis between dementia subtypes (Artero et al., 2003; Johnstone et al., 2002), distinguishing between age-related cognitive decline from other psychiatric disturbances like depression and anxiety disorder (Hodges et al., 1999; Libon et al., 2009), monitoring course of the disease, and measurement of functional potential, recovery, and treatment response.

Use of cognitive tests toward diagnosis of cognitive impairment in clinical settings poses a series of challenges in global populations:

1. Cognitive tests are developed mainly for the English-speaking Western population, which might not factor into the various sociodemographic factors (such as education, linguistic diversity, culture, etc.) that characterize societies across the world
2. Normative data for cognitive tests for a certain sociodemographic group/society might be unavailable
3. There remains a challenge in standardization and harmonization of the available cognitive tests or development of educationally fair and culture-free tests

Dementia diagnosis in societies characterized by linguistic, educational, and sociocultural heterogeneity is challenging. Most sociodemographically diverse societies have multiple spoken languages that are structurally diverse in terms of phonology, grammar, lexicon, and scripts. Neuropsychological evaluation in these linguistically diverse societies should have adapted tests in the target language to detect language difficulties. Culture also plays a key role in the development of cognitive stimuli based on semantic concepts (food, lifestyle, tools, clothing, etc.). Evidence suggests that variations in culture, values, experiences, and cognitive styles of the population with respect to which the test is primarily developed and standardized can impact cognitive test performance (Arnold et al., 1994; Flores et al., 2017). Due to differences in sociocultural characteristics, normative data developed in one country cannot be generalized to another. Hence, tests that are culturally relevant should be used for diagnosis of cognitive impairment. Furthermore, nearly half of the world's population is bilingual (Edwards et al., 2013). There is also evidence suggesting bilingualism influences language and cognitive processing. Bilingualism should therefore be considered as an important sociodemographic factor during neuropsychological testing in patients with cognitive impairment.

Low education levels and illiteracy exist in the majority world, which complicates the adaptation and development of cognitive tests. While neuropsychological tests adapted for low literacy are available in many countries, assessment of individuals with low education but complex occupations with superior expertise in complex-intricate skills (such as craftsmen, weavers, etc.) are not available. They need to be assessed with appropriate tests that are not just adapted to low education, but also tap into the complex cognitive domains such as perceptual motor and visuospatial skills. It is a challenge to accomplish translations of existing standardized tests, adapting tests for cultural relevance, or development of new tests that are educationally, culturally, and linguistically appropriate.

Neuropsychological testing is typically carried out using paper-pencil methods. However, the COVID-19 pandemic has accelerated the use of telemedicine and telerehabilitation for diagnosis and management of persons with dementia. The benefits of the digitization approach are that a standardized approach toward cognitive test administration without the clinician's influence leads to highly reliable data. There are, however, a few concerns that are encountered while using modern technology: certain geographic locations and socioeconomic groups may not have access to the necessary technology, digital literacy of individuals will need to be determined, and an educated clinician with significant expertise in administration of neuropsychological tests is irreplaceable.

The increasing number of dementia patients from the non-Western populations necessitates the cross-cultural adaptation and validation of the currently available instruments for diverse populations (Ardila et al., 1989, 2010; Finlayson-Pitts & Pitts Jr., 1997; Nielsen & Waldemar, 2016; Sisco et al., 2015). The best approach for detecting dementia in global societies is to develop or adapt/translate the currently available tools and scales and further validate them for the local patient population. Various sociodemographic factors such as language and culture, education, literacy, and bilingualism considerably affect the performance on cognitive tests, especially in the majority world.

Neuropsychological Testing for Dementia Assessment in Linguistically Diverse Contexts

Neuropsychological testing typically starts with a structured interview of the patient and caregiver, during which pertinent information on the onset and progression of the condition, speech and language abilities, behavior, awareness, and attitude toward the condition will be elicited; followed by administering the standardized tests and questionnaires. Cognitive tests are designed to assess general cognitive functions as well as specific cognitive domains like attention, memory, language, visuospatial ability, and executive functions. In certain societies, structured interview and administration of cognitive testing might not be feasible as the target population is unaware of neuropsychological examination. Therefore, to make the testing more acceptable, it may be important to clarify what to expect during testing, to correct preconceived misunderstandings, and to reduce feelings of apprehension or nervousness, if any (Aghvinian et al., 2021).

Screening, diagnosis, and classification of dementia subtypes necessitates detailed neuropsychological testing, laboratory tests, and neuroimaging. The clinical features, imaging, pathology, and diagnostic markers of different subtypes of dementia are detailed in Table 17-1. This chapter aims to give an introduction for professionals working in this sector by describing the most widely used neuropsychological tests (screening and diagnostic) and batteries, as well as severity, functionality, neuropsychiatric symptoms, and behavioral scales.

Assessment of General Cognitive Abilities

General cognitive assessments are done using brief screening or comprehensive tests. Mini-Mental State Examination (MMSE; Folstein et al., 1975), the Montreal Cognitive Assessment (MoCA; Nasreddine et al., 2005), and the Addenbrooke's Cognitive Examination (ACE; Hsieh et al., 2013; Mathuranath et al., 2000; Mioshi et al., 2006) are the most widely used tests and have been adapted and validated in several languages globally. These tests are easy to administer and are frequently used as part of standard clinical practice to detect the presence of cognitive impairment. Educational and sociocultural biases may occur, but have been overcome by following standardized adaptation and validation of these commonly used tests into multiple languages (Carvalho et al., 2010; Costa et al., 2012; dos Santos Kawata et al., 2012; Freitas et al., 2013; Fujiwara et al., 2010; Habib & Stott, 2019; Hsieh et al., 2013; Kan et al., 2019; Lee et al., 2008; Lifshitz et al., 2012; Lu et al., 2011; Memória et al., 2013; Muñoz-Neira et al., 2014; Nasreddine et al., 2005; Takenoshita et al., 2019; Wang et al., 2017, 2019; Zhou et al., 2014).

Table 17-1
Characteristics of Major Types of Dementia

FEATURES	ALZHEIMER'S DISEASE	VASCULAR DEMENTIA	FRONTOTEMPORAL DEMENTIA	LEWY BODY DEMENTIA
Clinical Symptoms	• Begins with memory problems and disorientation • Later, deficits in language and visuospatial skills	• Variable, focal neurological symptoms • Similar to Alzheimer's disease (AD), fewer memory problems	• Changes in personality and behavior • Speech and language deficits	• Fluctuating cognition, visual hallucinations • REM sleep behavior disorder
Motor Symptoms	Apraxia in severe stages	Focal weakness	Frontal release signs	Parkinsonism
Imaging	Hippocampal and generalized atrophy, temporal and parietal hypometabolism	Strokes, lacunar infarcts	Frontal/temporal atrophy and hypometabolism	Generalized atrophy, less hippocampal atrophy than AD, occipital hypometabolism
Pathology	Neurofibrillary tangles and amyloid plaques	Arterioles with thickened vessel wall	Tau inclusions and Pick bodies in the cortex	Alpha-synuclein Lewy bodies in the cortex and midbrain
Specific Diagnostic Criteria	• National Institute of Neurological and Communicative Disorders and Stroke-Alzheimer's Disease and Related Disorders Work Group (NINCDS-ADRDA) • National Institute on Aging and Alzheimer's Association (NIA-AA)	• National Institute of Neurological Diseases and Stroke (NINDS); Association Internationale pour la Recherche et l'Enseignement en Neurosciences (AIREN)	• International consensus criteria for diagnosis and classification of behavioral variant frontotemporal dementia (Rascovsky et al., 2011) • International consensus criteria for clinical diagnosis and classification of primary progressive aphasia (Gorno-Tempini et al., 2011)	• The revised criteria for the clinical diagnosis of dementia with Lewy bodies (DLB; McKeith et al., 2017)

Apart from the brief screening instruments, comprehensive tests are also available to assess global cognition. As the comprehensive tests are lengthy and time-consuming, they are not used as part of routine clinical practice. The Alzheimer's Disease Assessment Scale (ADAS-Cog; Rosen et al., 1984) is the most widely used tool specifically developed for AD, and is a sensitive and reliable comprehensive tool for documenting the progression of cognitive symptoms due to which it is generally used in drug trials (Hayes et al., 2009; Rockwood et al., 2007). The Cambridge Assessment of Memory and Cognition (CAMCOG; Roth et al., 1986) has also been proven to have excellent psychometric properties to diagnose dementia (Huppert et al., 1996; Lindeboom et al., 1993). Details of global cognition tests used for assessment of dementia is listed in Table 17-2.

Neuropsychological Test Batteries

Neuropsychological test batteries are used for detailing cognitive profiling and for differential diagnosis of various subtypes of dementia. There have been a few efforts toward developing comprehensive neuropsychological test batteries for use in different languages and countries. The Wechsler Adult Intelligence Scale (WAIS; Wechsler, 1955) is a widely used neuropsychological assessment battery in most nations despite its origin as an intelligence test because of its exceptional psychometric properties. The National Institutes of Health Cognitive Battery Toolbox (NIHTB-CB; Weintraub et al., 2013) is a quick, comprehensive, efficient, and easily available standard measure in neuroscience research that also has good psychometric qualities (Gershon et al., 2013). It assesses seven cognitive subdomains, including attention, processing speed, executive processes, language, working memory, and episodic memory. The Consortium to Establish a Registry for Alzheimer's Disease (CERAD; Morris et al., 1989) is a test battery developed specifically for individuals with suspected dementia (Bertolucci et al., 2001; Emre, 2003; Fillenbaum et al., 2008; Rossetti et al., 2010; Unverzagt et al., 1999). It also allows comprehensive neuropsychological evaluation of all types of dementias, and has been translated into many languages (Fillenbaum et al., 2008). The Cambridge Neuropsychological Test Automated Battery (CANTAB) is another well-known and widely used computerized neuropsychological battery that includes a number of nonverbal cognitive assessments that can be used in a variety of linguistic and cultural settings.

The 10/66 Dementia Research Group has developed and validated a battery with education and culture-neutral psychometric properties that could be used in the majority world (Prince et al., 2003). Another internationally recognized, valid, and reliable battery for comprehensive cognitive examination of vascular cognitive impairment is the National Institute of Neurological Disorders and Stroke (NINDS) and Canadian Stroke Network (CSN) battery (Hachinski et al., 2006). It has established standards for various age and educational groups (Strauss et al., 2006) and is useful in both English and non–English-speaking populations (Chen et al., 2015; Lin et al., 2016; Yu et al., 2013). In an effort to develop a battery that is suitable for the sociolinguistically diverse Indian context, the ICMR-Neurocognitive Toolbox (ICMR-NCTB; Iyer et al., 2020) was developed and validated in five different languages in India, allowing it to be useful to test cognitive function in various languages and educational levels. A list of neuropsychological test batteries used for assessment and diagnosis of dementia is listed in Table 17-2.

Table 17-2
Brief Screening Instruments, Comprehensive Long Tests of Global Cognition, and Neuropsychological Test Batteries for Assessment of Dementia

NAME OF THE TEST	AUTHOR (YEAR)	LANGUAGE AVAILABLE	COGNITIVE FUNCTIONS AND DOMAINS
Brief Screening of Global Cognition			
Philadelphia Brief Assessment of Cognition	Libon et al. (2007)	English	Working memory/executive control, lexical retrieval/language, visuospatial/visuoconstructional operations, verbal/visual episodic memory, and behavior/social attitude
Montreal Cognitive Assessment (MoCA)	Nasreddine et al. (2005)	English, French, Swahili, Sinhalese, Spanish, Chinese, Filipino, Korean, Malay, Japanese, Thai, German, Polish, Portuguese, Dutch, Turkish, Hebrew, Afrikaans, Amharic, Arabic, Armenian, Azerbaijani, Bengali, Bosnian, Bulgarian, Croatian, Czech, Danish, Finnish, Georgian, Gujarati, Hindi, Hungarian, Indonesian, Italian, Kannada, Marathi, Marathi, Persian, Russian, Urdu, Taiwanese	Executive functions, visuoconstructive skills, naming, memory, attention, sentence repetition, verbal fluency, abstraction, and orientation
Mini-Cog	Borson et al. (2003)	English, Turkish, Urdu, Thai, German, Portuguese, Croatian, Arabic, Persian, Czech, Spanish, Dutch, Korean, Hebrew, Norwegian, Vietnamese, Japanese, Tagalog, French	Visuospatial abilities, memory
The General Practitioner Assessment of Cognition (GPCOG)	Brodaty et al. (2002)	English, Arabic, Burmese, Cantonese, Dutch, Farsi, French, German, Greek, Hungarian, Italian, Korean, Maltese, Mandarin, Polish, Portuguese, Romanian, Russian, Sinhalese, Spanish, Thai, Urdu, Vietnamese, Welsh	Patient examination (name and address for subsequent recall, time orientation, visuospatial functioning, information recall), and informant interview

(continued)

Table 17-2 (continued)
Brief Screening Instruments, Comprehensive Long Tests of Global Cognition, and Neuropsychological Test Batteries for Assessment of Dementia

NAME OF THE TEST	AUTHOR (YEAR)	LANGUAGE AVAILABLE	COGNITIVE FUNCTIONS AND DOMAINS
Addenbrooke's Cognitive Examination (ACE)	Mathuranath et al. (2000)	English, Spanish, Korean, Czech, Persian, Danish, Arabic, Brazilian, Malayalam, French, Hebrew, Portuguese, Slovak, Lithuanian, Italian, Hindi, Telugu, Tamil, Kannada, Urdu, Gujarati, Greek, Korean, Malay, German, Sinhalese, Japanese, Chinese, Italian, Swahili	Orientation, attention, memory, verbal fluency, language, and visuospatial ability
Mini-Mental State Examination (MMSE)	Folstein et al. (1975)	English, Afrikaans, Albanian, Arabic, Armenian, German, Dutch, French, Bengali, Bosnian, Portuguese, Bulgarian, Spanish, Chinese, Croatian, Czech, Danish, Farsi, Filipino, Finnish, Georgian, Greek, Gujarati, Hebrew, Hindi, Hungarian, Italian, Japanese, Kannada, Korean, Malay, Malayalam, Marathi, Norwegian, Polish, Punjabi, Romanian, Russian, Swedish, Tamil, Telugu, Thai, Turkish, Urdu, Vietnamese, Yoruba	Orientation, memory, attention, calculation, language, visuoconstructive skills, and writing
Comprehensive Long Tests of Global Cognition			
Cambridge Cognitive Examination (CAMCOG)	Roth et al. (1986)	English, Chinese, Bangla, Finnish, French, Dutch, Gujarati, Italian, Japanese, Hindi, Korean, Malay, Sinhalese, Turkish, Portuguese, Bengali	Orientation, language, memory, attention, praxis, calculation, abstract thinking, and perception
Alzheimer's Disease Assessment Scale—Cognitive Subscale (ADAS-Cog)	Rosen et al. (1984)	English, Arabic, French, Italian, Hungarian, Greek, Chinese, Tamil, Hindi, Cantonese, German, Malayalam, Marathi, Spanish, Dutch, Mandarin, Bangla, Punjabi, Urdu, Japanese, Korean	Memory, praxis, language, and orientation

(continued)

Table 17-2 (continued)
Brief Screening Instruments, Comprehensive Long Tests of Global Cognition, and Neuropsychological Test Batteries for Assessment of Dementia

NAME OF THE TEST	AUTHOR (YEAR)	LANGUAGE AVAILABLE	COGNITIVE FUNCTIONS AND DOMAINS
Neuropsychological Test Batteries			
National Institute of Neurological Disorders and Stroke and the Canadian Stroke Network (NINDS-CSN) neuropsychological battery	Hachinski et al. (2006)	American English, Spanish, Mandarin Chinese, Taiwanese, Korean, French, German	Execution/attention, language, visuomotor speed, visuoconstruction, and memory
Kolkata screening battery	Das et al. (2006)	Bengali, Hindi	Verbal fluency, naming, calculation, memory, and visuospatial construction
NIMHANS Neuropsychological Battery	Rao et al. (2004)	English	Attention, memory, executive functions, language, visuospatial construction
10/66 Dementia Research Group battery	Prince et al. (2003)	English, Spanish, Arabic, Korean, Chinese, Portuguese, Tamil, Mandarin	Global cognition, attention, orientation, language, memory, executive function, and visuospatial abilities
Neuropsychological Assessment Battery (NAB)	Stern & White (2003)	English, German, Portuguese	Attention, language, spatial, memory, and executive function
Wechsler Abbreviated Scale of Intelligence (WASI)	Wechsler (1999)	English	Vocabulary, block design, similarities, and matrix reasoning
NEUROPSI	Ostrosky-Solís et al. (1997)	Spanish, English	Orientation, attention, memory, language, visuoperceptual abilities, and executive functions

(continued)

Table 17-2 (continued)

Brief Screening Instruments, Comprehensive Long Tests of Global Cognition, and Neuropsychological Test Batteries for Assessment of Dementia

NAME OF THE TEST	AUTHOR (YEAR)	LANGUAGE AVAILABLE	COGNITIVE FUNCTIONS AND DOMAINS
Consortium to Establish a Registry for Alzheimer's Disease—Clinical Assessment Battery (CERAD-Clinical Battery)	Morris et al. (1989)	English, Bulgarian, Chinese, French, Finnish, German, Hebrew, Italian, Japanese, Korean, Norwegian, Spanish, Portuguese, Cantonese, Estonian	Memory, language, constructional praxis, and intellectual status
Cambridge Neuropsychological Test Automated Battery (CANTAB)	Sahakian et al. (1988)	English	Attention, semantic/verbal memory, working memory, visual memory, executive function, planning, decision making, and response control
Wechsler Adult Intelligence Scale (WAIS)	Wechsler (1955)	English, Spanish, French, German, Chinese, Dutch, Arabic, Indonesian, Afrikaans, Korean, Finnish, Swedish, Norwegian, Danish, Scandinavian, Russian	General intellect, attention, visuospatial construction, language, and guided observation in other areas
Wechsler Memory Scale (WMS)	Wechsler (1945)	English, Spanish, Dutch, Portuguese, Norwegian, Chinese	Verbal memory, visual memory, general memory, attention/concentration, and delayed recall

Assessment of Specific Cognitive Domains

Thorough neuropsychological examinations are required to assess specific cognitive domains such as attention, processing speed, executive functions, memory, language, and visuospatial ability. Decline of specific cognitive domains needs to be addressed to track the progression of mild cognitive impairment (MCI) into dementia. Multiple test administration for a single domain assessment may be required at times to monitor the progress and to estimate the effectiveness of treatment strategies. Generally, one or more of these cognitive domains are impaired in individuals with MCI, ADRD, and other neurological conditions and an expert clinician can select the most reliable and valid test considering the underlying neurological condition. Among the neuropsychological tests that assess specific cognitive domains, the tests for attention, executive functions, and visuospatial construction are similar globally except for the tests for language and memory. The major cognitive domains and the commonly used valid and reliable tests under each cognitive domain are discussed below (Table 17-3).

Attention and Processing Speed

Poor concentration ability, getting easily distracted, and an inability to perform daily activities are some of the symptoms noted in MCI and ADRD patients which suggests that individuals with cognitive impairment might have attention deficits (Perry & Hodges, 1999). More specifically deficits in sustained attention and divided attention are exhibited by AD (McGuinness et al., 2010) and patients with Lewy body dementia often show fluctuating attention that impairs their functional abilities (Ballard et al., 2002; Bradshaw et al., 2004). Reduced speed of information processing is one of the primary symptoms of other dementias with Parkinson's disease: progressive supranuclear palsy and small vessel vascular disease due to disruption in frontal-subcortical circuits (Karantzoulis & Galvin, 2011; Kobylecki et al., 2015; Prins et al., 2005; Sawamoto et al., 2002). Traditional paper-pencil tasks, verbal tasks, and computerized tasks are used universally to understand attention abilities in dementia.

Memory and Learning

Memory impairment is the cardinal symptom and reliable indicator of dementia. Dementia patients often report short-term memory loss (i.e., inability to recall recent events compared to remote events in the early stage of dementia). They manifest repeating the same thing, forgetting conversations and appointments. During the middle stage of dementia, the memory impairment affects daily activities and, along with memory deficits, thinking, problem-solving, and constructional abilities are also lost (Storandt, 1994). As the disease progresses, the ability to recall events from the past is gradually lost (Albert et al., 1989; Butters et al., 1995; Storandt, 1994). Early pathological changes in Alzheimer's disease have been documented in the medial temporal regions, which are critical for episodic memory (Braak & Braak, 1991). This results in episodic memory deficits in the early stages of AD (Ergis & Eusop-Roussel, 2008; Greene et al., 1996; Salmon et al., 2000). When illness extends to the frontal, temporal, and parietal association areas, semantic memory problems are common in AD according to Braak and Braak (1991). Aphasic symptoms such as poor performance on confrontation naming, semantic categorization, verbal fluency, and difficulties recalling overlearned items are signs of semantic memory problems (Chan et al., 1993; Hodges & Patterson, 1995; Nebes, 1989). Deficits in working memory are also typical in dementia patients (Baddeley et al., 1986; Kessels et al., 2011). Clinically available memory tests can be classified as verbal and nonverbal memory tests (Cullum & Rosenberg, 1998).

Table 17-3
Tests of Specific Cognitive Domains for Dementia

NAME OF THE TEST	AUTHOR (YEAR)	LANGUAGES AVAILABLE	AREAS OF ASSESSMENT
Attention and Processing Speed			
Visual Search and Attention Test (VSAT)	Trenerry et al. (1989)	English	Visual search and selective attention
Paced Auditory Serial Addition Test (PASAT)	Gronwall & Sampson (1974)	English, French, Deutsch, Italian, Spanish, Arabic	Rate of information processing and sustained and divided attention
Symbol Digit Modalities Test (SDMT)	Smith (1973)	English	Divided attention, visual scanning, and motor speed
Digit Symbol Substitution Test (DSST)	Wechsler (1955)	English, Spanish, French, German, Chinese, Dutch, Arabic, Indonesian, Afrikaans, Korean, Finnish, Swedish, Norwegian, Danish, Scandinavian, Russian	Attention and psychomotor speed
Trail-Making Test (A and B)	Partington & Leiter (1949)	English, Japanese, Swedish, Italian, Dutch, Portuguese, Bulgarian, Czech, Danish, Slovak, Turkish, Ukrainian, Finnish, Hungarian, Japanese, Norwegian, Polish, Russian, Arabic, Spanish, Greek, French, German, Hindi, Bengali, Telugu, Kannada, Malayalam	Selective attention, divided attention, visual search speed, and scanning
Memory and Learning			
Rey Auditory Verbal Learning Test (immediate and delayed recall)	Schmidt (1996)	English, French, Czech, Persian, Portuguese, German, Arabic, Malay, Venezuelan, Spanish, Greek, Xhosa	Long-term auditory/verbal memory, learning strategy, interference, retention of information, learning and retrieval performance
Hopkins Verbal Learning Test (HVLT)	Brandt (1991)	English, Spanish, Arabic, French, Chinese, Indonesian, Xhosa, Korean, Japanese, Greek, Czech	Immediate memory span, new verbal learning, susceptibility to interference, delayed free recall, and recognition memory

(continued)

Table 17-3 (continued)
Tests of Specific Cognitive Domains for Dementia

NAME OF THE TEST	AUTHOR (YEAR)	LANGUAGES AVAILABLE	AREAS OF ASSESSMENT
Continuous Visual Memory Test (CVMT)	Trahan & Larrabee (1988)	English	Visual learning and memory
California Verbal Learning Test (CVLT)	Delis et al. (1987)	English, German, Norwegian, Greek, Korean, Italian, Chinese, Spanish, Japanese, Portuguese, Polish, Dutch	Immediate memory span, new verbal learning, susceptibility to interference, delayed free recall, and recognition memory
Benton Visual Retention Test (BVRT-Memory)	Benton (1974)	English	Visual memory, visual perception, and visuospatial construction ability
Digit Span (forward and backward)	Wechsler (1955)	English, Spanish, French, German, Chinese, Dutch, Arabic, Indonesian, Afrikaans, Korean, Finnish, Swedish, Norwegian, Danish, Scandinavian, Russian	Short-term auditory memory, working memory, and attention
Logical Memory Test	Wechsler (1945)	English, Spanish, French, German, Chinese, Dutch, Arabic, Indonesian, Afrikaans, Korean, Finnish, Swedish, Norwegian, Danish, Scandinavian, Russian	Short-term memory, long-term verbal memory, and executive features of memory processing
Language			
Boston Naming Test (BNT)	Kaplan, et al. (1983)	English, Spanish, Finnish, Greek, Swedish, Maltese, Dutch, French, Chinese, Tongan, Portuguese, Danish, Japanese	Confrontation naming
Snodgrass & Vanderwart Naming Test	Snodgrass & Vanderwart (1980)	English	Confrontation naming
Western Aphasia Battery (WAB)	Kertesz (1979)	English, Korean, Cantonese, Tagalog, Telugu, Kannada, Malayalam, Bengali, Nepali, Tamil, Hindi, Hungarian, French, Portuguese, Hebrew, Persian, Japanese	Spontaneous speech, auditory verbal comprehension, repetition, naming and word-finding, reading, writing, apraxia, visuospatial construction and calculation tasks, supplemental writing and reading tasks (WAB-R only)
Boston Diagnostic Aphasia Examination (BDAE)	Goodglass & Kaplan (1972)	English, Finnish, Spanish, Thai, Greek, Hindi, Portuguese	Fluency, auditory comprehension, naming, reading, automatic speech, reading comprehension, and writing

(continued)

Table 17-3 (continued)
Tests of Specific Cognitive Domains for Dementia

NAME OF THE TEST	AUTHOR (YEAR)	LANGUAGES AVAILABLE	AREAS OF ASSESSMENT
Controlled Oral Word Association (COWA)	Borkowski et al. (1967)	English, Spanish, Hindi, Chinese, Portuguese, German, Swedish, French	Verbal fluency
Token Test	De Renzi & Vignolo (1962)	English, Spanish, French, German, Chinese, Dutch, Arabic, Indonesian, Afrikaans, Korean, Finnish, Swedish, Norwegian, Danish, Scandinavian, Russian	Auditory verbal comprehension
Executive Functions			
Delis–Kaplan Executive Function System (D-KEFS)	Delis et al. (2001)	English	Cognitive flexibility, motor sequencing, category fluency, letter fluency, problem solving, planning, response inhibition, reasoning, and abstraction
Frontal Assessment Battery	Dubois et al. (2000)	Swedish, Spanish, Chilian, Japanese, German, Persian, Italian, Chinese, Turkish	Conceptualization, cognitive flexibility, motor sequencing, sensitivity to interference and environmental stimuli, and inhibitory control
Verbal Fluency Test	Benton et al. (1989)	English, Portuguese, Spanish, Swedish, Icelandic, Turkish, Arabic, Chinese, Italian, Hebrew, Dutch, Finnish, Greek, Lakota, Malayalam, Russian, Vietnamese	Lexical access, cognitive flexibility, ability to use strategies and self-monitor
Behavioral Assessment of Dysexecutive Syndrome (BADS)	Wilson et al. (1996)	English, Spanish, Chinese, Japanese, Portuguese, Hebrew	Inhibitory control, planning, behavior, problem solving, and cognitive flexibility
Wisconsin Card-Sorting Test	Grant & Berg (1948)	English, Russian, German, Hindi, Punjabi, Spanish	Reasoning, cognitive flexibility, and abstraction
Raven's Progressive Matrices	Raven (1938)	English	Nonverbal logical reasoning
Stroop Test	Stroop (1935)	English, Greek, Italian, Xhosa, Czech, Portuguese, Hebrew, Catalan, Spanish, Arabic, Russian	Inhibitory control and selective attention

(continued)

Table 17-3 (continued)
Tests of Specific Cognitive Domains for Dementia

NAME OF THE TEST	AUTHOR (YEAR)	LANGUAGES AVAILABLE	AREAS OF ASSESSMENT
Visuospatial-Constructive Abilities			
Clock Drawing Test	Brodaty & Moore (1997)	English, Afrikaans, Albanian, Arabic, Armenian, German, Dutch, French, Bengali, Bosnian, Portuguese, Bulgarian, Spanish, Chinese, Croatian, Czech, Danish, Farsi, Filipino, Finnish, French, Georgian, Greek, Gujarati, Hebrew, Hindi, Hungarian, Italian, Japanese, Kannada, Korean, Malay, Malayalam, Marathi, Norwegian, Polish, Punjabi, Romanian, Russian, Swedish, Tamil, Telugu, Thai, Turkish, Urdu, Vietnamese	Visuospatial and praxis abilities, visuospatial planning, and retrieval of clock time representation
Rey Complex Figure Test Copy (RCFT)	Meyers & Meyers (1995)	English, Spanish, French, German, Chinese, Dutch, Arabic, Indonesian, Xhosa, Korean, Finnish, Swedish, Norwegian, Danish, Scandinavian, Russian, Portuguese, Hebrew	Visuoconstruction and visual memory
Benton Visual Retention Test Copy (BVRT-Copy)	Benton (1945)	English	Visuoperception and visual memory
Koh's Block Design Test	Kohs (1923)	English, Spanish, French, German, Chinese, Dutch, Arabic, Indonesian, Afrikaans, Korean, Finnish, Swedish, Norwegian, Danish, Scandinavian, Russian	Developed as an intelligence test, widely used for assessment of visuospatial and motor skill

Language

Language impairment is most common in Alzheimer's dementia and primary progressive aphasias and is studied extensively by researchers (Price et al., 1993; Taler & Phillips, 2008). Early-stage AD often exhibits "empty speech" which is characterized by abundant circumlocutions, words with limited ideas, and non-specific language (Nicholas et al., 1985). When the disease progresses to moderate-severe stage, language comprehension (Bickel et al., 2000) and production (Kemper et al., 2001) deficits are pertinent which results in communication breakdown. The advanced stage of AD is characterized by echolalia and stereotypic utterances or complete loss of verbal communication (Ferris & Farlow, 2013).

Various neuropsychological tools offer detailed language evaluation, which helps for differential diagnosis and intervention. Profiling of language abilities is also essential for differential diagnosis of different types of primary progressive aphasia (PPA) namely nonfluent/agrammatic, semantic variant, and logopenic PPA. Several language assessment batteries are available to evaluate specific aspects of language.

Executive Functions

Executive functions include higher cognitive abilities such as response inhibition, set-shifting, problem solving, judgment, emotional management, planning, organizing, and self-monitoring. These functions represent the integrity of frontal lobe functioning (Alvarez & Emory, 2006; Stuss, 2011). Executive function deficits are the initial symptoms of behavioral variant of frontotemporal dementia (Harciarek & Cosentino, 2013; Hornberger et al., 2008; Possin et al., 2013). Various executive function deficits are also seen in Parkinson's disease, progressive supranuclear palsy (PSP), and vascular dementia caused by disrupted frontal-subcortical circuits (Krishnan et al., 2006; Santangelo et al., 2018). Executive function deficits like self-monitoring set-shifting, sequencing, and set-shifting are also reported in the early stage of AD (Lafleche & Albert, 1995; Perry & Hodges, 1999).

Visuospatial and Constructional Abilities

Visuospatial tests evaluate the ability to process simple and complex visual stimuli. Studies have shown that visuospatial and visuoconstructive deficits are salient features of AD and Lewy Body Dementia. This has been evidenced in visual perception, visual search, simple and complex two-dimensional figure drawing, and visuoconstructional tasks (Hamilton et al., 2008). Mendez et al. (1990) reported object recognition and spatial localization deficits which indicates complex visual-spatial disturbances in AD. Caine and Hodges (2001) had also demonstrated visuospatial deficits along with episodic memory and semantic deficits that indicated occipitoparietal lesions in early AD. There are a number of standardized tests that can be used to assess visuospatial perception and constructional ability.

Social Cognition

Social cognition impairment has been consistently demonstrated in dementia and its subtypes. Impaired emotion recognition and empathy have also been reported in patients with PPA. The standard tests used in the assessment of emotion recognition include Pictures of Facial Affect (POFA), the Florida Affect Battery, and the Interpersonal Reactivity Index to evaluate empathy.

Scales and Questionnaires

Severity Scales

Severity scales are used to measure the severity of the disease and track global cognitive decline over time. These instruments are administered to the patient or family member or any other informant through semi-structured interviews. The severity ratings will be measured based on signs, symptoms, functional abilities, and other behaviors elicited during the interview. The Global Deterioration Scale (GDS; Reisberg et al., 1982) and the Clinical Dementia Rating Scale (CDR; Hughes et al., 1982) are the two widely used severity instruments. These two scales have been culturally and linguistically adapted into many languages globally by rewording items to commonly used words or adding words/phrases to clarify a concept.

Activities of Daily Living

ADRD is characterized by a significant loss of functional abilities. To assess everyday functionality in dementia, a semi-structured interview with caregivers is required (Waldemar et al., 2007). These scales will determine the capacity of the individual to carry out self-care routines which helps to make treatment decisions. The majority of these scales are rated based on how well they functioned prior to the onset of dementia. These instruments measure activities of daily living (ADLs) and instrumental activities of daily living (IADLs). Many ADL and IADL scales have been adapted for diverse contexts (Fillenbaum et al., 1999; Mathuranath et al., 2005). IADL and ADL scales, combined with cognitive screening results, allow for an accurate diagnosis of dementia and MCI (Gold, 2012; Rodakowski et al., 2014).

Behavior

Depression, hallucinations, delusions, and agitation are some of the noncognitive, neuropsychiatric symptoms associated with dementia (Marin et al., 1997; Mok et al., 2004; Rainer et al., 1999). While not as common as memory impairment, these noncognitive symptoms are present in the later stages of dementia (Aalten et al., 2005; Steinberg et al., 2004; Tariot et al., 1995). The presence of these symptoms indicates the disease progression, reflects the caregiver's distress, and highlights the need for implementing pharmacological interventions. The Neuropsychiatric Inventory (NPI; Cummings et al., 1994) is a widely used instrument to assess the neuropsychiatric symptoms in the geriatric population.

Quality of Life

Quality of life (QOL) questionnaires assess how people perceive daily life when they have dementia. QOL measures are vital and are required as part of health outcome appraisals. There are both generic and dementia-specific QOL measures. QOL assessment determines the impact of health care when cure is not possible, generally on the following domains: material and physical well-being, relationships with other people, social, community and civic activities, personal development and fulfilment, and recreation.

Caregiver Burden

Dementia is a source of concern not only for the general population but also for family members. Researchers have developed many scales to evaluate the distress and burden of the caregivers, as it requires equal attention as dementia illness. Scales and questionnaires for assessing severity/staging, ADLs, neuropsychiatric symptoms, QOL, and caregiver burden for dementia are detailed in Table 17-4.

Neuropsychological Testing for Dementia Assessment in Educationally Diverse Contexts

According to UNESCO (2013), one in every five individuals in the world are low literate or illiterate, and most of the older adults who are illiterate reside in the South and West Asia. The currently available tools underestimate the cognitive abilities of low-literate or illiterate individuals, leading to overestimating cognitive pathology (Mandyla et al., 2021). The ability to read and write changes the way in which the information is conceptualized and memorized (Vygotsky & Cole, 1978)

The widely used screening instruments (e.g., MMSE, Clock Drawing Test, Mini-COG, MoCA, ADAS-Cog) are not appropriate for testing illiterate people and individuals with low education since all these tests include copying, drawing, reading, and writing. Hence, it is important to administer tests without education bias such as Picture-Based Memory Impairment Screen (PMIS; Verghese et al., 2012), Category Fluency Test, TNI-93 (Maillet et al., 2016), Fuld Object Memory Evaluation (Chung, 2009), and Cognitive State Test (COST; Babacan-Yildiz et al., 2013). Traditional attention and visuospatial construction tests, like Digit Span, Clock Drawing Test, and the Trail Making Test, are developed and widely used for the Western population and are ineffective for the low-educated non-Western population. Tests like Stick Design Test, Five-Digit, Color Trail Test, and Indian Trail Making Test can be used for the low-literate population (Franzen et al., 2020; Iyer et al., 2020). Taking into account the older person's age, lifestyle, and educational level, modifications in test instructions and procedures are recommended (Reisberg et al., 2001).

Neuropsychological Testing for Dementia Assessment in Bilingual Contexts

Three-quarters of the world population consider bilingualism a natural phenomenon (Crystal, 2007). Furthermore, 17% of the global population is multilingual. Hence, bilingualism is an important demographic factor that needs to be considered for neuropsychological assessment along with age, gender, educational level, and literacy. It is evidenced that the continuous usage and monitoring of two or more languages enables bilingual speakers to perform better in executive functions including working memory, inhibiting irrelevant messages, conflict resolution, and task switching (Bialystok, 2010; Gollan et al., 2005; Kerrigan et al., 2017; Rosselli et al., 2016; Singh & Mishra, 2013). On the contrary, bilingual costs on verbal tasks including picture naming and verbal fluency tasks

Table 17-4
Scales and Questionnaires for Assessing Severity/Staging, Activities of Daily Living, Neuropsychiatric Symptoms, Quality of Life, and Caregiver Burden

NAME OF THE TEST	AUTHOR (YEAR)	LANGUAGES AVAILABLE	DESCRIPTION OF RATING
Staging Scales			
Clinicians Global Impression of Change (CIBIC Plus)	Schneider et al. (1997)	English, Japanese, Korean, Spanish, Swedish, Danish, Russian	7-point rating scale (1 = very much improved, 2 = much improved, 3 = minimally improved, 4 = no change, 5 = minimally worse, 6 = much worse, 7 = very much worse)
Clinical Dementia Rating (CDR)	Hughes et al. (1982)	English, Portuguese, Spanish, Korean, Chinese, Persian, French, Vietnamese, Arabic, Danish, Bulgarian, Dutch, Finnish, German, Italian, Japanese, Korean, Hindi, Bengali, Telugu, Kannada, Malayalam	5-point scale (0.5 = questionable dementia, 1 = mild, 2 = moderate, 3 = severe) used to characterize six domains (memory, orientation, judgment and problem solving, community affairs, home and hobbies, and personal care)
Global Deterioration Scale (GDS)	Reisberg (1982)	English	7 stage (1 = no cognitive decline), 2 = very mild cognitive decline (age-associated memory impairment), 3 = mild cognitive decline (MCI), 4 = moderate cognitive decline (mild dementia), 5 = moderately severe cognitive decline (moderate dementia), 6 = severe cognitive decline (moderately severe dementia), 7 = very severe cognitive decline (severe dementia)

(continued)

Table 17-4 (continued)
Scales and Questionnaires for Assessing Severity/Staging, Activities of Daily Living, Neuropsychiatric Symptoms, Quality of Life, and Caregiver Burden

NAME OF THE TEST	AUTHOR (YEAR)	LANGUAGES AVAILABLE	DESCRIPTION OF RATING
Activities of Daily Living Scales			
Alzheimer's Disease Cooperative Study—Activities of Daily Living MCI (ADCS/ADL/MCI)	Pedrosa et al. (2010)	English, Turkish, Portuguese, Japanese, Korean, Mandarin, Chinese	Check ADLs in MCI
Bristol Activities of Daily Living Scale	Bucks et al. (1996)	English, Greek, Czech, Portuguese, Arabic, Sinhalese	20-item questionnaire including activities such as dressing, preparing food, and using transport
Disability Assessment for Dementia Scale (DAD)	Gelinas & Gauthier (1994)	English, French, Chinese, Spanish, Turkish, Persian, Portuguese, Korean	Check ADLs in community-dwelling dementia patients, including basic ADLs, IADLs, leisure activities, initiation, planning and organization, effective performance
Instrumental Activities of Daily Living (IADL)	Lawton & Brody (1969)	English, Hindi, Kannada, Telugu, Bengali, Malayalam, Spanish, Chinese, Korean, Persian, Sinhalese, Malay	Eight complex daily living tasks such as telephone use, shopping, housekeeping, and finances as assessed
Barthel Index	Mahoney & Barthel (1965)	English, Portuguese, British, Dutch, German, Taiwanese, Turkish, Chinese, Persian, Italian, Iranian, Sinhalese, Urdu, Danish	Focuses on physical disability, scores 10 variables evaluating ADL and mobility

(continued)

Table 17-4 (continued)

Scales and Questionnaires for Assessing Severity/Staging, Activities of Daily Living, Neuropsychiatric Symptoms, Quality of Life, and Caregiver Burden

NAME OF THE TEST	AUTHOR (YEAR)	LANGUAGES AVAILABLE	DESCRIPTION OF RATING
Assessment of Neuropsychiatric Symptoms			
Neuropsychiatric Inventory (NPI)	Cummings et al. (1994)	English, Norwegian, Chinese, Turkish, Portuguese, Swedish, Dutch, Korean, Hellenic, Danish, Lebanese, Icelandic, Malay, Spanish, Thai, Hindi, Bengali, Telugu, Kannada, Malayalam	Identify the frequency and severity of neuropsychiatric symptoms (delusions, agitation, depression, irritability, and apathy) and their impact on the caregiver
Frontal Behavioral Inventory (FBI)	Kertesz et al. (1997)	English, Italian, Korean, Polish, Portuguese	24-item questionnaire to the caregiver, differentiate frontotemporal dementia from other dementia subtypes
Cornell Scale for Depression in Dementia (CSDD)	Alexopoulos (1988)	English, Korean, Portuguese, Persian, Chinese, Arabic, Greek, Japanese, Dutch, Norwegian, Thai, German	Detect signs and symptoms (mood-related signs, behavioral disturbances, physical signs, cyclic function, and ideational disturbance) of depression in dementia and healthy individuals
Behavioral Pathology in Alzheimer's Disease Rating Scale (BEHAVE-AD)	Reisberg et al. (1987)	English, French, Malayalam, Icelandic, Chinese, Korean, Thai, German, Turkish, Japanese, Hebrew	Measure behavioral and psychological symptoms of AD (paranoid and delusional ideation, hallucinations, activity disturbances, aggressive behavior, sleep disturbance, affective symptoms, anxiety, and phobias)
Geriatric Depression Scale—15 items (GDS-15)	Yesavage et al. (1983)	English, Taiwanese, Igbo, Chinese, Turkish, Malay, Spanish, French, Japanese, Italian, Greek, Hindi, Bengali, Telugu, Kannada, Malayalam	Short form of GDS to screen, diagnose, and evaluate depression in older individuals

(continued)

Table 17-4 (continued) Scales and Questionnaires for Assessing Severity/Staging, Activities of Daily Living, Neuropsychiatric Symptoms, Quality of Life, and Caregiver Burden

NAME OF THE TEST	AUTHOR (YEAR)	LANGUAGES AVAILABLE	DESCRIPTION OF RATING
Montgomery–Asberg Depression Rating Scale (MADRS)	Montgomery & Asberg (1979)	English, Bangla, Portuguese, Japanese, Malay, Persian, French, Spanish, Thai, Dutch, Arabic, Spanish, Swedish, Serbian, German, Korean	Measure the severity of depressive episodes in patients with mood disorders
Hamilton Rating Scale for Depression (HAM-D24)	Hamilton (1960)	English, Persian	Clinician-rated scale to assess 24 depressive symptoms
Quality of Life Measures			
Dementia Quality of Life Measure (DEMQOL)	Smith et al. (2005)	English, Spanish, Japanese, Italian, Chinese, Sinhalese, Portuguese, Swedish, German, Greek	Includes daily activities and looking after oneself, health and well-being, cognitive functioning, social relationships, and self-concept
Quality of Life-AD (QOL-AD)	Logsdon et al. (1999)	English, Portuguese, French, Mandarin, Japanese, Chinese, Spanish, German, Polish, Czech, Greek, Hindi, Bengali, Telugu, Kannada, Malayalam	Disease-specific QOL rated for 13 items (i.e., physical health, energy, mood, living situation, memory)
Short Form-36	Ware & Sherbourne (1992)	English, Spanish, Swedish, Hindi, Bengali, Telugu, Kannada, Malayalam, Arabic, Chinese, French, Italian, Korean, Greek, Portuguese, German, Polish, Japanese, Czech	Generic questionnaire for overall health-related QOL. Includes eight sections (vitality, physical functioning, bodily pain, general health perceptions, physical role functioning, emotional role functioning, social role functioning, mental health)
EuroQol measure	Group (1990)	English, Spanish, Dutch, Catalan, Croatian, French, Finnish, Danish, German, Hungarian, German, Japanese, Peruvian, Polish, Portuguese, Turkish, Venezuelan, Xhosa	Generic questionnaire including five dimensions (mobility, self-care, usual activities, pain/discomfort, and anxiety/depression)

(continued)

Table 17-4 (continued)

Scales and Questionnaires for Assessing Severity/Staging, Activities of Daily Living, Neuropsychiatric Symptoms, Quality of Life, and Caregiver Burden

NAME OF THE TEST	AUTHOR (YEAR)	LANGUAGES AVAILABLE	DESCRIPTION OF RATING
Caregiver Burden Scales			
General Health Questionnaire	Goldberg & Williams (1988)	English, Portuguese, Turkish, Iranian, Slovak, Zulu, Spanish, Urdu, Vietnamese, Japanese, Persian, Maltese, Chinese, Indonesian, Finnish, Russian, German, Polish	Brief 12-item questionnaire for common mental health disorders to measure psychiatric well-being
Zarit Burden Interview	Zarit et al. (1980)	English, Hausa, Portuguese, Chinese, French, Japanese, German, Hebrew, Spanish, Korean, Hindi, Hebrew, Italian	A 22-item self-report instrument of the burden of the caregivers of adults with dementia

due to interlanguage interference have also been reported (Anderson et al., 2017; Fernandes et al., 2007; Gollan et al., 2005; Sandoval et al., 2010). This indicates that the effects of bilingualism on the verbal or nonverbal cognitive tasks must be considered during assessment of cognitive disturbances in dementia.

In a bilingual context, it is essential to interpret the standard neuropsychological test scores by considering various factors such as language of test administration (Mungas et al., 2010), language proficiency of the patient (Artiola i Fortuny & Mullaney, 1998; Pontón, 2001; Rosselli et al., 2002), language proficiency of the examiner, and responses produced in various languages (Paplikar et al., 2021). The following recommendations for neuropsychological testing in bilingual speakers have been put forth that can be used in bilingual communities across societies (Paplikar et al., 2021): (1) evaluating patient's linguistic proficiency; (2) evaluating the examiner's language proficiency; (3) cognitive testing to be administered in the patient's native language; and (4) considering borrowed and language mixed words while interpreting the cognitive test scores. According to Paplikar et al. (2021), responses obtained in both native and other spoken languages should be considered while interpreting the cognitive test scores. However, researchers are yet to establish clear criteria and norms for scoring responses from nontarget languages. In a bi/multilingual setting, the neuropsychological evaluation team should coordinate and avail competent bilingual examiners in the clinics, to provide standard evaluation and care to the non-English speakers.

Specific Issues Related to Global Populations

Most countries do not have the facility of multidisciplinary memory clinics and experts (neurologists and neuropsychologists) as part of the health care workforce for dementia diagnosis and management. The size and skill of the dementia care workforce are insufficient considering the escalating demand in both developed and developing countries. Hence, there is an emergent demand to have capacity-building programs and improve health literacy on dementia, especially in the majority world, with limited resources for timely diagnosis and care of dementia considering the growing figures of the dementia population. Multiple dementia education programs need to be initiated for the health care workforce to ensure adequate and quality health care support and care for people living with dementia in these countries.

Currently, the dementia-specific continued education programs organized by national level dementia societies and medical councils offer only training for neurologists, geriatricians, and geriatric psychiatrists, which explains the existing diagnosis and treatment gap and highlights the importance of training professionals across multiple levels of the health care system starting from primary care.

To address the issue, regional training programs using common physician training modules for dementia must be implemented. These programs should ensure the participation of medical and allied health professionals involved in dementia diagnosis and care. The professionals should have the minimum standard training for providing quality service, and the outcomes need to be monitored by the experts. Expert-led focus groups can also be held to exchange and update information on current dementia care trends. Dementia education can also be endorsed in curricula of undergraduate and postgraduate medical and allied professions. Community-level health workers could be educated to screen for dementia as a support mechanism to deal with the impact on diagnosis due to the expert shortage.

Conclusion

Dementia diagnosis for heterogenous populations is challenging. Various factors such as culture and language, education, and bilingualism affect the cognitive test performance. This chapter provided an overview of different neuropsychological tests suitable for diverse populations that are routinely used to assess global cognition, specific cognitive domains, and various scales for severity rating, ADLs, QOL, and neuropsychiatric symptoms. It is also important to follow recommendations for neuropsychological testing in bilingual speakers. Due to scarcity in experienced health care professionals and resources, there is a need to have physician training modules for dementia diagnosis and care. These tests must be tailored to an individual patient and standardized for use in specific populations, taking into account different factors such as language and culture, education, and bilingualism.

References

Aalten, P., de Vugt, M. E., Jaspers, N., Jolles, J., & Verhey, F. R. J. (2005). The course of neuropsychiatric symptoms in dementia. Part I: Findings from the two-year longitudinal Maasbed study. *International Journal of Geriatric Psychiatry, 20*(6), 523-530.

Aghvinian, M., Santoro, A. F., Gouse, H., Joska, J. A., Linda, T., Thomas, K. G. F., & Robbins, R. N. (2021). Taking the test: A qualitative analysis of cultural and contextual factors impacting neuropsychological assessment of Xhosa-Speaking South Africans. *Archives of Clinical Neuropsychology, 36*(6), 976-980.

Albert, M. S., Moss, M. B., & Milberg, W. (1989). Memory testing to improve the differential diagnosis of Alzheimer's disease. *Progress in Clinical and Biological Research, 317*, 55-69.

Alexopoulos, G. S., Abrams, R. C., Young, R. C., & Shamoian, C. A. (1988). Cornell scale for depression in dementia. *Biological Psychiatry, 23*(3), 271-284.

Alladi, S., & Hachinski, V. (2018). World dementia: One approach does not fit all. *Neurology, 91*(6), 264-270.

Alvarez, J. A., & Emory, E. (2006). Executive function and the frontal lobes: A meta-analytic review. *Neuropsychology Review, 16*(1), 17-42.

American Psychiatric Association. (2013). *Diagnostic and statistical manual of mental disorders* (5th ed.). https://doi.org/10.1176/appi.books.9780890425596

Anderson, J. A. E., Saleemi, S., & Bialystok, E. (2017). Neuropsychological assessments of cognitive aging in monolingual and bilingual older adults. *Journal of Neurolinguistics, 43*, 17-27.

Ardila, A., Bertolucci, P. H., Braga, L. W., Castro-Caldas, A., Judd, T., Kosmidis, M. H., Matute, R., Nitrini, R., Ostrosky-Solis, F., & Rosselli, M. (2010). Illiteracy: The neuropsychology of cognition without reading. *Archives of Clinical Neuropsychology, 25*(8), 689-712.

Ardila, A., Rosselli, M., & Rosas, P. (1989). Neuropsychological assessment in illiterates: Visuospatial and memory abilities. *Brain and Cognition, 11*(2), 147-166.

Arnold, B. R., Montgomery, G. T., Castañeda, I., & Longoria, R. (1994). Acculturation and performance of Hispanics on selected Halstead-Reitan neuropsychological tests. *Assessment, 1*(3), 239-248.

Artero, S., Tierney, M. C., Touchon, J., & Ritchie, K. (2003). Prediction of transition from cognitive impairment to senile dementia: A prospective, longitudinal study. *Acta Psychiatrica Scandinavica, 107*(5), 390-393.

Artiola i Fortuny, L., & Mullaney, H. A. (1998). Assessing patients whose language you do not know: Can the absurd be ethical? *The Clinical Neuropsychologist, 12*(1), 113-126.

Babacan-Yildiz, G., Isik, A. T., Ur, E., Aydemir, E., Ertas, C., Cebi, M., Soysal, P., Gursoy, E., Kolukisa, M., & Kocaman, G. (2013). COST: Cognitive State Test, a brief screening battery for Alzheimer disease in illiterate and literate patients. *International Psychogeriatrics, 25*(3), 403-412.

Baddeley, A., Logie, R., Bressi, S., Sala, S. della, & Spinnler, H. (1986). Dementia and working memory. *Quarterly Journal of Experimental Psychology Section A, 38*(4), 603-618.

Ballard, C. G., Aarsland, D., McKeith, I., O'Brien, J., Gray, A., Cormack, F., Burn, D., Cassidy, T., Starfeldt, R., & Larsen, J.-P. (2002). Fluctuations in attention: PD dementia vs DLB with parkinsonism. *Neurology, 59*(11), 1714-1720.

Benton, A. L. (1945). A visual retention test for clinical use. *Archives of Neurology & Psychiatry, 54*(3), 212-216.

Benton, A. L. (1974). *Revised Visual Retention Test: Clinical and experimental applications.* Psychological Corporation.

Benton, A. L., Hamsher, K. d, & Sivan, A. (1989). Multilingual Aphasia Examination. *Neuropsychology, Blocking, Schizophrenia, 59.*

Bertolucci, P. H. F., Okamoto, I. H., Brucki, S. M. D., Siviero, M. O., Toniolo Neto, J., & Ramos, L. R. (2001). Applicability of the CERAD neuropsychological battery to Brazilian elderly. *Arquivos de Neuro-Psiquiatria, 59,* 532-536.

Bialystok, E. (2010). Global–local and trail-making tasks by monolingual and bilingual children: Beyond inhibition. *Developmental Psychology, 46*(1), 93.

Bickel, C., Pantel, J., Eysenbach, K., & Schröder, J. (2000). Syntactic comprehension deficits in Alzheimer's disease. *Brain and Language, 71*(3), 432-448.

Borkowski, J. G., Benton, A. L., & Spreen, O. (1967). Word fluency and brain damage. *Neuropsychologia, 5*(2), 135-140.

Borson, S., Scanlan, J. M., Chen, P., & Ganguli, M. (2003). The Mini-Cog as a screen for dementia: Validation in a population-based sample. *Journal of the American Geriatrics Society, 51*(10), 1451-1454.

Braak, H., & Braak, E. (1991). Neuropathological stageing of Alzheimer-related changes. *Acta Neuropathologica, 82*(4), 239-259.

Bradshaw, J., Saling, M., Hopwood, M., Anderson, V., & Brodtmann, A. (2004). Fluctuating cognition in dementia with Lewy bodies and Alzheimer's disease is qualitatively distinct. *Journal of Neurology, Neurosurgery & Psychiatry, 75*(3), 382-387.

Brandt, J. (1991). The Hopkins Verbal Learning Test: Development of a new memory test with six equivalent forms. *The Clinical Neuropsychologist, 5*(2), 125-142.

Brodaty, H., & Moore, C. M. (1997). The Clock Drawing Test for dementia of the Alzheimer's type: A comparison of three scoring methods in a memory disorders clinic. *International Journal of Geriatric Psychiatry, 12*(6), 619-627.

Brodaty, H., Pond, D., Kemp, N. M., Luscombe, G., Harding, L., Berman, K., & Huppert, F. A. (2002). The GPCOG: A new screening test for dementia designed for general practice. *Journal of the American Geriatrics Society, 50*(3), 530-534.

Bucks, R. S., Ashworth, D. L., Wilcock, G. K., & Siegfried, K. (1996). Assessment of activities of daily living in dementia: Development of the Bristol Activities of Daily Living Scale. *Age and Ageing, 25*(2), 113-120.

Butters, N., Delis, D. C., & Lucas, J. A. (1995). Clinical assessment of memory disorders in amnesia and dementia. *Annual Review of Psychology, 46*(1), 493-523.

Caine, D., & Hodges, J. R. (2001). Heterogeneity of semantic and visuospatial deficits in early Alzheimer's disease. *Neuropsychology, 15*(2), 155.

Carvalho, V. A., Barbosa, M. T., & Caramelli, P. (2010). Brazilian version of the Addenbrooke Cognitive Examination-revised in the diagnosis of mild Alzheimer disease. *Cognitive and Behavioral Neurology, 23*(1), 8-13.

Chan, A. S., Butters, N., Paulsen, J. S., Salmon, D. P., Swenson, M. R., & Maloney, L. T. (1993). An assessment of the semantic network in patients with Alzheimer's disease. *Journal of Cognitive Neuroscience, 5*(2), 254-261.

Chen, X., Wong, A., Ye, R., Xiao, L., Wang, Z., Lin, Y., Yang, F., Li, H., Feng, T., & Duan, L. (2015). Validation of NINDS-CSN neuropsychological battery for vascular cognitive impairment in Chinese stroke patients. *BMC Neurology, 15*(1), 1-6.

Chung, J. C. C. (2009). Clinical validity of Fuld Object Memory Evaluation to screen for dementia in a Chinese society. *International Journal of Geriatric Psychiatry: A Journal of the Psychiatry of Late Life and Allied Sciences, 24*(2), 156-162.

Costa, A. S., Fimm, B., Friesen, P., Soundjock, H., Rottschy, C., Gross, T., Eitner, F., Reich, A., Schulz, J. B., & Nasreddine, Z. S. (2012). Alternate-form reliability of the Montreal Cognitive Assessment Screening test in a clinical setting. *Dementia and Geriatric Cognitive Disorders, 33*(6), 379-384.

Crystal, D. (2007). *How language works.* Penguin Publishers.

Cullum, C. M., & Rosenberg, R. N. (1998). Memory loss—When is it Alzheimer disease? *Journal of the American Medical Association, 279*(21), 1689-1690.

Cummings, J. L., Mega, M., Gray, K., Rosenberg-Thompson, S., Carusi, D. A., & Gornbein, J. (1994). The Neuropsychiatric Inventory: Comprehensive assessment of psychopathology in dementia. *Neurology, 44*(12), 2308.

Das, S. K., Biswas, A., Roy, T., Banerjee, T. K., Mukherjee, C. S., Raut, D. K., & Chaudhuri, A. (2006). A random sample survey for prevalence of major neurological disorders in Kolkata. *Indian Journal of Medical Research, 124*(2), 163.

de Renzi, A., & Vignolo, L. A. (1962). Token test: A sensitive test to detect receptive disturbances in aphasics. *Brain: A Journal of Neurology.*

Delis, D. C., Kaplan, E., & Kramer, J. H. (2001). *Delis-Kaplan executive function system.*

Delis, D. C., Kramer, J. H., Kaplan, E., & Ober, B. A. (1987). *California Verbal Learning Test.* The Psychological Corporation.

dos Santos Kawata, K. H., Hashimoto, R., Nishio, Y., Hayashi, A., Ogawa, N., Kanno, S., Hiraoka, K., Yokoi, K., Iizuka, O., & Mori, E. (2012). A validation study of the Japanese version of the Addenbrooke's Cognitive Examination-Revised. *Dementia and Geriatric Cognitive Disorders Extra, 2*(1), 29-37.

Dubois, B., Slachevsky, A., Litvan, I., & Pillon, B. (2000). The FAB: A frontal assessment battery at bedside. *Neurology, 55*(11), 1621-1626.

Edwards, J., Bhatia, T. K., Ritchie, W. C., & Wiley, J. (2013). *The handbook of bilingualism and multilingualism.* Wiley.

Emre, M. (2003). Dementia associated with Parkinson's disease. *The Lancet Neurology, 2*(4), 229-237.

Ergis, A. M., & Eusop-Roussel, E. (2008). Early episodic memory impairments in Alzheimer's disease. *Revue Neurologique, 164,* S96-S101.

Fernandes, M. A., Craik, F., Bialystok, E., & Kreuger, S. (2007). Effects of bilingualism, aging, and semantic relatedness on memory under divided attention. *Canadian Journal of Experimental Psychology/Revue Canadienne de Psychologie Expérimentale, 61*(2), 128.

Ferri, C. P., Prince, M., Brayne, C., Brodaty, H., Fratiglioni, L., Ganguli, M., Hall, K., Hasegawa, K., Hendrie, H., & Huang, Y. (2005). Global prevalence of dementia: A Delphi consensus study. *The Lancet, 366*(9503), 2112-2117.

Ferris, S. H., & Farlow, M. (2013). Language impairment in Alzheimer's disease and benefits of acetylcholinesterase inhibitors. *Clinical Interventions in Aging, 8,* 1007.

Fillenbaum, G. G., Chandra, V., Ganguli, M., Pandav, R., Gilby, J. E., Seaberg, E. C., Belle, S., Baker, C., Echement, D. A., & Nath, L. M. (1999). Development of an activities of daily living scale to screen for dementia in an illiterate rural older population in India. *Age and Ageing, 28*(2), 161-168.

Fillenbaum, G. G., van Belle, G., Morris, J. C., Mohs, R. C., Mirra, S. S., Davis, P. C., Tariot, P. N., Silverman, J. M., Clark, C. M., & Welsh-Bohmer, K. A. (2008). Consortium to Establish a Registry for Alzheimer's Disease (CERAD): The first twenty years. *Alzheimer's & Dementia, 4*(2), 96-109.

Finlayson-Pitts, B. J., & Pitts Jr, J. N. (1997). Tropospheric air pollution: Ozone, airborne toxics, polycyclic aromatic hydrocarbons, and particles. *Science, 276*(5315), 1045-1051.

Folstein, M. F., Folstein, S. E., & McHugh, P. R. (1975). "Mini-Mental State": A practical method for grading the cognitive state of patients for the clinician. *Journal of Psychiatric Research, 12*(3), 189-198.

Flores, I., Casaletto, K. B., Marquine, M. J., Umlauf, A., Moore, D. J., Mungas, D., Gershon, R. C., Beaumont, J. L., & Heaton, R. K. (2017). Performance of Hispanics and non-Hispanic Whites on the NIH Toolbox Cognition Battery: The roles of ethnicity and language backgrounds. *The Clinical Neuropsychologist, 31*(4), 783-797.

Franzen, S., van den Berg, E., Goudsmit, M., Jurgens, C. K., van de Wiel, L., Kalkisim, Y., Uysal-Bozkir, Ö., Ayhan, Y., Nielsen, T. R., & Papma, J. M. (2020). A systematic review of neuropsychological tests for the assessment of dementia in non-western, low-educated or illiterate populations. *Journal of the International Neuropsychological Society, 26*(3), 331-351.

Freitas, S., Simões, M. R., Alves, L., & Santana, I. (2013). Montreal Cognitive Assessment: Validation study for mild cognitive impairment and Alzheimer disease. *Alzheimer Disease & Associated Disorders, 27*(1), 37-43.

Fujiwara, Y., Suzuki, H., Yasunaga, M., Sugiyama, M., Ijuin, M., Sakuma, N., Inagaki, H., Iwasa, H., Ura, C., & Yatomi, N. (2010). Brief screening tool for mild cognitive impairment in older Japanese: Validation of the Japanese version of the Montreal Cognitive Assessment. *Geriatrics & Gerontology International, 10*(3), 225-232.

Gélinas, I., & Gauthier, L. (1994). Disability Assessment for Dementia (DAD). *Canadian Medical Association Journal, 150*(3), 387.

Gershon, R. C., Wagster, M. v, Hendrie, H. C., Fox, N. A., Cook, K. F., & Nowinski, C. J. (2013). NIH toolbox for assessment of neurological and behavioral function. *Neurology, 80*(11 Suppl. 3), S2-S6.

Gold, D. A. (2012). An examination of instrumental activities of daily living assessment in older adults and mild cognitive impairment. *Journal of Clinical and Experimental Neuropsychology, 34*(1), 11-34.

Goldberg, D. P., & Williams, P. (1988). *A user's guide to the General Health Questionnaire.* NFER-Nelson.

Gollan, T. H., Montoya, R. I., Fennema-Notestine, C., & Morris, S. K. (2005). Bilingualism affects picture naming but not picture classification. *Memory & Cognition, 33*(7), 1220-1234.

Goodglass, H., & Kaplan, E. (1972). *The assessment of aphasia and related disorders.* Lea & Febiger.

Grant, D. A., & Berg, E. A (1948). A behavioral analysis of degree of reinforcement and ease of shifting to new responses in a Weigl-type card-sorting problem. *Journal of Experimental Psychology, 38*(4), 404-411.

Greene, J. D. W., Baddeley, A. D., & Hodges, J. R. (1996). Analysis of the episodic memory deficit in early Alzheimer's disease: Evidence from the doors and people test. *Neuropsychologia, 34*(6), 537-551.

Gronwall, D. M., & Sampson, H. (1974). *The psychological effects of concussion.* Auckland University Press/ Oxford University Press.

Group, T. E. (1990). EuroQol: A new facility for the measurement of health-related quality of life. *Health Policy, 16*(3), 199-208.

Hachinski, V., Iadecola, C., Petersen, R. C., Breteler, M. M., Nyenhuis, D. L., Black, S. E., Powers, W. J., DeCarli, C., Merino, J. G., & Kalaria, R. N. (2006). National Institute of Neurological Disorders and Stroke–Canadian stroke network vascular cognitive impairment harmonization standards. *Stroke, 37*(9), 2220-2241.

Habib, N., & Stott, J. (2019). Systematic review of the diagnostic accuracy of the non-English versions of Addenbrooke's Cognitive Examination–Revised and III. *Aging & Mental Health, 23*(3), 297-304.

Hamilton, M. (1960). A rating scale for depression. *Journal of Neurology, Neurosurgery, and Psychiatry, 23*(1), 56.

Hamilton, J. M., Salmon, D. P., Galasko, D., Raman, R., Emond, J., Hansen, L. A., Masliah, E., & Thal, L. J. (2008). Visuospatial deficits predict rate of cognitive decline in autopsy-verified dementia with Lewy bodies. *Neuropsychology, 22*(6), 729.

Harciarek, M., & Cosentino, S. (2013). Language, executive function and social cognition in the diagnosis of frontotemporal dementia syndromes. *International Review of Psychiatry, 25*(2), 178-196.

Harvey, P. D. (2022). Clinical applications of neuropsychological assessment. *Dialogues in Clinical Neuroscience.*

Hayes, T. L., Larimer, N., Adami, A., & Kaye, J. A. (2009). Medication adherence in healthy elders: Small cognitive changes make a big difference. *Journal of Aging and Health, 21*(4), 567-580.

Hodges, J. R., & Patterson, K. (1995). Is semantic memory consistently impaired early in the course of Alzheimer's disease? Neuroanatomical and diagnostic implications. *Neuropsychologia, 33*(4), 441-459.

Hodges, J. R., Patterson, K., Ward, R., Garrard, P., Bak, T., Perry, R., & Gregory, C. (1999). The differentiation of semantic dementia and frontal lobe dementia (temporal and frontal variants of frontotemporal dementia) from early Alzheimer's disease: A comparative neuropsychological study. *Neuropsychology, 13*(1), 31.

Hornberger, M., Piguet, O., Kipps, C., & Hodges, J. R. (2008). Executive function in progressive and nonprogressive behavioral variant frontotemporal dementia. *Neurology, 71*(19), 1481-1488.

Hsieh, S., Schubert, S., Hoon, C., Mioshi, E., & Hodges, J. R. (2013). Validation of the Addenbrooke's Cognitive Examination III in frontotemporal dementia and Alzheimer's disease. *Dementia and Geriatric Cognitive Disorders, 36*(3-4), 242-250.

Hughes, C. P., Berg, L., Danziger, W., Coben, L. A., & Martin, R. L. (1982). A new clinical scale for the staging of dementia. *British Journal of Psychiatry, 140*(6), 566-572.

Huppert, F. A., Jorm, A. F., Brayne, C., Girling, D. M., Barkley, C., Beardsall, L., & Paykel, E. S. (1996). Psychometric properties of the CAMCOG and its efficacy in the diagnosis of dementia. *Aging, Neuropsychology, and Cognition, 3*(3), 201-214.

Iyer, G. K., Paplikar, A., Alladi, S., Dutt, A., Sharma, M., Mekala, S., Kaul, S., Saroja, A. O., Divyaraj, G., & Ellajosyula, R. (2020). Standardising dementia diagnosis across linguistic and educational diversity: Study design of the Indian Council of Medical Research-Neurocognitive Tool Box (ICMR-NCTB). *Journal of the International Neuropsychological Society, 26*(2), 172-186.

Johnstone, B., Hogg, J. R., Schopp, L. H., Kapila, C., & Edwards, S. (2002). Neuropsychological deficit profiles in senile dementia of the Alzheimer's type. *Archives of Clinical Neuropsychology, 17*(3), 273-281.

Kan, K. C., Subramaniam, P., Shahrizaila, N., Kamaruzzaman, S. B., Razali, R., & Ghazali, S. E. (2019). Validation of the Malay Version of Addenbrooke's Cognitive Examination III in detecting mild cognitive impairment and dementia. *Dementia and Geriatric Cognitive Disorders Extra, 9*(1), 66-76.

Kaplan, E., Goodglass, H., & Weintraub, S. (1983). *The Boston Naming test.* Lea & Febiger.

Karantzoulis, S., & Galvin, J. E. (2011). Distinguishing Alzheimer's disease from other major forms of dementia. *Expert Review of Neurotherapeutics, 11*(11), 1579-1591.

Kemper, S., Thompson, M., & Marquis, J. (2001). Longitudinal change in language production: Effects of aging and dementia on grammatical complexity and propositional content. *Psychology and Aging, 16*(4), 600.

Kerrigan, L., Thomas, M. S. C., Bright, P., & Filippi, R. (2017). Evidence of an advantage in visuo-spatial memory for bilingual compared to monolingual speakers. *Bilingualism: Language and Cognition, 20*(3), 602-612.

Kertesz, A. (1979). *Aphasia and associated disorders: Taxonomy, localization, and recovery.* Holt Rinehart & Winston.

Kertesz, A., Davidson, W., & Fox, H. (1997). Frontal behavioral inventory: Diagnostic criteria for frontal lobe dementi. *Canadian Journal of Neurological Sciences, 24*(1), 29-36.

Kessels, R. P. C., van Doormaal, A., & Janzen, G. (2011). Landmark recognition in Alzheimer's dementia: Spared implicit memory for objects relevant for navigation. *PLoS ONE, 6*(4), e18611.

Kobylecki, C., Langheinrich, T., Hinz, R., Vardy, E. R. L. C., Brown, G., Martino, M.-E., Haense, C., Richardson, A. M., Gerhard, A., & Anton-Rodriguez, J. M. (2015). 18F-florbetapir PET in patients with frontotemporal dementia and Alzheimer disease. *Journal of Nuclear Medicine, 56*(3), 386-391.

Kohs, S. C. (1923). *Intelligence measurement: A psychological and statistical study based upon the block-design tests.* Macmillan.

Krishnan, S., Mathuranath, P. S., Sarma, S., & Kishore, A. (2006). Neuropsychological functions in progressive supranuclear palsy, multiple system atrophy and Parkinson's disease. *Neurology India, 54*(3), 268.

Lafleche, G., & Albert, M. S. (1995). Executive function deficits in mild Alzheimer's disease. *Neuropsychology, 9*(3), 313.

Lawton, M. P., Brody, E. M., & Médecin, U. (1969). Instrumental activities of daily living (IADL). *The Gerontologist, 9*, 179-186.

Lee, J.Y., Lee, D. W., Cho, S.-J., Na, D. L., Jeon, H. J., Kim, S.-K., Lee, Y. R., Youn, J.-H., Kwon, M., & Lee, J.-H. (2008). Brief screening for mild cognitive impairment in elderly outpatient clinic: Validation of the Korean version of the Montreal Cognitive Assessment. *Journal of Geriatric Psychiatry and Neurology, 21*(2), 104-110.

Libon, D. J., Massimo, L., Moore, P., Coslett, H. B., Chatterjee, A., Aguirre, G. K., Rice, A., Vesely, L., & Grossman, M. (2007). Screening for frontotemporal dementias and Alzheimer's disease with the Philadelphia Brief Assessment of Cognition: A preliminary analysis. *Dementia and Geriatric Cognitive Disorders, 24*(6), 441-447.

Libon, D. J., McMillan, C., Gunawardena, D., Powers, C., Massimo, L., Khan, A., Morgan, B., Farag, C., Richmond, L., & Weinstein, J. (2009). Neurocognitive contributions to verbal fluency deficits in frontotemporal lobar degeneration. *Neurology, 73*(7), 535-542.

Lifshitz, M., Dwolatzky, T., & Press, Y. (2012). Validation of the Hebrew version of the MoCA test as a screening instrument for the early detection of mild cognitive impairment in elderly individuals. *Journal of Geriatric Psychiatry and Neurology, 25*(3), 155-161.

Lin, H.-F., Chern, C.-M., Chen, H.-M., Yeh, Y.-C., Yao, S.-C., Huang, M.-F., Wang, S.-J., Chen, C.-S., & Fuh, J.-L. (2016). Validation of NINDS-VCI neuropsychology protocols for vascular cognitive impairment in Taiwan. *PLOS ONE, 11*(6), e0156404.

Lindeboom, J., ter Horst, R., Hooyer, C., Dinkgreve, M., & Jonker, C. (1993). Some psychometric properties of the CAMCOG. *Psychological Medicine, 23*(1), 213-219.

Logsdon, R. G., Gibbons, L. E., McCurry, S. M., & Teri, L. (1999). Quality of life in Alzheimer's disease: Patient and caregiver reports. *Journal of Mental Health and Aging, 5*, 21-32.

Lu, J., Li, D., Li, F., Zhou, A., Wang, F., Zuo, X., Jia, X.-F., Song, H., & Jia, J. (2011). Montreal cognitive assessment in detecting cognitive impairment in Chinese elderly individuals: A population-based study. *Journal of Geriatric Psychiatry and Neurology, 24*(4), 184-190.

Mahoney, F. I., & Barthel, D. W. (1965). Functional evaluation: The Barthel Index: a simple index of independence useful in scoring improvement in the rehabilitation of the chronically ill. *Maryland State Medical Journal.*

Maillet, D., Matharan, F., le Clésiau, H., Bailon, O., Pérès, K., Amieva, H., & Belin, C. (2016). TNI-93: A new memory test for dementia detection in illiterate and low-educated patients. *Archives of Clinical Neuropsychology, 31*(8), 896-903.

Mandyla, M.-A., Yannakoulia, M., Hadjigeorgiou, G., Dardiotis, E., Scarmeas, N., & Kosmidis, M. H. (2021). Identifying appropriate neuropsychological tests for uneducated/illiterate older individuals. *Journal of the International Neuropsychological Society*, 1-14.

Marin, D. B., Green, C. R., Schmeidler, J., Harvey, P. D., Lawlor, B. A., Ryan, T. M., Aryan, M., Davis, K. L., & Mohs, R. C. (1997). Noncognitive disturbances in Alzheimer's disease: Frequency, longitudinal course, and relationship to cognitive symptoms. *Journal of the American Geriatrics Society, 45*(11), 1331-1338.

Mathuranath, P. S., George, A., Cherian, P. J., Mathew, R., & Sarma, P. S. (2005). Instrumental activities of daily living scale for dementia screening in elderly people. *International Psychogeriatrics, 17*(3), 461-474.

Mathuranath, P. S., Nestor, P. J., Berrios, G. E., Rakowicz, W., & Hodges, J. R. (2000). A brief cognitive test battery to differentiate Alzheimer's disease and frontotemporal dementia. *Neurology, 55*(11), 1613-1620.

McGuinness, B., Barrett, S. L., Craig, D., Lawson, J., & Passmore, A. P. (2010). Attention deficits in Alzheimer's disease and vascular dementia. *Journal of Neurology, Neurosurgery & Psychiatry, 81*(2), 157-159.

Memória, C. M., Yassuda, M. S., Nakano, E. Y., & Forlenza, O. V. (2013). Brief screening for mild cognitive impairment: validation of the Brazilian version of the Montreal cognitive assessment. *International Journal of Geriatric Psychiatry, 28*(1), 34-40.

Mendez, M. F., Turner, J., Gilmore, G. C., Remler, B., & Tomsak, R. L. (1990). Balint's syndrome in Alzheimer's disease: Visuospatial functions. *International Journal of Neuroscience, 54*(3-4), 339-346.

Meyers, J. E., & Meyers, K. R. (1995). Rey complex figure test under four different administration procedures. *Clinical Neuropsychologist, 9*(1), 63-67.

Mioshi, E., Dawson, K., Mitchell, J., Arnold, R., & Hodges, J. R. (2006). The Addenbrooke's Cognitive Examination Revised (ACE-R): A brief cognitive test battery for dementia screening. *International Journal of Geriatric Psychiatry: A Journal of the Psychiatry of Late Life and Allied Sciences, 21*(11), 1078-1085.

Mok, W. Y. W., Chu, L. W., Chung, C. P., Chan, N. Y., & Hui, S. L. (2004). The relationship between non-cognitive symptoms and functional impairment in Alzheimer's disease. *International Journal of Geriatric Psychiatry, 19*(11), 1040-1046.

Montgomery, S. A., & Åsberg, M. (1979). A new depression scale designed to be sensitive to change. *British Journal of Psychiatry, 134*(4), 382-389.

Morris, J. C., Mohs, R. C., & Rogers, H. (1989). Consortium to establish a registry for Alzheimer's disease (CERAD) clinical and neuropsychological. *Psychopharmacology Bulletin, 24*(3-4), 641.

Mungas, D., Beckett, L., Harvey, D., Tomaszewski Farias, S., Reed, B., Carmichael, O., Olichney, J., Miller, J., & DeCarli, C. (2010). Heterogeneity of cognitive trajectories in diverse older persons. *Psychology and Aging, 25*(3), 606.

Muñoz-Neira, C., Henríquez Chaparro, F., Delgado, C., Brown, J., & Slachevsky, A. (2014). Test your memory—Spanish version (TYM-S): A validation study of a self-administered cognitive screening test. *International Journal of Geriatric Psychiatry, 29*(7), 730-740.

Nasreddine, Z. S., Phillips, N. A., Bédirian, V., Charbonneau, S., Whitehead, V., Collin, I., Cummings, J. L., & Chertkow, H. (2005). The Montreal Cognitive Assessment, MoCA: A brief screening tool for mild cognitive impairment. *Journal of the American Geriatrics Society, 53*(4), 695-699.

Nebes, R. D. (1989). Semantic memory in Alzheimer's disease. *Psychological Bulletin, 106*(3), 377.

Nicholas, M., Obler, L. K., Albert, M. L., & Helm-Estabrooks, N. (1985). Empty speech in Alzheimer's disease and fluent aphasia. *Journal of Speech, Language, and Hearing Research, 28*(3), 405-410.

Nielsen, T. R., & Waldemar, G. (2016). Effects of literacy on semantic verbal fluency in an immigrant population. *Aging, Neuropsychology, and Cognition, 23*(5), 578-590.

Ostrosky, F., Ardila, A., & Rosselli, M. (1997). *NEUROPSI: Una batera neuropsicològica breve* [NEUROPSI; A brief neuropsychological test battery]. Laboratorios Bayer.

Paplikar, A., Alladi, S., Varghese, F., Mekala, S., Arshad, F., Sharma, M., Saroja, A. O., Divyaraj, G., Dutt, A., & Ellajosyula, R. (2021). Bilingualism and its implications for neuropsychological evaluation. *Archives of Clinical Neuropsychology, 36*(8), 1511-1522.

Partington, J. E., & Leiter, R. G. (1949). *Partington's Pathways Test.* Psychological Service Center Journal.

Pedrosa, H., de Sa, A., Guerreiro, M., Maroco, J., Simoes, M. R., Galasko, D., & de Mendonça, A. (2010). Functional evaluation distinguishes MCI patients from healthy elderly people—the ADCS/MCI/ADL scale. *Journal of Nutrition, Health & Aging, 14*(8), 703-709.

Perry, R. J., & Hodges, J. R. (1999). Attention and executive deficits in Alzheimer's disease: A critical review. *Brain, 122*(3), 383-404.

Pontón, M. O. (2001). Research and assessment issues with Hispanic populations. In M. O. Pontón & J. León-Carrión (Eds.), *Neuropsychology and the Hispanic patient: A clinical handbook* (pp. 39-58). Lawrence Erlbaum Associates Publishers.

Possin, K. L., Feigenbaum, D., Rankin, K. P., Smith, G. E., Boxer, A. L., Wood, K., Hanna, S. M., Miller, B. L., & Kramer, J. H. (2013). Dissociable executive functions in behavioral variant frontotemporal and Alzheimer dementias. *Neurology, 80*(24), 2180-2185.

Price, B. H., Gurvit, H., Weintraub, S., Geula, C., Leimkuhler, E., & Mesulam, M. (1993). Neuropsychological patterns and language deficits in 20 consecutive cases of autopsy-confirmed Alzheimer's disease. *Archives of Neurology, 50*(9), 931-937.

Prince, M., Acosta, D., Chiu, H., Scazufca, M., Varghese, M., & Group, 10/66 Dementia Research. (2003). Dementia diagnosis in developing countries: a cross-cultural validation study. *The Lancet, 361*(9361), 909-917.

Prince, M. J., Wimo, A., Guerchet, M. M., Ali, G. C., Wu, Y.-T., & Prina, M. (2015). *World Alzheimer report 2015: The global impact of dementia: An analysis of prevalence, incidence, cost and trends.*

Prins, N. D., van Dijk, E. J., den Heijer, T., Vermeer, S. E., Jolles, J., Koudstaal, P. J., Hofman, A., & Breteler, M. M. B. (2005). Cerebral small-vessel disease and decline in information processing speed, executive function and memory. *Brain, 128*(9), 2034-2041.

Rainer, M., Mucke, H. A., Masching, A., & Haushofer, M. (1999). Non-cognitive symptom profiles in dementia-experience from psychiatric services and memory clinics. *Psychiatrische Praxis, 26*(2), 71-75.

Rao, S. L., Subbakrishna, D. K., & Gopukumar, K. (2004). *NIMHANS neuropsychological battery manual.* National Institute of Mental Health and Neurosciences.

Raven, J. C., & Court, J. H. (1938). *Raven's Progressive Matrices.* Western Psychological Services.

Reisberg, B., Borenstein, J., Franssen, E., Salob, S., Steinberg, G., Shulman, E., Ferris, S. H., & Georgotas, A. (1987). BEHAVE-AD: A clinical rating scale for the assessment of pharmacologically remediable behavioral symptomatology in Alzheimer's disease. In *Alzheimer's Disease* (pp. 1-16). Springer.

Reisberg, B., Ferris, S. H., de Leon, M. J., & Crook, T. (1982). The Global Deterioration Scale for assessment of primary degenerative dementia. *American Journal of Psychiatry, 139*(9), 1136-1139. doi:10.1176/ajp.139.9.1136

Reisberg, B., Finkel, S., Overall, J., Schmidt-Gollas, N., Kanowski, S., Lehfeld, H., Hulla, F., Sclan, S. G., Wilms, H.-U., & Heininger, K. (2001). The Alzheimer's disease activities of daily living international scale (ADL-IS). *International Psychogeriatrics, 13*(2), 163-181.

Rockwood, K., Moorhouse, P. K., Song, X., MacKnight, C., Gauthier, S., Kertesz, A., Montgomery, P., Black, S., Hogan, D. B., & Guzman, A. (2007). Disease progression in vascular cognitive impairment: cognitive, functional and behavioural outcomes in the Consortium to Investigate Vascular Impairment of Cognition (CIVIC) cohort study. *Journal of the Neurological Sciences, 252*(2), 106-112.

Rodakowski, J., Skidmore, E. R., Reynolds III, C. F., Dew, M. A., Butters, M. A., Holm, M. B., Lopez, O. L., & Rogers, J. C. (2014). Can performance on daily activities discriminate between older adults with normal cognitive function and those with mild cognitive impairment? *Journal of the American Geriatrics Society, 62*(7), 1347-1352.

Rosen, W. G., Mohs, R. C., & Davis, K. L. (1984). A new rating scale for Alzheimer's disease. *American Journal of Psychiatry, 141*(11), 1356-1364. doi:10.1176/ajp.141.11.1356

Rosselli, M., Ardila, A., Lalwani, L. N., & Vélez-Uribe, I. (2016). The effect of language proficiency on executive functions in balanced and unbalanced Spanish–English bilinguals. *Bilingualism: Language and Cognition, 19*(3), 489-503.

Rosselli, M., Ardila, A., Salvatierra, J., Marquez, M., Luis, M., & Weekes, V. A. (2002). A cross-linguistic comparison of verbal fluency tests. *International Journal of Neuroscience, 112*(6), 759-776.

Rossetti, H. C., Cullum, C. M., Hynan, L. S., & Lacritz, L. (2010). The CERAD Neuropsychological Battery total score and the progression of Alzheimer's disease. *Alzheimer Disease and Associated Disorders, 24*(2), 138.

Roth, M., Tym, E., Mountjoy, C. Q., Huppert, F. A., Hendrie, H., Verma, S., & Goddard, R. (1986). CAMDEX: A standardised instrument for the diagnosis of mental disorder in the elderly with special reference to the early detection of dementia. *The British Journal of Psychiatry, 149*(6), 698-709.

Sahakian, B. J., Morris, R. G., Evenden, J. L., Heald, A., Levy, R., Philpot, M., & Robbins, T. W. (1988). A comparative study of visuospatial memory and learning in Alzheimer-type dementia and Parkinson's disease. *Brain, 111*(3), 695-718.

Salmon, E., Collette, F., Degueldre, C., Lemaire, C., & Franck, G. (2000). Voxel-based analysis of confounding effects of age and dementia severity on cerebral metabolism in Alzheimer's disease. *Human Brain Mapping, 10*(1), 39-48.

Sandoval, T. C., Gollan, T. H., Ferreira, V. S., & Salmon, D. P. (2010). What causes the bilingual disadvantage in verbal fluency? The dual-task analogy. *Bilingualism: Language and Cognition, 13*(2), 231-252.

Santangelo, G., Cuoco, S., Pellecchia, M. T., Erro, R., Barone, P., & Picillo, M. (2018). Comparative cognitive and neuropsychiatric profiles between Parkinson's disease, multiple system atrophy and progressive supranuclear palsy. *Journal of Neurology, 265*(11), 2602-2613.

Sawamoto, N., Honda, M., Hanakawa, T., Fukuyama, H., & Shibasaki, H. (2002). Cognitive slowing in Parkinson's disease: A behavioral evaluation independent of motor slowing. *Journal of Neuroscience, 22*(12), 5198-5203.

Schmidt, M. (1996). *Rey Auditory Verbal Learning test: A handbook* (Vol. 17). Western Psychological Services.

Schneider, L. S., Olin, J. T., Doody, R. S., Clark, C. M., Morris, J. C., Reisberg, B., Ferris, S. H., Schmitt, F. A., Grundman, M., & Thomas, R. G. (1997). Validity and reliability of the Alzheimer's Disease Cooperative Study-Clinical global impression of change (ADCS-CGIC). In *Alzheimer Disease* (pp. 425-429). Springer.

Singh, N., & Mishra, R. K. (2013). Second language proficiency modulates conflict-monitoring in an oculomotor Stroop task: Evidence from Hindi-English bilinguals. *Frontiers in Psychology, 4*, 322.

Sisco, S., Gross, A. L., Shih, R. A., Sachs, B. C., Glymour, M. M., Bangen, K. J., Benitez, A., Skinner, J., Schneider, B. C., & Manly, J. J. (2015). The role of early-life educational quality and literacy in explaining racial disparities in cognition in late life. *Journals of Gerontology Series B: Psychological Sciences and Social Sciences, 70*(4), 557-567.

Smith, A. (1973). *Symbol Digit Modalities test*. Western Psychological Services.

Smith, S. C., Lamping, D. L., Banerjee, S., Harwood, R., Foley, B., Smith, P., Cook, J. C., Murray, J., Prince, M., & Levin, E. (2005). Measurement of health-related quality of life for people with dementia: development of a new instrument (DEMQOL) and an evaluation of current methodology. *Health Technology Assessment (Winchester, England), 9*(10).

Snodgrass, J. G., & Vanderwart, M. (1980). A standardized set of 260 pictures: Norms for name agreement, image agreement, familiarity, and visual complexity. *Journal of Experimental Psychology: Human Learning and Memory, 6*(2), 174.

Steinberg, M., Tschanz, J. T., Corcoran, C., Steffens, D. C., Norton, M. C., Lyketsos, C. G., & Breitner, J. C. S. (2004). The persistence of neuropsychiatric symptoms in dementia: The Cache County Study. *International Journal of Geriatric Psychiatry, 19*(1), 19-26.

Stern, R. A., & White, T. (2003). *Neuropsychological Assessment Battery: Administration, scoring, and interpretation manual*. Psychological Assessment Resources.

Storandt, M. (1994). General principles of assessment of older adults. In M. Storandt & G. R. VandenBos (Eds.), *Neuropsychological assessment of dementia and depression in older adults: A clinician's guide* (pp. 7-32). American Psychological Association. https://doi.org/10.1037/10157-002

Strauss, E., Sherman, E. M. S., & Spreen, O. (2006). *A compendium of neuropsychological tests: Administration, norms, and commentary*. American Chemical Society.

Stroop, J. R. (1935). The basis of Ligon's theory. *American Journal of Psychology, 47*(3), 499-504.

Stuss, D. T. (2011). Traumatic brain injury: Relation to executive dysfunction and the frontal lobes. *Current Opinion in Neurology, 24*(6), 584-589.

Takenoshita, S., Terada, S., Yoshida, H., Yamaguchi, M., Yabe, M., Imai, N., Horiuchi, M., Miki, T., Yokota, O., & Yamada, N. (2019). Validation of Addenbrooke's Cognitive Examination III for detecting mild cognitive impairment and dementia in Japan. *BMC Geriatrics, 19*(1), 1-8.

Taler, V., & Phillips, N. A. (2008). Language performance in Alzheimer's disease and mild cognitive impairment: A comparative review. *Journal of Clinical and Experimental Neuropsychology, 30*(5), 501-556.

Tariot, P. N., Mack, J. L., Patterson, M. B., Edland, S. D., Weiner, M. F., Fillenbaum, G., Blazina, L., Teri, L., Rubin, E., & Mortimer, J. A. (1995). The behavior rating scale for dementia of the consortium to establish a registry for Alzheimer's disease. *American Journal of Psychiatry, 152*(9), 1349-1357. https://doi.org/10.1176/ajp.152.9.1349

Trahan, D. E., & Larrabee, G. J. (1983). *Continuous Visual Memory test*. Psychological Assessment Resources.

Trenerry, M. R., Crosson, B., DeBoe, J., & Leber, W. R. (1990). *Visual Search and Attention test: Professional manual*. PAR Psychological Assessment Resources.

UNESCO Institute for Statistics. (2013). *Adult and youth literacy*. Published online.

Unverzagt, F. W., Morgan, O. S., Thesiger, C. H., Eldemire, D. A., Luseko, J., Pokuri, S., Hui, S. I. U. L., Hall, K. S., & Hendrie, H. C. (1999). Clinical utility of CERAD neuropsychological battery in elderly Jamaicans. *Journal of the International Neuropsychological Society, 5*(3), 255-259.

Verghese, J., Noone, M. L., Johnson, B., Ambrose, A. F., Wang, C., Buschke, H., Pradeep, V. G., Abdul Salam, K., Shaji, K. S., & Mathuranath, P. S. (2012). Picture-based memory impairment screen for dementia. *Journal of the American Geriatrics Society, 60*(11), 2116-2120.

Vygotsky, L. S., & Cole, M. (1978). *Mind in society: Development of higher psychological processes*. Harvard University Press.

Waldemar, G., Phung, K. T. T., Burns, A., Georges, J., Hansen, F. R., Iliffe, S., Marking, C., Rikkert, M. O., Selmes, J., Stoppe, G., & Sartorius, N. (2007). Access to diagnostic evaluation and treatment for dementia in Europe. *International Journal of Geriatric Psychiatry, 22*(1), 47-54.

Wang, B., Ou, Z., Gu, X., Wei, C., Xu, J., & Shi, J. (2017). Validation of the Chinese version of Addenbrooke's Cognitive Examination III for diagnosing dementia. *International Journal of Geriatric Psychiatry, 32*(12), e173-e179.

Wang, B.-R., Zheng, H.-F., Xu, C., Sun, Y., Zhang, Y.-D., & Shi, J.-Q. (2019). Comparative diagnostic accuracy of ACE-III and MoCA for detecting mild cognitive impairment. *Neuropsychiatric Disease and Treatment, 15,* 2647.

Ware Jr, J. E., & Sherbourne, C. D. (1992). The MOS 36-item short-form health survey (SF-36): I. Conceptual framework and item selection. *Medical Care,* 473-483.

Wechsler, D. (1945). A standardized memory scale for clinical use. *Journal of Psychology, 19*(1), 87-95.

Wechsler, D. (1955). Wechsler Adult Intelligence Scale. *Archives of Clinical Neuropsychology.*

Wechsler, D. (1999). *Wechsler abbreviated scale of intelligence.* APA PsycTests.

Weintraub, S., Dikmen, S. S., Heaton, R. K., Tulsky, D. S., Zelazo, P. D., Bauer, P. J., Carlozzi, N. E., Slotkin, J., Blitz, D., & Wallner-Allen, K. (2013). Cognition assessment using the NIH Toolbox. *Neurology, 80*(11 Suppl. 3), S54-S64.

Wilson, B. A., Evans, J. J., Alderman, N., Burgess, P. W., & Emslie, H. (1997). Behavioural assessment of the dysexecutive syndrome. *Methodology of Frontal and Executive Function, 239,* 250.

World Health Organization (2018). *The global dementia observatory reference guide.* Author.

Yesavage, J. A., Brink, T. L., Rose, T. L., Lum, O., Huang, V., Adey, M., & Leirer, V. O. (1982). Development and validation of a geriatric depression screening scale: a preliminary report. *Journal of Psychiatric Research, 17*(1), 37-49.

Yu, K.-H., Cho, S.-J., Oh, M. S., Jung, S., Lee, J.-H., Shin, J.-H., Koh, I.-S., Cha, J.-K., Park, J.-M., & Bae, H.-J. (2013). Cognitive impairment evaluated with Vascular Cognitive Impairment Harmonization Standards in a multicenter prospective stroke cohort in Korea. *Stroke, 44*(3), 786-788.

Zarit, S. H., Reever, K. E., & Bach-Peterson, J. (1980). Relatives of the impaired elderly: Correlates of feelings of burden. *The Gerontologist, 20*(6), 649-655.

Zhou, S., Zhu, J., Zhang, N., Wang, B., Li, T., Lv, X., Ng, T. P., Yu, X., & Wang, H. (2014). The influence of education on Chinese version of Montreal cognitive assessment in detecting amnesic mild cognitive impairment among older people in a Beijing rural community. *The Scientific World Journal, 2014,* 689456. doi:10.1155/2014/689456

Glossary

accent: Linguistic variation at the speech sound level. Usually perceived in terms of difference from the normative dialect (in North America, Standard American English). May be heard in speakers of English as a second language (i.e., a foreign accent), or in speakers of a dialect other than Standard American English. As an example, a speaker from Texas may produce ride as "rahd," or get as "git." Accents are to be distinguished from variation at other levels of language, e.g., at the level of grammar (such as ain't for isn't).

accommodation: A common dynamic in human interaction, where speakers tend to become more similar on all levels of language while talking to each other.

activity: The component of the *International Classification of Functioning, Disability and Health* that represents the capacity to carry out a behavior or skill in a situation in which the effect of the context is absent or made irrelevant (e.g., in a standardized evaluation setting).

adjunct: A part of a sentence that specifies additional information, in English usually as a prepositional phrase (e.g., The sun rose slowly <u>over the city</u> [adjunct underlined]).

affix: Umbrella term for prefix and suffix.

affricate: A double consonant sound that begins with a plosive and turns into a fricative. Examples in English include the sounds written as ch and j.

A-FROM (Aphasia Framework for Outcome Measurement): A framework for outcome measurement in aphasia, based on the *International Classification of Functioning Disability and Health.*

agitation: A psychiatric condition in which a person becomes restless and irritable. It is common in cognitive disorders such as Alzheimer's disease, frontotemporal dementia, vascular dementia, and other dementias. Severe agitation impairs social functioning and daily functionality, which requires medical care.

Bortz, M. (Ed.). *A Guide to Global Language Assessment: A Lifespan Approach* (pp. 355-369).
DOI: 10.4324/9781003524472

agrammatic primary progressive aphasia (PPA): A subtype of PPA is also referred to as progressive non-fluent aphasia. This type of PPA occurs due to neurodegeneration in the left inferior frontal and anterior-superior temporal areas, characterized by effortful, nonfluent speech. They will have difficulty to process the grammatical aspects of language.

agraphia: An acquired writing disorder due to brain injury.

alexia: An acquired reading disorder due to brain injury. Alexia can include an impairment of oral reading and/or an impairment of reading comprehension.

Amerindians: The Indigenous people of Caribbean who were the main inhabitants of Guyana at the time of European contact.

Anglo: A shorthand term for White North Americans of Anglo-Saxon descent; may also be used for other White North Americans who have assimilated into the Anglo mainstream. In a broader sense, Anglo serves as a prefix to refer to English origin in general. (*See* **Anglophone**.)

Anglophone: A geographical area or a population where/for whom English is the primary language.

anxiety disorder: A psychiatric condition in which a person has intense and persistent anxiety, worry, or fear about daily situations that interfere with ADLs and social functioning.

APA: American Psychological Association.

apathy: Lack of interest or motivation to social or emotional situations around oneself.

aphasia: An impairment of language affecting speech comprehension, production, naming, repetition, reading, and writing caused by damage in the brain areas related to language processing.

approximant: A speech sound that, by virtue of its acoustics, falls in between consonants and vowels. In English, this refers to the liquids (the sounds written as l, r) and the glides (the sounds written as y, w). Approximants are usually classified as consonants because they can form an acoustic boundary between two vowels; but unlike in regular consonants, airflow out of the mouth is not blocked (partially or fully).

ASD: Autism spectrum disorder.

ASHA: American Speech-Language-Hearing Association.

aspects (of language): In the chapter, when used to refer to language specifically (as opposed to aspects of communication), the same as components of language.

association: In the chapter, any kind of connection between mental representations.

attention: A cognitive process that involves actively focusing on specific stimuli or aspects of the environment while ignoring the other details.

automatic speech recognition (ASR): The automatic translation of speech into text using machine learning applications.

auxiliary: Any form of the verbs to be, to do, or to have that accompanies a main verb to specify its tense, e.g., I am running or Paul didn't call me (auxiliaries underlined).

base: *See* **word base.**

behavioral variant of frontotemporal dementia: One of the variants of frontotemporal dementia that involves changes in personality and behavior. Typical symptoms include behavioral disinhibition, apathy, loss of empathy, perseverations, executive function deficits, and changes in eating habits.

bilingual: A speaker or speech community who habitually relies on two languages for communication.

bilingualism: Ability to use two languages for communication in everyday life.

borrowed word: Also called a *loan word.* It is adapted from a source language to another language with or without modifications.

bound morpheme: A morpheme that cannot stand by itself. Also known as prefix or suffix, depending on its position with regard to the word base.

capacity: What a person can do in a standardized, controlled environment.

cardinal vowels: The vowels that are produced when the mouth is wide open (ah), or almost closed with or without rounding of the lips and backing of the tongue (oo and ee). Any other vowel quality falls somewhere between these three.

category: *See* **semantic categorization.**

Category Fluency Test: Important part of neuropsychological tests administered for individuals with brain damage. This test assesses the ability to retrieve as many words as possible from a specific category within a given time.

CDC: Centers for Disease Control and Prevention.

circumlocutions: A word is substituted by a phrase. It is a characteristic feature of anomic aphasia and some forms of dementia.

clausal density: Average number of clauses per utterance.

click sound: A consonant produced by "clucking" the tongue instead of pushing air out from the mouth. Clicks are found in various African languages.

Clock Drawing Test: A nonverbal screening test for detecting cognitive impairment. It assesses executive function and visuospatial function.

codemixing: The use of more than one language in a conversation by alternating languages within utterances, or inserting words from one language while speaking another language. Usually occurs in speech communities where bilingualism is the norm. *(See also* **translanguaging**.)

codeswitching: A multilingual speaker's practice of alternating between two or more languages in conversation. Can also be the practice of changing one's communication (language or dialect) when entering a speech community that is not one's own. May overlap with differences in cultural power, and be accompanied by feelings of "selling out."

cognition: A technical term for thinking, or more broadly for conscious information processing.

cognitive impairment: Any impairment in one or more cognitive domains involving sensory-perceptual, attention, learning, memory, language, thinking, and judgment skills. Dementia and mild cognitive impairment are common age-related cognitive impairments.

colonialism: The ideology and practice of European countries (with Britain in the lead) subduing a vast majority of the world's cultures for power and profit. At its height from the 1700s to the mid-1900s, colonialism has resulted in today's globalized and interconnected world, and in the prevalence of European languages (with English in the lead) in a multitude of speech communities around the globe.

Color Trail Test: A neuropsychological test analogous to the Trail Making Test used for assessing frontal or executive function abilities. It is designed to reduce culture bias and language bias.

communication: A complex, multifaceted process of transmitting information. For the purposes of the chapter, communication refers only to face-to-face interaction between humans, although it also occurs in non-face-to-face and nonsynchronous forms (e.g., in texting or writing books), and between nonhuman entities (animals or computerized devices). In face-to-face interaction between humans, communication comprises nonverbal, extralinguistic, and verbal aspects, as well as the intention(s) of the persons involved, and their interpretation of the other person's communicative actions.

communicative action: Any action by a speaker and/or hearer during face-to-face interaction that is intended or can be interpreted as part of the ongoing communication.

community-based research (CBR): CBR always focuses on a topic that has been identified as relevant in a given community by the community itself. It has a partnership approach and always involves community members, researchers, and other organizational representatives in all stages of the research process.

components (of language): The five traditional levels or aspects of language (all three terms are used interchangeably in the chapter) that scholars arrive at when they analyze language. Components include pragmatics (the use of language), semantics (the meaningful content of language), syntax (the structure of sentences), morphology (the meaning-related structure of words), and phonology (the sound structure of words). The latter three are subsumed under the form of language, yielding a threefold partition into use, content, and form. The term levels imply a hierarchy among components; it is commonly assumed that pragmatics is the highest-ranking among them, as the intended use of one's verbal expression shapes both content and all aspects of form. Phonology is considered the lowest level, since its units of analysis—phonemes and syllables—are devoid of meaning, as opposed to units of analysis at the other levels. Morphology ranks below semantics and syntax, as its unit of analysis, i.e., morphemes, includes the internal structure of the words that form sentences. Syntax is ranked below semantics, as sentences have meaning but meaning can be encoded in an array of other verbal communicative actions, from whole discourses (encompassing multiple sentences) to single-word utterances.

concentration: A cognitive process allowing a person to selectively pay attention to external stimuli while ignoring others for an extended period of time.

concept: The mental representation of a word's meaning.

confrontation naming: Involves identifying an object that is visually presented or represented in a line drawing. It is generally included as part of the neuropsychological assessment to check word retrieval ability. Commonly used picture naming tests assess confrontation naming.

connotation: The emotional aspects of an individual's mental representation of a word.

connotative: *See* **connotation**.

consonant: Any speech sound produced by closing the mouth so that the air pushed out from the lungs becomes turbulent *(see* **fricative**) or gets stopped completely *(see* **plosive**). Note: Approximants are considered consonants even though they do not meet these criteria *(see* **vowel**), so are clicks.

consonant cluster: An occurrence of two consonants in direct vicinity. Examples are found in words of the following shapes: stem, cart, cakes, baked, told, etc. (clusters underlined).

Contextual Factors: The component of the *International Classification of Functioning, Disability and Health* that represents the personal and environmental factors that influence an individual's life.

conversation analysis: A qualitative approach to the study of social interactions that uses detailed micro-analysis of spoken language, gesture, embodied action, and gaze. Data are often collected through video recording and analyzed to show how participants respond to one another in moment-by-moment sequences, shaping the unfolding interaction in both predictable and unexpected ways.

copula: Any form of the verb to be that functions as the only verb in a sentence, e.g., in I am a doctor or Paul was not at home (copulas underlined).

creole: A natural language that develops when children are born in a pidgin-speaking community and the pidgin becomes their native language, fulfilling all their communicative needs.

creole continuum: A dialect continuum of varieties of a creole language, ranging between the variety that is most distinct from the lexifier or superstrate language and the variety that most closely resembles the lexifier or superstrate language.

cross-linguistic comparison: Comparing abilities in domains of language, such as vocabulary or grammar, in multilingual speakers across all of their languages.

cross-linguistic influences: The influence of language-specific features of an individual's language, such as syntactic, morphological, or phonotactic rules, on their other language.

culture: The customs, arts, social institutions, and achievements of a particular nation, people, or other social group.

declarative knowledge: What we know about something. My declarative knowledge may include the various plants referred to by the word tree, that America was founded in 1776, or that in a North American context a male staring at another male intends to convey contempt or aggression. Declarative knowledge is distinguished from procedural knowledge, which comprises the how-to of performing actions.

deficit discourses: Modes of speaking, writing, or constructing policy that frame people's disadvantages as resulting from their own deficiencies or failures. Deficit discourses can seem benevolent, but are deeply embedded in racism, classism, patriarchy, and/or ableism. The notion of a "word gap" is a deficit discourse currently popular in the United States that suggests children from minoritized and stigmatized communities could do better in school if only their parents would speak differently to them in early childhood.

deictic: A communicative action (gestural or verbal) that derives its meaning, at least partly, from the speaker's physical and cognitive orientation, and hence changes meaning when used by another speaker. As an example, the deictic gesture of pointing needs to be adjusted depending on the direction from which the speaker is pointing at an object of interest. By contrast, nondeictic gestures such as flapping of arms to indicate a bird do not change their meaning based on speaker orientation.

delusion: A psychotic symptom characterized by a rigid, idiosyncratic, and false belief that is against reality.

dementia: General term used for progressive decline in attention, orientation, memory, language, thinking and judgement from a previous level of functioning that severely interfere with activities of daily living.

depression: A common mental disorder characterized by a persistent feeling of sadness, hopelessness, and loss of interest in activities severe enough to interfere with daily functioning.

determiner: A word that "determines" the reference scope of a noun. For the purposes of the chapter, we use determiner exclusively to mean "a" and "the" (and their equivalents in other languages). Under this definition, it "determines" that the referent object of the noun in question is singular, countable, and newly introduced in a conversation (e.g., I saw a good movie last night). By contrast, the covers both singular and plural of countable referents (the movie versus the movies), and implies that the referent is known to both speakers in the conversation (e.g., The movie was good). These intertwined layers of meaning make determiners hard to acquire for speakers of languages with different systems.

developmental language disorder (DLD): A condition that is diagnosed when a child's language skills (oral, written, and sign) are persistently below the level expected for the child's age and interfere with their ability to communicate effectively with other people; the condition occurs in the absence of a known biomedical condition such as autism spectrum disorder or Down syndrome.

Developmental Sentence Scoring (DSS): A composite measure to quantify and evaluate the grammatic complexity of children's expressive language.

DHR: *Declaration of Human Rights.*

dialect: A form of language variety. From a scholarly standpoint, a system of linguistic communication is called a dialect of [language X] when it is mutually intelligible with other dialects of the same language. This applies to African American English, Southern White English, and Standard American English (dialects of American English), or to Received Pronunciation, Cockney, and Liverpool Scouse (dialects of British English). For sociocultural and political rather than scientific reasons, however, dialects are frequently perceived as (inferior and/or "homely") variations on a conventional "standard" such as SAE or RP. Clinicians are asked to adopt the scholarly view.

differential diagnosis: A systematic process of determining a disorder or condition from other disorders or conditions exhibiting similar symptoms.

Digit Span: A test of verbal short-term working memory that includes forward and backward span. Forward span assesses the number of digits one can repeat immediately following the presentation in the same order, and backward span assess the number of digits one can repeat immediately following the presentation in the reverse order.

diphthong: A speech sound composed of two vowels that are joined in one continuous mouth movement. Standard American English has the following diphthongs: *i* as in bite, *ow* as in house, *oy* as in boy, *ey* as in bay, and *o* as in boat. The first three are fairly common across the world's languages, while the latter two are less frequent. In addition, they are produced using a subtler movement. Both factors may make them harder to learn for speakers from a non-English background.

disproportionality: A group's representation in a particular category that exceeds expectations for that group, or differs substantially from the representation of others in that category.

divided attention: Attention allocated to one or more channels of information concurrently, allowing one to simultaneously perform multiple tasks.

domain: In the chapter, we use the term domain to mean topic areas. For reasons unrelated to language background (e.g., personal, professional, or cultural ones), speakers may be very knowledgeable in one domain—and hence able to talk about it in depth in the language in which they have acquired their knowledge—but less knowledgeable in another. As an example, individuals from India or Nigeria may have acquired much of their academic knowledge in English, their proficiency in academic language may therefore be well ahead of their pragmatic competence in everyday communication.

DSM-5: *Diagnostic and Statistical Manual of Mental Disorders, Fifth Edition.*

dual-language learners (DLL): Children who are acquiring two or more languages at the same time or are learning a second language while developing their first (typically the home language along with the majority language of a country).

dynamic assessment: An assessment process that uses an active teaching process where a clinician will assess a child's perception, learning, thinking, and problem solving using specific tasks

echolalia: Uncontrolled repetition of words and phrases of others. It is a common symptom in childhood autism, dementia, aphasia, and traumatic brain injury.

ecological validity: Measures how generalizable findings gained in speech and language assessment are to the real communicative abilities of children in everyday communication.

Educational Assessment and Resource Centre (EARC): In Kenya, EARCs are community centers for children with disabilities where they can be assessed to determine appropriate school placement, to obtain referrals to health and rehabilitation professionals, and can receive (re)habilitative therapy.

empathy: Ability to be sensitive and understand other people's feelings, thoughts, and experiences within their frame of reference.

encoding: A process by which a socially shared meaning is given a linguistic form.

English learner (EL) or English language learner (ELL): An individual who has limited proficiency in the English language and typically requires specialized or modified instruction in both the English language and in their academic courses.

entrenchment: The process by which a mental representation (especially of the procedural kind) gets "etched" into a speaker's cognitive system, so that the speaker is able to access it even subconsciously and/or in situations where their system is taxed by various demands.

episodic memory: It is a type of long-term explicit memory that involves memory of events, situations, and personal experiences. Impairment in episodic memory is the most common symptom of Alzheimer's disease.

ethnographic assessment: An evaluation of speech and language that considers the child's familial and environmental culture though the use of nonbiased evaluation materials.

ethnography: A qualitative research approach that emphasizes long-term participation in the life of a specific community. Ethnographic research aims to describe the practices and perspectives of those being studied, shedding light on how they make meaning out of events and what motivates their actions. Ethnographers use a variety of methods to gather data such as participant observation, interviewing, review of documents, or video recording.

executive function: Executive function refers to the higher-order cognitive processes such as attention, inhibition, working memory, task switching, problem solving, reasoning, and planning. These all help to perform goal-directed behaviors in everyday life.

executive function skills: A set of high-level cognitive processes, for example, inhibition, set shifting, and attention, that support planning and executing a variety of behaviors and mental activities.

extralinguistic: Refers to aspects of the communication process that are neither verbal nor nonverbal. In this book we use the term mainly to mean the same as paralinguistic behaviors or conventions.

facial affect: Essential part of nonverbal communication in which emotions are expressed through the face.

false friends: Words from different languages whose form is similar but who have a quite different meaning. Examples include English exit and Spanish éxito ("success"), or French joli ("pretty, beautiful") and English jolly. False friends occur almost exclusively between closely related languages, and typically pose problems for more advanced speakers of both idioms in question.

fast science: Fast science directly builds on previously published research, and its aims are defined by previously produced knowledge. Hence, if any disparity or iniquity is present in a research line, fast science will reinforce those. Fast science can be contrasted with CBR that is always motivated by a specific community's need and does not directly build on previous research.

filler: A communicative action that "fills" speakers' pauses and is also used for hearer feedback, that is, for actions produced by listeners to let the speaker know they are listening. Examples in English include uh-huh, ok, head nods, and the like.

focus group: Small group of professionals with similar backgrounds who share their ideas, beliefs, and practices on a particular area of interest.

form: In linguistics, the outer structure of linguistic productions, that is, the levels of syntax, morphology, and phonology. Form is distinguished from the content *(see* **semantics**) and use aspects of language *(see* **pragmatics**).

frequency: As an aspect of prosody, frequency means the same as pitch—that is, the alternation between "lower" and "higher" voice in normal speaking. *See also* **intonation**.

fricative: A speech sound produced by closing the mouth just enough so that the airflow becomes turbulent and produces audible friction. Examples in English include /f/, /v/, /s/, /z/, /ʃ/, /θ/, /ð/, /h/, and /ʒ/.

frontal lobe function: Executive functions involving higher-order cognitive skills such as attention, working memory, inhibition, planning, organization, thinking, reasoning and problem solving, emotional control, self-monitoring, and execution of voluntary movements are referred to as frontal lobe functions.

frontal subcortical circuits: They link the regions of the frontal lobe and subcortical structures that mediate motor activity and behaviors in humans. There are five parallel frontal subcortical circuits that connect the frontal lobe with the striatum, basal ganglia, and thalamus. The motor circuit originates in the supplementary motor area, occulomotor circuit in the frontal eye fields, and three circuits in the prefrontal cortex (dorsolateral prefrontal cortex, lateral orbital cortex, and anterior cingulate cortex).

frontotemporal dementia: A subtype of dementia caused by progressive neurodegeneration primarily in the frontal and temporal areas of the brain affecting personality, behavior, and language.

functional communication: A communication approach focused on getting the message across, rather than on use of grammatical and complete language production.

genealogy: In linguistics, the study of the ways languages are related to each other.

general-purpose verbs: High-frequency verbs that are not tied to specific actions.

gestural communication: *See* **gesture**.

gesture: A communicative action done with one's body or a part thereof. Examples include hand movements for emphasis, pointing, nodding "yes," "thumbs up," etc.

graduated prompting: A type of dynamic assessment that entails the clinician going through a prompt hierarchy to determine how much prompting or how many prompts the client needs to be successful or to grasp the desired skill.

grammar: In linguistics, an umbrella term for syntax and morphology.

hallucination: A psychotic symptom characterized by the perception of sensory stimuli (visual/auditory/tactile/gustatory/proprioceptive) that are not really present.

heuristic: A "mental shortcut" to quickly arrive at a mental representation (however preliminary) of how facts are related to other facts.

high-context culture: A culture in which a large part of communication occurs via subtle nonverbal signals and through mutually assumed shared understanding of the situational context. Examples include many non-Western cultures, e.g., Japanese culture, where subtle shifts in eye gaze may communicate as much information as entire sentences in English. *(See also* **low-context culture.**)

Hindustani: The umbrella term for Hindi and Urdu, the main languages of Northern India and Pakistan, respectively. Linguistically speaking, Hindi and Urdu are dialects of each other, but politically they are official languages of two inimical nations.

honorifics: Bits of language used to indicate the social status of the speaker vis-à-vis the listener. Examples include Japanese, where affixes are attached to a listener's name to indicate their rank with regard to the speaker, or French and German, which use the second person singular pronoun when speakers are familiar with one another but the second (French) and third (German) person plural, respectively, when there is social distance between speakers.

ICD-10: *International Classification Disorders-10.*

idiom: Used in the chapter as a synonym for "individual language" (such as English, Kiswahili, or Tamil).

illiteracy: Lack of ability to read and write.

Index of Productive Syntax (IPSyn): A composite measure to quantify and evaluate the grammatic complexity of children's expressive language.

intensity: As an aspect of prosody, intensity means "loudness."

interference: In this book, it means the same as transfer; any linguistic behavior that deviates from the intended or target production and can be traced back to the speaker's underlying system.

interlanguage interference: A linguistic phenomenon in which words and phrases from the dominant language (L1) interfere with the nondominant language (L2). This often occurs in unbalanced bilinguals where the second language is less proficient than the first.

interlocutor: An umbrella term for speaker and listener during conversation.

International Classification of Functioning, Disability and Health (ICF): A framework developed by the World Health Organization to provide a common language to describe health and disability by giving detailed operational definitions of different functions that constitute health.

International Phonetic Alphabet (IPA): An alphabetic system of phonetic notation based primarily on the Latin script.

intonation: In prosody, the combination of frequency (pitch) and duration aspects of spoken language, resulting in a language- and speaker-specific "up-and-down" over time.

Kiswahili: Also known as Swahili, Kiswahili is an East African language that serves as a lingua franca throughout Eastern Africa.

knowledge translation (KT): KT includes various activities that ensure research results generated and disseminated within academic settings reach the general public and/or organizations for practical use.

language disorder: A disorder of spoken and written language skills that may impact an individual's vocabulary, grammar, sentence structure, pragmatic, and phonological skills not associated with intellectual disabilities or other conditions.

language family: A group of languages that have a common ancestor language. Examples include the Romance languages (such as French, Spanish, Italian, and Romanian), which are all descended from Latin; or the Sino-Tibetan languages (such as Tibetan, Mandarin Chinese, Cantonese, or Burmese), which can all be traced back to a shared ancestor (termed Proto-Sino-Tibetan). Language families can also be part of larger families; for example, the Romance languages are part of the larger Indo-European family, which includes the Germanic family (with English and German, among others) and the Indo-Iranian family (with Persian and Hindustani as prominent members).

language mixed word: Often referred to as codemixing at the word level. A word from another known language is mixed with the original language spoken.

language mixing: The use of more than one language in a conversation or within an utterance.

language mode: Multilingual individuals can communicate in a predominantly monolingual mode, using one of their languages without any language mixing; or can communicate in a multilingual mode, using all their languages. Language mode is considered to be a continuum.

language proficiency: Level of mastery in comprehending, expressing, and using a particular language for communication purposes in daily life.

language socialization: A focus of research in anthropology, developmental psychology, and allied fields that examines how young children or novices become competent communicators within a particular community of practice. Language socialization researchers look at how linguistic, social, and cultural competency emerge together through engagement in embodied interactions and everyday routines.

language typology: The classification of different languages according to their structural features.

levels (of language): *See* **components of language**.

Lewy body dementia: A subtype of progressive dementia characterized by abnormal protein (Lewy bodies) in the brain areas involved in memory, reasoning, thinking, and movement. Alpha-synuclein is the major component of Lewy bodies. Distinguishing features include altered attention, alertness, visual hallucinations, sleep disturbances, bradykinesia, tremors, and rigidity.

lexeme: A lexicon entry, that is, a speaker's mental representation of an individual word. Also used for individual words of a language. Lexemes may consist of one or more free morphemes (compare house—1 morpheme—versus dollhouse—2 morphemes).

lexeme base: *See* **word base**.

lexical diversity: The range of different words used in a text or by a person in oral communication.

lexicon: A store of words from the vocabulary and knowledge of an individual; the entirety of a language's individual words. The words in lexicon are referred to as *lexemes.*

lexifier language: A language that provides the majority lexical items or vocabulary of a pidgin or creole language, often referred to as the *superstrate language.*

lingua franca: A language that serves as a shared idiom between native speakers of different languages, usually over a larger geographical region, during a specific period of time, or for a particular population. Examples include Kiswahili in East Africa, Latin for medieval European scholars and administrators, Sabir for medieval Mediterranean traders, and English for much of the world today.

linguistic competence: The system of knowledge that one has unconsciously about a language which enables them to produce and understand sentences, and to differentiate between grammatical and ungrammatical sentences.

liquid: A speech sound produced with partial closure of the mouth but does not feature turbulent ("noisy") sound or stoppage of sound. English liquids include the sounds written as r and l, respectively. *(See* **approximant**.)

logopenic PPA: A variant of primary progressive aphasia also known as phonological progressive aphasia. The speech is characterized by a slow rate, long pauses associated with word-finding difficulties, phonological paraphasias, and sentence repetition difficulties.

low-context culture: A culture in which communication does not rely on mutually assumed shared understanding of the situational context, and hence uses explicit, direct verbal statements rather than nonverbal signals or indirect verbal hints. Examples include many Western cultures, particularly American middle-class culture. *(See also* **high-context culture**.)

macrostructure (of a language): Overall, global meanings of discourse.

majority-world countries: Majority world is an alternative term for Global South or Third World. It includes countries in Africa, Asia, South, and Central America and the Caribbean.

mass noun: A noun that cannot take an indefinite determiner or the plural form. For an example, consider butter: it is not grammatically accurate to say a butter, and while butters can be used as a shorthand for packs or servings of butter, it cannot refer to the object itself.

mean length of utterances: A measure of linguistic productivity in children. It is calculated by dividing the number of words or morphemes by the number of utterances.

mediated learning: The social and quality interactions or exchanges between a clinician and the client with the purpose of providing enrichment of the student's learning experience.

memory: A cognitive process that entails encoding, storing, and retrieval of information learned in the past.

mental representation: Any piece of knowledge stored in a person's mind. Usually distinguished into declarative (semantic knowledge) and procedural (knowledge of skills).

microstructure (of a language): The local structures of words, clauses, sentences, or turns in conversation.

mild cognitive impairment: The transitional phase between normal aging and dementia is referred as mild cognitive impairment. It is characterized by a slight decline in one or more cognitive domains from a previous level of functioning, but not severe enough to affect instrumental activities of daily living.

modal verb: A verb that "modifies" a main verb with regard to the speaker's relationship to the action expressed in the main verb. Examples include must, which indicates an obligation; can, which refers to an ability; or would, which indicates a conditional potentiality. Grammatically speaking, modal verbs stand out among other verbs of English as they do not take a third person singular -s (as in he must, she can, or it would).

modalities of language: The four main forms of language: oral receptive language (auditory comprehension), oral expressive language (talking), reading, and writing.

modality: Any format in which linguistic communication is used. Examples include the spoken modality, either face-to-face or mediated by technology; the written modality in its various digital and paper-based forms; or the signed modality, as in the various sign languages of Deaf communities around the world.

modifiability: The strategies the student uses when learning new skills, the amount and types of prompts (e.g., scaffolding) the students require in response to the interventions provided, and an analysis of the types of gains the student made during the interventions.

monolingual: A speaker or speech community who habitually relies on only one language for communication.

morpheme: Any smallest unit of meaning in a given language. Morphemes can be distinguished into free and bound morphemes. Free morphemes are single words that can stand by themselves, such as book, happy, or swim; bound morphemes are affixes that cannot, such as the plural -s in books, the un- in unhappy, or the -ing in swimming. Depending on their position in the word, bound morphemes are further classified into prefixes and suffixes.

morphology: The component of language concerned with word structure, that is, the study of morphemes.

morphosyntactic features: The linguistic units having both morphological (relating to word structure and formation) and syntactic (relating to the combination of words and phrases in a sentence) properties.

motor skills: The technical term for the ability to produce precise, effective, and efficient movements.

Moving-Average Type/Token Ratio (MATTR): A calculatory variant of Type/Token Ratio.

Mughal: A dynasty of warrior kings from Central Asia who conquered and ruled over much of India from the 1500s to the 1800s.

multilingual: A speaker or speech community who habitually relies on more than two languages for communication. The term may also be used to include bilinguals.

multilingual individuals: People who use more than one language in their daily communication.

narrative: The technical term for stories and accounts of personal experience.

nasal: A type of speech sound produced with the airflow coming out from the nose, rather than the mouth. English nasals include /n/, /m/, and /ŋ/.

neurocognitive disorder: A group of disorders which is characterized by a decline in the previous level of cognitive functioning caused due to brain dysfunction. According to DSM-5, mild cognitive impairment is considered a minor neurocognitive disorder and dementia is considered as a major neurocognitive disorder.

neuropsychological testing: In-depth assessment using a group of tests specially designed for assessing global cognition; specific cognitive domains such as intelligence, attention, memory, language, visuospatial functions; and executive functions to infer about brain functioning. They are systematically administered in a formal environment by well-trained neuropsychologists.

nondeictic: *See* **deictic.**

nonfluent PPA: *See* **agrammatic PPA.**

nonstandardized assessment: An assessment that does not include a standardized test.

nonverbal: An umbrella term for aspects of communication that do not directly involve spoken words. Examples include gestures, facial expressions, head nods, and the like.

nonverbal memory: Ability to encode, store and retrieve nonverbal information (other than spoken and written). This includes retaining visual experiences, images, faces, shapes, smells, tastes, feelings, etc.

normative: Establishing, relating, or deriving from a standard norm.

normative: Something considered "normal." Normativity can be helpful or harmful when a client exhibits communicative actions not in line with prevalent norms. In a North American context, for example, Standard American (that is, White, middle-class, Anglo) communication norms include eye contact on part of the listener and subdued gestures on part of the speaker. In many African American speech communities, by contrast, eye contact while listening is considered disrespectful, and emphatic gesturing while speaking is the norm. Clinicians working with individuals from this culture can use normativity helpfully, using their knowledge of African American conventions to correctly understand individuals' actions as tokens of respect, attentiveness, and engagement. Or they can use normativity in a harmful way, penalizing or pathologizing actions that are not in line with White, Anglo norms.

noun: A type of word that refers to "things in the world" (including abstract "things"). Most nouns can take a plural form (compare house and houses).

object: In syntax, the sentence element that refers to an entity impacted by the action expressed in the main verb (as in, The boy threw <u>the ball</u>, object underlined).

object recognition: In cognitive psychology, it is the ability to recognize an object based on its physical (shape, size, color, texture) and semantic attributes (use and previous experience).

omission: The technical term for leaving something out.

overgeneralization: A type of production where a speaker takes a general linguistic rule and uses it where it does not apply. Examples in English include past tense *-ed* applied to irregular verbs (catched, runned), or plural *-s* applied to nouns with irregular plural, or to mass nouns (mouses, stuffs).

overlap: The event of two or more speakers talking at the same time.

paralinguistic: Refers to aspects of verbal communication that are neither actual words nor fall under nonverbal communication, includes loudness *(see* **volume**), rate of speech, and prosody.

Parkinson's disease: A progressive neurological disorder primarily affecting the motor unit causing bradykinesia, resting tremor, rigidity, and loss of postural reflexes. Nonmotor symptoms including dementia appear after more than a year of onset leading to difficulties in memory and thinking.

participation: The component of the *International Classification of Functioning, Disability and Health* that involves being actively engaged in tasks, activities, and routines at home, school, and community that are typical for persons of that age.

past tense: The grammatical form of verbs that expresses the event referred to by the verb took place in the past. English has both regular and irregular past tense forms (compare bak-ed, play-ed, wound-ed to ran, taught, lost, was).

PECS: Picture Exchange Communication System.

performance: What a person actually does in their daily environment.

phoneme: The smallest unit of language that, when exchanged for another such unit, changes a word's (or morpheme's) meaning. As an example, exchanging /p/ for /b/ creates a meaning difference in many languages (compare English pin versus bin). Phonemes are considered abstract units of language that may be produced in varying ways when used in spoken language. Variations occur based on a speaker's rate or articulatory proficiency, phonemic context within the utterance, and speaker's language status. A speaker of a non-standard dialect or from a different language background is likely to produce some phonemes differently than would be expected in the Standard dialect. *(See* **accent**.)

phonemic segment: An alternative term for phoneme.

phonetic inventory: An index of the different sounds and sound sequences children use across all word positions.

phonetic overlap: The shared phonemes of two or more languages.

phonetic symbols: Symbols representing sounds of a language.

phonology: A branch of linguistics to study speech sounds, their patterns, distribution, and organization within and across languages; the study of phonemes.

phrase: A syntactic unit of language that does not have a subject and predicate but can, in certain contexts, stand on its own. Examples include the man (noun phrase), running around the house (verb phrase) or around the house (prepositional phrase).

pidgin: A combination of two or more languages generally used for limited communication, but importantly where participants need a common language, for example, in contexts of trade.

pilot study: A pilot study is a small-scale preliminary study conducted before a full-scale study. The goal of a pilot study is to evaluate the feasibility of the planned research and to potentially improve study design.

PIR: Package of Interventions for Rehabilitation.

pitch: The alternation between "lower" and "higher" voice in normal speaking.

plosive: A speech sound produced by blocking the airflow coming out of the mouth and releasing it in a sudden burst. Examples in English include /t/, /p/, /k/, /d/, /b/, and /g/.

pragmatics: The component of language concerned with cultural conventions about speaking. Of the five traditional components of language, pragmatics is the broadest, encompassing a vast range of areas from general rules about taboo topics in conversation all the way to subtle distinctions of politeness (e.g., in requesting, consider the difference between may I ...? and can I ...?). Nonverbal and paralinguistic aspects of communication, as well as proxemics, are technically not part of pragmatics, but they are often treated as such for practical reasons. Together, these aspects of communication are perceived most readily by interlocutors and used to form rapid initial impressions of the speaker. If the speaker's pragmatics and nonverbals do not match the listener's cultural expectations, those impressions may well turn out negative, impacting subsequent interaction.

predicate: The part of a sentence that informs the listener what the speaker wants to say about the sentence's subject. As an example, consider the sentence Paul is a doctor. "Is a doctor" is what the listener learns about Paul, that is, the predicate.

prefix: A bound morpheme attached to the beginning of a word. Examples in English include *un-* as in unhappy, *de-* as in depart, or *mis-* as in mistreat.

preposition: A type of word that indicates a real world or abstract or grammatical relationship. As an example, it can refer to spatial configurations such as in the bowl, or abstractions from those such as in due time. To can mean toward or in order to, but also have a purely grammatical function such as in I want to leave.

prevalence: The proportion of the population with a particular disease, condition, or attribute at a particular point in time.

primary progressive aphasia (PPA): A neurological syndrome caused by focal degeneration of language areas mainly in the frontotemporal regions in the left hemisphere. There is progressive deterioration in the language including in understanding, speaking, and naming abilities.

procedural knowledge: Our how-to knowledge for motor and mental actions. My procedural knowledge may include how to ride a bike, how to form a sentence, or how to produce a word including all the correct speech sounds. Procedural knowledge is distinguished from declarative knowledge, which comprises the knowledge about things and phenomena.

production: What comes out of a speaker's mouth. Quite literally, what they produce when using language.

proficiency: The technical term for level of competence in any given language.

progressive supranuclear palsy: A rare chronic and progressive neurological disorder causing problems in movement, balance, vision, speech, swallowing, and cognition. It is caused by an accumulation of abnormal tau protein in the brain.

pronoun: A word that refers to or replaces a noun (or a proper name). Examples in Standard American English are I, you, he, she, it, they (first, second, and third persons singular); and we, you, they (first, second, and third persons plural). To distinguish the second persons singular and plural, Southern and African American English use y'all for the latter.

prosody: The duration, intensity, and frequency aspects of verbal communication—in other words, the speaker's intonation (the combination of rate and pitch) and volume (loudness).

proxemics: Cultural rules regarding distance between speakers.

PRT: Pivotal Response Treatment.

psychometric properties: They are particular intrinsic features of a test that include reliability and validity and indicate how well the test can evaluate the construct of interest. A good quality test should be reliable, valid, and have normative data.

pulmonary (sound): A speech sound produced with the help of airflow coming from the lungs and exiting the mouth or nose. Most speech sounds are pulmonary, but some languages feature sounds that are produced in different ways. *(See also* **click sound**.)

rate (of speech): The speed at which verbal language is produced.

recall: A mental process that involves recalling any previously learned information and bringing it into conscious awareness. If information is retrieved without any cue, it is referred to as free recall; if it is retrieved with a cue (partial information), it is referred to as cued recall.

reference dialect: The dialect of a language that clinicians, teachers, etc. use, consciously or unconsciously, to compare a speaker's productions against what is "normal." In the North American context, the reference dialect is Standard American English, which encompasses both the adult productions and the developmental aspects of White, professional-level communication. *(See also* **normative**.)

response inhibition: A cognitive process, specifically an executive function, which inhibits the habitually occurring, natural, dominant behavioral response to a stimulus that helps to perform adaptive goal-directed responses.

Sabir: A Romance language variety used for communication between traders around the Mediterranean. In use from the 11th to the 19th century, Sabir was also called lingua franca ("the language of the Franks," i.e., of the Europeans); this term was later extended to other idioms that serve similar purposes.

salient: The technical term for "standing out" or "being readily accessible/perceptible."

schematic association: The connection of the core meaning of a concept with extended meanings and with other core and extended meanings. As an example, the concept "dog" may be associated with scary for some speakers, but with a human's best friend for others. *(See also* **semantics**.)

schwa: The vowel sound produced in the very center of the mouth (e.g., the very first sound in "about").

screening: A systematic process of detecting the presence or absence of a condition/disease in people who are at risk for a specific disorder or condition using brief and less time-consuming instruments, measures, or tests. This helps in the early detection of the disease and further prevention and risk reduction management.

segmental features: Features of a language, such as consonant and vowel sounds or phonemes.

self-monitoring: A metacognitive ability to monitor and regulate one's own behaviors appropriate to the context. It is a function of the prefrontal cortex.

semantic categorization: The way individual languages structure declarative knowledge, typically in forms of taxonomies. An example would be the food category, which in most languages includes different types of foods such as vegetables, fruits, or meats that in turn comprise various concrete foods (e.g., carrot, apple, or pork). Both the content and the structure of such taxonomies varies by language and dialect, according to culture. For example, the meat category in SAE does not include grasshopper or squirrel. The same is not true for the languages of Southeast Asian cultures, where grasshoppers are considered a delicacy; or for Cajun English spoken in South Louisiana, where squirrels are regularly hunted for game. Wholesale taxonomic differences may be encountered in the realm of illness, where certain ailments may be considered spiritual rather than medical issues.

semantic memory: One type of long-term memory that deals with factual and conceptual information.

semantic variant of PPA: A subtype of PPA also referred to as semantic dementia is characterized by progressive loss of semantic knowledge despite other language and cognitive abilities being well preserved. Patients with a semantic variant of PPA have problems with naming and single-word comprehension.

semantics: The meaning component of language. In terms of mental representation, usually thought of as a central concept with an extended schema. As an example, together with the phonological representation for tree, speakers are thought to possess a general, abstract representation of trees (concept), as well as of the "place" of trees in the larger world and of the ways the word tree is used in language (extended schema).

sensitivity: The percentage of persons with the condition who are correctly identified by the test.

Sepedi: An Indigenous language that is the main member of the Sesotho language group, forming part of South Africa's 11 official languages.

set-shifting: Ability to unconsciously shift attention between two tasks or mental sets. It is one of the executive function processes that is also referred to as task-switching. It is a measure of mental flexibility.

short-term memory: Capacity to retain a limited amount of information for a short period of time.

small vessel vascular disease: Pathological condition causing the small end arteries, arterioles, venules, and capillaries to be narrowed causing reduced oxygenation in the heart.

social cognition: It is the unique ability of humans to interpret social information and behave appropriately according to the social context. This involves perceiving, processing, interpreting, and responding to social stimuli. More specifically, it encompasses processing facial expressions, joint attention, theory of mind, empathy, and moral processing.

socioeconomic status (SES): SES indicates an individual's or family's economic access to resources. It is often measured by education, income, or occupation.

sociolinguist: A linguist who studies the interrelation of language use and language variation on the one hand, and sociological phenomena on the other.

sociopsychological: The joint dynamics of social interaction and inner responses to the former.

South Asia: The Indian subcontinent and adjacent regions.

spatial localization: Locating an external stimulus (auditory, visual, or audiovisual) within the spatial map.

specificity: The percentage of persons without the condition who are correctly excluded by the test.

speech community: A group of people who share a common way of talking and communicating.

Standard American English (SAE): The dialect of the professional, college-educated, White, middle-class population in the United States. SAE serves as the normative or reference dialect in North America (with some regional variation).

standardized assessment: An assessment that uses a test that has been normed by age or population. It has strict administration and scoring guidelines.

standardized tests: Examinations administered and scored in a predetermined, standard manner, which include consistency in test materials, use of specific administration procedures, and use of specific and consistent scoring rules.

stereotypic utterances: Repetitive utterances which are either lexical forms or neologisms. Stereotypic utterances are common in aphasia and in frontotemporal dementia.

story grammar: The integral components of a story and the relationships among these parts.

subject: The part of a sentence about which the listener is informed by the speaker. As an example, consider the sentence: Paul is a doctor. "Paul" is what the listener is informed about, that is, the subject.

substitution: The technical term for exchanging something for something else.

suffix: A bound morpheme attached to the end of a word. Examples in English include *-s* as in tables, *-ing* as in swimming, or *-ed* as in baked.

suprasegmental features: Also called prosodic features, these are features of a language that accompany or add over speech sounds such as stress, tone, or word juncture.

sustained attention: Ability to attend or focus on a specific stimulus for an extended period of time.

syntax: The study of sentence elements. Typically recognized elements include subject and predicate, with the predicate potentially containing a verb, object, and adjunct. Alternatively, sentences may also be analyzed into phrases.

tap: A sound produced by briefly "tapping" the tip of the tongue against the roof of the mouth. Fairly common across the world's languages, this sound is commonly used by foreign speakers of English to replace the liquid English r.

TEACCH: Treatment and Education of Autistic and Related Communication Handicapped Children.

telepractice: The use of telecommunication technology to deliver health care services.

tense: The linguistic term for time; specifically, for the way time is expressed in a given language's structure. All languages have ways of doing so, mainly through a mix of dedicated lexemes (such as today or tomorrow) and morphemes (such as -ed to indicate past, or will to indicate future).

Tense and Agreement Productivity (TAP): A composite measure for language sample analysis of children drawing.

Tense Marker Total (TMT): A composite measure of tense/agreement diversity.

Test-Teach-Retest: A type of dynamic assessment in which a clinician identifies areas impeding effective learning of a learner through assessment and subsequently provides explicit instruction for the identified area, the clinician then reassesses the client's understanding of what was taught.

Testing the Limits: A type of dynamic assessment in which a clinician gauges a client's skills during the assessment or an intervention trial.

topic-associating: The default structure for narratives in African American culture. Topic-associating narratives are less explicit and sequentially structured than topic-centered narratives, and hence require a more active listener. They consist in telling several episodes of events in which the main character/problem/event are left implicit for the listener to infer. Because of their structural differences to the Anglo narrative structure normative in schooling, topic-associating stories may not be valued or understood by teachers.

topic-centered: The default structure for narratives in many Western cultures, such as White (Anglo) American culture. Topic-centered narratives include a main character and a problem (or difficulty) that is overcome by the main character or a description of events that centers on a main event and follows a sequential order.

Trail Making Test: A paper-pencil neuropsychological test of visual attention, visual search, cognitive flexibility, and speed of processing. In the first part, one has to connect the numbers from 1 to 25 written in black dots in the forward sequence. In the second part, one has to connect the numbers from 1 to 25 and switch the color of the dots. The time taken to complete the task and errors are the output measures in the Trail Making Test.

transfer: In Chapter 3, the same as interference: any linguistic behavior that deviates from the intended or target production and can be traced back to the speaker's underlying system.

translanguaging: A more recent term for codemixing; that is, the interweaving of two (or more) languages in everyday conversation within one speech community. Usually occurs in speech communities where bilingualism is the norm. As an example, a Hispanic South Texan may produce utterances such as *Voy a trabajar now, see y'all later* ("I'm going to work now …"). Translanguaging as a way of life within a community is to be distinguished from codeswitching, where a speaker in a community not their own defers to the other community's normative standards in order to avoid sociopsychological repercussions.

triadic interactions: Interactions that take place between three people. Research on child language development has primarily focused on dyadic interactions (typically, face-to-face exchanges between a mother and her infant), but language socialization researchers show that many communities around the world favor a triadic or multi-party participation structure, while dyadic "conversations" between an adult and an infant are comparatively rare.

trill: A sound produced as a very rapid succession of taps.

turn at talk: A chunk of verbal communicative actions by one speaker in a conversation. Turns are counted from the moment a speaker starts talking to the moment they finish and another speaker takes a turn.

Type/Token Ratio (TTR): A measure of lexical diversity, calculated by the ratio of different unique word stems (types) to the total number of words (tokens).

utterance: A verbal communicative action that communicates a single thought. As thoughts can be simple or complex, utterances range from single-word productions such as yes and no, all the way to complex sentences.

variety: When used to mean "variety of a language," this term indicates a rule-based system that differs systematically from the normative variety. In North America, SAE is typically considered the standard (normative) variety; other varieties include African American English, Southern White English, or Hispanic English.

verb: A type of word that refers to an action or event (e.g., "slept" in The children slept).

verb group: A cluster of multiple verbs. Verb groups minimally feature an auxiliary and a main verb, as in Paul <u>was sleeping</u> (verb group underlined).

verbal: In linguistics, this term means "involving spoken words."

verbal communication: A type of communication in which messages are transmitted through written or spoken words.

verbal fluency: A neuropsychological test in which the person is asked to retrieve as many words possible from a specific category within a given time.

verbal memory: Ability to encode, store, and retrieve verbal or phonological information (spoken).

visual search: A perceptual process involving actively searching and detecting target stimuli among distractor stimuli.

visuospatial construction: The ability to see an image or object and construct the exact replica of the same. It is also referred to as constructional praxis.

visuospatial skills: Ability to identify visual and spatial relationships of objects within the environment that requires visually perceiving, analyzing, and manipulating objects.

volume: The technical term for "loudness."

vowel: Any speech sound produced by expelling air from the mouth unimpeded by closure so that the airflow is smooth (neither turbulent nor stopped). Approximants, while typically classified as consonants due to their function in syllable structure, meet this definition; they are therefore also called semivowels.

WEIRD Societies: Societies that are Western, Educated, Industrialized, Rich, and Developed. This acronym was coined by the psychologists Henrich, Heine, and Norezayan in a 2010 paper in which they pointed out that most research in the behavioral sciences was based solely on participants from such societies. They reviewed a wider range of comparative research and argued that WEIRD participants are outliers, not a reliable basis for generalizations about human cognition and behavior.

WHO: World Health Organization.

WHO region: A largely arbitrary subdivision of the world into six regions for administrative purposes within the World Health Organization.

word base: For present purposes, we define word base simply as any free morpheme(s) that form the core of a lexeme in question, and to which bound morphemes may be attached. Thus, when we speak of word bases, we mean the free morpheme house in houses, or dollhouse in dollhouses.

working memory: A part of short-term memory that stores and avails a small amount of information for a brief period while performing mental operations related to that information.

Financial Disclosures

Suvarna Alladi, DM Neurology reported no financial or proprietary interest in the materials present herein.

Kyriakos Antoniou, PhD is the coauthor of Chapter 15, of which the writing of this chapter has been supported by an award from the Cyprus Research and Innovation Foundation (CULTURE/AWARD-YR/0421B/0005) to the first and last authors.

Juan Bornman, PhD reported no financial or proprietary interest in the materials present herein.

Mellissa Bortz, PhD, CCC-SLP reported no financial or proprietary interest in the materials present herein.

Maria Christopoulou, EdD has not disclosed any relevant financial relationships.

Keziah Conrad, PhD, MS, CCC-SLP reported no financial or proprietary interest in the materials present herein.

Elise Davis-McFarland, PhD, CCC-SLP, ASHA Honors reported no financial or proprietary interest in the materials present herein.

Tamirand Nnena De Lisser, PhD reported no financial or proprietary interest in the materials present herein.

Jill de Villiers, PhD receives royalties as an author of the DREAM assessments.

Lisa Domby, MS, CCC-SLP reported no financial or proprietary interest in the materials present herein. The Brillo Assessment of Spanish Grammar and Personal Narratives is free-access material for use by credentialed speech-language therapists in Guatemala.

Hanna Ehlert, PhD reported no financial or proprietary interest in the materials present herein.

Lynn Ellwood, MHSc, S-LP(C), Reg. CASLPO reported no financial or proprietary interest in the materials present herein.

Elizabeth E. Galletta, PhD, CCC-SLP has not disclosed any relevant financial relationships.

Rachael Gibson reported no financial or proprietary interest in the materials present herein.

Mira Goral, PhD, CCC-SLP reported no financial or proprietary interest in the materials present herein.

Teresa Hutchings, MEd, CCC-SLP reported financial interests via royalties in the assessments and training materials described in their chapter.

Yvette D. Hyter, PhD, CCC-SLP, ASHA Honors reported no financial or proprietary interest in the materials present herein.

Maria Elizabeth Jaramillo, MS, MPH, CCC-SLP received a $600 travel award from the UNC Graduate and Professional Student Federation for activities related to development of the Brillo Assessment of Spanish Grammar and Personal Narratives.

Tobias A. Kroll, PhD, CCC-SLP reported no financial or proprietary interest in the materials present herein.

Wendy Lee, MS, CCC-SLP received compensation as an employee of Boao Bethel International Medical Center during the development of the assessments.

Xueman Lucy Liu, AuD/CCC-A/FAAA, MS/CCC-SLP receives royalties as an author of the DREAM assessments.

Ulrike Lüdtke, PhD reported no financial or proprietary interest in the materials present herein.

Monika Molnar, PhD reported no financial or proprietary interest in the materials present herein.

Giselle Núñez, PhD, CCC-SLP reported no financial or proprietary interest in the materials present herein.

Florence Omolo reported no financial or proprietary interest in the materials present herein.

Avanthi Paplikar, PhD, SLP reported no financial or proprietary interest in the materials present herein.

Kakia Petinou, PhD, SLP is the coauthor of Chapter 15, of which the writing of this chapter has been supported by an award from the Cyprus Research and Innovation Foundation (CULTURE/AWARD-YR/0421B/0005) to the first and last authors.

David K. Rochus reported no financial or proprietary interest in the materials present herein.

Eric Rolfhus, PhD has financial interests via royalties in the assessments and training materials described in Chapter 12.

Sulare Telford Rose, PhD, CCC-SLP reported no financial or proprietary interest in the materials present herein.

Lebogang Sehako reported no financial or proprietary interest in the materials present herein.

Jeannie van der Linde, PhD reported no financial or proprietary interest in the materials present herein.

Carla van Nieuwenhuizen reported no financial or proprietary interest in the materials present herein.

Christina Valenti, MA, CF-SLP, TSSLD reported no financial or proprietary interest in the materials present herein.

Anna Monina M. Vanta, MS, CCC-SLP reported no financial or proprietary interest in the materials present herein.

Aparna Venugopal, MSc, SLP reported no financial or proprietary interest in the materials present herein.

Samantha Washington, EdD, CCC-SLP reported no financial or proprietary interest in the materials present herein.

Carol Westby, PhD, CCC-SLP reported no financial or proprietary interest in the materials present herein.

Marleen F. Westerveld, PhD, FSPA, CPSP reported no financial or proprietary interest in the materials present herein.

Dr. phil. Jan Wohlgemuth, MA is faculty at Universitas Indonesia (a state-funded university) and is funded by DAAD (German Academic Exchange Service; funded by the German Federal Government).

Index

activities of daily living, dementia assessment, 338
adult language assessment, 305–354
adults application of language disorders in *International Classification of Functioning, Disability and Health,* 40
alternative methods of language assessment, 19
aphasia, 307–321
  assessment, 309–310
    nonstandardized assessment, 310
    standardized assessment, 310
  assessment in monolingual/multilingual people, 309–312
  assessment in multilingual contexts, 310–312
    nonstandardized assessment, 312
    standardized assessment, 310–312
  guide to clinicians/clinical researchers, 313–319
    examiners/language mode, 313–314
    interpreters, working with, 315–316
    interpreting results, 316–319
    materials, 313
    monolingual *vs.* multilingual sessions/examiners, 314–315
  multilingualism, 308–309
assessment of creole languages, 223–245
assessment methods, 67–153
asylum seekers, global context, 9
augmentative/alternative communication, 275–288
  as voice, 281–283
  deciding on augmentative/alternative communication system, 283–286

defining, 278–281
autism spectrum disorder, 289–303
assessment tools, 297–298
clinical markers, 298
expressive vocabulary/receptive vocabulary, 297
narrative skills, 298
observation scales, 298
phonological skills, 297
questionnaires, 298
bilingualism-multilingualism-multicultural, theoretical/empirical aspects, 292–295
characteristics, 290
children with
challenges, 291
characteristics of, 291
communication skills, 291
from diverse backgrounds, assessment tools/resources for, 296
multilingual/multicultural backgrounds, management of individuals with, 291–292
multilingual/multicultural perspective, assessment in, 295–298
prevalence, 290
sentence repetition tasks for, 267
terminology, 290
automation for language sample analysis, multilingual children, 124–126

background, 1–66
bi-multilingual cultures, 50–53
codeswitching, 52–53
proficiency in bi-/multilingual speakers, 52
translanguaging, 50–53
translanguaging (codemixing), 52–53
body functions/body structures, *International Classification of Functioning, Disability and Health,* 31–32

caregiver burden, dementia assessment, 339
challenge of language assessment, developmental language disorder, 26–27
diagnosis of, 27–30
children
automation for language sample analysis, 124–126
bilingual, narrative skills of, 144–145
communication disorders, ethnographic analysis, 95
assessment, 91–109
assessing language structure/use, 94
assessment process, 100–101
case study, 98–101
ethnographic assessment, 105–107
ethnographic interview, 101–107
ethnographic interview in new place, 105
in international settings, 97–98
interviewing children, 103–104
language sampling, 93–98
nonbiased assessments, 92–93
standardized tests, 92
steps for conducting interview, 102–103
unbiased approach to information gathering, 101–102
with culturally/linguistically different children, 95–97
culturally/linguistically different, language sampling with, 95–97
from culturally/linguistically diverse backgrounds, narrative skills, 143–145
fictional narratives, 143
narrative skills of bilingual children, 144–145
personal narratives, 143–144
early language socialization, 179–180
ethnographic assessment for communication disorders, 91–109
interviewing, 103–104
Mandarin speaking, in China, standardized assessments/screeners, 247–262
multilingual, automation for language sample analysis, 124–126
sentence repetition tasks for, 265–267
autism spectrum disorder, 267
developmental language disorder, 265–266
second language acquisition, 266–267
sentence repetition tasks as measure of working memory, 267
socialization, language, research, 179–180
with autism spectrum disorder, 291

China, Mandarin-speaking children in, standardized language, assessments/ screeners, 247–262. *See also* Mandarin-speaking children in
assessing assessment, 253–254
assessments for youngest/most delayed, 254–256
children, designing for, 252
experts, collaboration among, 248
lessons learned, 248–260
linguistic differences, 249–251
multiple assessments, 254
risk potential, screeners to gauge, 254
sample for population, 252
special circumstances of China, 247–248
technology, advantages of, 256–259
training/guidance, 259–260
codemixing, 52–53
codeswitching, 52–53
coding/analysis, multilingual samples, 118–124
collaboration, 20–22
cross-linguistic team work, 21
interprofessional teams for developing language assessments, 20
networking, 21
university repositories, 21
community-based research
time-consuming process, Western Kenya, 206
Western Kenya
defining goals, 207
equipment, 207–208
ethics, 208
funding, 208
participant recruitment/incentives, 207
research methods, 207–208
contextual factors, *International Classification of Functioning, Disability and Health,* 36–37
creole languages in absence of norms
assessment, 240–242
alternatives to standardized tests, 241
language samples, 241–242
case study, 242–243
client background, 242
language sample, 243
creole continuum, 230–233
education/literacy, 231–233
general cultural norms/values/beliefs, 231
differences between languages, Creoles, dialects/accents, 225–226
Guyanese Creole, 223–245
linguistic discrimination, Creoles, 226–227
morphosyntactic features, 233–240
morphosyntactic features of Guyanese, 233–234
plural marking, 236
prepositions, 236–240
pronouns, 236
serial verb construction, 236
tense, mode/aspect, 234–235
pidgins/Creoles, background on, 224–225
speech-language pathology in Guyana, 228–230
description of country/people, 228–229
Guyanese Creole, 229–230
cultural communication differences, 47
cultural/linguistic diversity in assessment, 11–15
cultural competence, 13–14
cultural diversity, deconstructing, 12–13
cultural humility, 14
cultural responsiveness, 14
developing cultural competence, responsiveness/humility, 13
historical/cultural perspective of assessment, 11–12
materials to develop cultural competence/ responsiveness/humility, 14–15
culturally/linguistically diverse individuals, 69–90
case studies, 88–89
dynamic assessment, 83–87
graduated prompting, 85–86
test-teach-retest, 83–85
testing limits, 86–87
types of, 72
research, 72–83
dynamic assessment, 73–77
measures of modifiability characteristics, 77–83
theories supporting use of dynamic assessment, 71
culture, socialization, language, research, 186–187

defining assessment, 3–4
dementia, neuropsychological assessment, 323–354
  attention, 332
  in bilingual contexts, 339–345
  in educationally diverse contexts, 339
  general cognitive abilities, assessment of, 325–327
  global populations, 345
  linguistically diverse contexts, 325–339
  memory/learning, 332
    constructional abilities, 337
    executive functions, 337
    language, 337
    social cognition, 337
    visuospatial ability, 337
  neuropsychological test batteries, 327–339
  processing speed, 332
  scales/questionnaires, 338–339
    activities of daily living, 338
    behavior, 338
    caregiver burden, 339
    quality of life, 338
    severity scales, 338
  specific cognitive domains, assessment of, 332–337
development of standardized language assessments and screeners for Mandarin-speaking children in China, 247–262
developmental communication, Western Kenya, 195–221
  caregiver questionnaire—Dholuo, 212–216
  caregiver questionnaire—English, 217–221
  challenges, 206–208
  community-based research
    defining goals, 207
    equipment, 207–208
    ethics, 208
    funding, 208
    participant recruitment/incentives, 207
    phone communication costs, 207–208
    research methods, 207–208
    time-consuming process, 206
    transportation, 207–208
  community-based research team, establishing, 199
    academic partners, 199
    community partners, 199
  conceptual framework guiding project, 198
  developing/implementing community-based research approach, 198–201
  guidelines, developing community-based research in communication disorders, 208–209
    early stages, 209
    late-stage considerations, 209
    once project underway, 209
  methodological approach/pilot, long-term plans, training teachers, 205
  methodological approach/pilot efforts, 201–205
    culturally appropriate questionnaires, 201–202
    data acquisition flow, 203
    long-term plans, 204–205
      analyses, 205
      educational material, 205
      participants, 204
      procedure, 204–205
    preliminary results, 203–204
  principles of community-based research, 200–201
  prior non-community-based research, 197–198
  project description, 196–198
    context, 196–197
    goals, 197
developmental language disorder, 26–27
  diagnosis of, 27–30
diagnosis of developmental language disorder, 27–30
  International Classification of Functioning, Disability and Health, 27–30
disability, socialization, language, research, 183–184
drawing on language socialization research to improve speech and language assessment, 177–194
dynamic assessments, 69–90
environment, social, socialization, language, research, 188–189
ethnographic interview, 101–107
  ethnographic assessment, 105–107
  ethnographic interview in new place, 105
  interviewing children, 103–104
  steps for conducting interview, 102–103
  unbiased approach to information gathering, 101–102

examples of global assessments, 155–272
executive functions, dementia,
neuropsychological assessment, 337
existing structures to devise language
assessment, 20

global assessment examples, 155–272
global context, 6–10
asylum seekers, 9
linguistic human rights, global contexts, 10
majority-world contexts, in minority-world
countries, 9
majority-world countries, 6
migrants, 9
minority-world countries, 6–9
refugees, 9
underserved/unserved populations, 9
graduated prompting, 85–86
Guatemala, partnering for community-based
measure of expressive language, 157–175
continuity, 159
designing impact assessment
adapting test, 161–165
coding responses, 166
cognitive interviews, 170
options, considering, 161
responsiveness results, 166–168
scenario, 165–166
steps for responsiveness, 161–170
supplemental assessor manual, 169
engaging host partners, 158
ethical concerns, 159–160
field testing, 169
focus groups, 168–169
mutuality, 159–160
reciprocity, 159–160
reflection, meaningful, ensuring, 171–173
sustainability, 159
U.S. and non-U.S. participants, support for,
170
feedback, eliciting, 170

historical perspective of language assessment
translation, 18–19

identifying developmental communication
milestones in Western Kenya, 195-221
interference/transfer, 53–62
in communication, 54–57
in language, 57–62
interference/transfer in communication,
54–57
interference/transfer in language, 57–62
*International Classification of Functioning,
Disability and Health*, 30–37
activity/participation, 32–36
activity, 32–34
participation, 34–36
adult application of language disorders in,
40
body functions/body structures, 31–32
case study application, 38–40
challenge of language assessment, 26–30
developmental language disorder,
26–27
diagnosis of developmental language
disorder, 27–30
contextual factors, 36–37
framework of, 25–43
student application of language disorders
in, 38–39
*International Classification of Functioning,
Disability and Health* framework and global
assessment, 25–43
interview, ethnographic, 101–107
ethnographic assessment, 105–107
ethnographic interview in new place, 105
interviewing children, 103–104
steps for conducting interview, 102–103
unbiased approach to information
gathering, 101–102

Kenya, Western, developmental communication.
See developmental communication

language, culture and, 47–48
language and language families, 45–66
bi-multilingual cultures/translanguaging,
50–53
codeswitching, 52–53
proficiency in bi-/multilingual
speakers, 52
translanguaging (codemixing), 52–53
interference/transfer, 53–62
interference/transfer in
communication, 54–57
interference/transfer in language,
57–62

languages around world, 46–50
cultural communication differences, 47
language, culture and, 47–48
language families, 49–50
structural differences unrelated to culture, 48–49
sources of linguistic information, 62–64
language sample analysis, 111–130
automation for language sample analysis, multilingual children, 124–126
coding/analysis of multilingual samples, 118–124
collection of samples, 113–115
transcription, 115–117
language socialization research, 177–194
assessment, 185
culture, 186–187
disability, 183–184
diversity, 186–187
early childhood, 179–180
at school, 180–183
social environment, 188–189
languages around world
cultural communication differences, 47
language and culture, 47–48
language families, 49–50
structural differences unrelated to culture, 48–49
learning, dementia, neuropsychological assessment, 332
executive functions, 337
language, 337
social cognition, 337
visuospatial ability, 337
linguistic diversity, 15–16
multilingualism, 15–16
translanguaging, 16

majority-/minority-world countries, cultural/linguistic diversity barriers, 11
Mandarin-speaking children in China, standardized language, assessments/screeners, 247–262
assessing assessment, 253–254
assessments for youngest/most delayed, 254–256
children, designing for, 252
experts, collaboration among, 248
lessons learned, 248–260
linguistic differences, 249–251
multiple assessments, 254
risk potential, screeners to gauge, 254
sample for population, 252
special circumstances of China, 247–248
technology, advantages of, 256–259
training/guidance, 259–260
memory
dementia, neuropsychological assessment, 332
executive functions, 337
language, 337
social cognition, 337
visuospatial ability, 337
working, sentence repetition tasks as measure of, 267
methods of assessment, 67–153
migrants, global context, 9
multilingualism, 15–16

narrative assessment, 131–153
analyzing fictional narrative skills, 139–142
assessment of fictional narratives, 136–139
examples of global initiatives, 146–148
adapting narrative protocols, 147
global *TALES*, 146
multilingual assessment instrument for narratives, 146–147
fictional narratives, 133, 136–142
narrative skills, children from culturally/linguistically diverse backgrounds, 143–145
fictional narratives, 143
narrative skills of bilingual children, 144–145
personal narratives, 143–144
personal narratives, 132, 134–136
analyzing personal narrative skills, 136
assessment of personal narratives, 134–135
neuropsychological assessment, dementia, 323–354
attention, 332
in bilingual contexts, 339–345
in educationally diverse contexts, 339
general cognitive abilities, assessment of, 325–327
global populations, 345
linguistically diverse contexts, 325–339

memory/learning, 332
constructional abilities, 337
executive functions, 337
language, 337
social cognition, 337
visuospatial ability, 337
neuropsychological test batteries, 327–339
processing speed, 332
scales/questionnaires, 338–339
activities of daily living, 338
behavior, 338
caregiver burden, 339
quality of life, 338
severity scales, 338
specific cognitive domains, assessment of, 332–337

partnering for community-based measure of expressive language, Guatemala, 157–175
continuity, 159
designing impact assessment
adapting test, 161–165
coding responses, 166
cognitive interviews, 170
interpreting results, 166–168
options, considering, 161
scenario, 165–166
steps for responsiveness, 161–170
supplemental assessor manual, 169
engaging host partners, 158
ethical concerns, 159–160
field testing, 169
focus groups, 168–169
mutuality, 159–160
reciprocity, 159–160
reflection, meaningful, ensuring, 171–173
sustainability, 159
U.S. and non-U.S. participants, support for, 170
feedback, eliciting, 170
preface, xvii–xxii
preschoolers, Setswana-speaking, assessment of passive in, 269
aims/hypothesis, 269
method, 269
setting, 269
prevention of language disorders, 4–5
protocols, narrative, adapting, 147

quality of life, demential assessment, 338
questionnaires, dementia, neuropsychological assessment, 338–339

ratio of clients to speech-language therapists, global context, 10
refugees, global context, 9
research, dynamic assessment, 72–83

sample analysis, 111–130
automation for language sample analysis, multilingual children, 124–126
coding/analysis of multilingual samples, 118–124
collection of samples, 113–115
transcription, 115–117
sampling language, 93–98
analysis, 95
assessing language structure/use, 94
with culturally/linguistically different children, 95–97
in international settings, 97–98
scales, dementia, neuropsychological assessment, 338–339
severity scales, 338
school, socialization, language, research, 180–183
sentence repetition tasks for culturally/ linguistically diverse clients, 263–272
adults, 268
children, 265–267
autism spectrum disorder, 267
developmental language disorder, sentence repetition tasks, 265–266
second language acquisition, 266–267
sentence repetition tasks as measure of working memory, 267
collaboration in development of cross-linguistic sentence repetition tasks, 268
considerations for developing sentence repetition tasks, 268
definitions of sentence repetition tasks, 263
sentence repetition tasks, 264
language disorder assessment, 273–303
measuring progress, 264
requirements of sentence repetition tasks, 270
discussion, 270
results, 270

Setswana-speaking preschoolers, assessment of passive in, 269
aims/hypothesis, 269
method, 269
setting, 269
social cognition, dementia, neuropsychological assessment, 337
socialization, language, research, 177–194
assessment, 185
at school, 180–183
culture, 186–187
disability, 183–184
early childhood, 179–180
social environment, 188–189
sources of linguistic information, 62–64
spectrum disorder, autism, 289–303
assessment tools, 297–298
clinical markers, 298
expressive vocabulary/receptive vocabulary, 297
narrative skills, 298
observation scales, 298
phonological skills, 297
questionnaires, 298
bilingualism-multilingualism-multicultural, theoretical/empirical aspects, 292–295
characteristics, 290
children with
challenges, 291
characteristics of, 291
communication skills, 291
from diverse backgrounds, assessment tools/resources for, 296
multilingual/multicultural backgrounds, management of individuals with, 291–292
multilingual/multicultural perspective, assessment in, 295–298
prevalence, 290
sentence repetition tasks for, 267
terminology, 290
speech-language professional
role in assessment, 5
speech-language therapy in global context, 6
standardized language assessment, 247–262
structural differences unrelated to culture, 48–49
student application of language disorders in *International Classification of Functioning, Disability and Health,* 38–39

transcription, 115–117
translanguaging, 16, 52–53

underserved/unserved populations, global context, 9

visuospatial ability, dementia, neuropsychological assessment, 337
voice, having, 275–288. *See also* augmentative/alternative communication

Western Kenya, developmental communication. *See* developmental communication
working memory, sentence repetition tasks as measure of, 267
World Health Organization *International Classification of Functioning, Disability and Health* model of health and disability, 27–43
World Health Organization regions/language families, 16–17

Printed in the United States
by Baker & Taylor Publisher Services